Key Heterocyclic Cores for Smart Anticancer Drug–Design

Part II

Edited by

Rajesh Kumar Singh

Department of Pharmaceutical Chemistry,
Shivalik College of Pharmacy,
Nangal IKG Punjab Technical University,
Jalandhar, Punjab, 140126,
India

Key Heterocyclic Cores for Smart Anticancer Drug–Design Part II

Editor: Rajesh Kumar Singh

ISBN (Online): 978-981-5040-04-3

ISBN (Print): 978-981-5040-05-0

ISBN (Paperback): 978-981-5040-06-7

First published in 2022.

need for a court order if at any point you breach any terms of this License Agreement. In no event will any delay or failure by Bentham Science Publishers in enforcing your compliance with this License Agreement constitute a waiver of any of its rights.

3. You acknowledge that you have read this License Agreement, and agree to be bound by its terms and conditions. To the extent that any other terms and conditions presented on any website of Bentham Science Publishers conflict with, or are inconsistent with, the terms and conditions set out in this License Agreement, you acknowledge that the terms and conditions set out in this License Agreement shall prevail.

Bentham Science Publishers Pte. Ltd.
80 Robinson Road #02-00
Singapore 068898
Singapore
Email: subscriptions@benthamscience.net

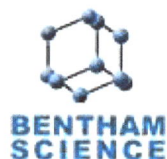

CONTENTS

FOREWORD

In the age of knowledge and technology, cancer is a disgrace on the face of humanity. Despite the fact that tremendous progress has been made in cancer therapy over the past 50 years, it remains a critical public health concern needing extensive research into new therapeutic strategies. Despite the availability of numerous anticancer drugs, issues such as multidrug resistance, diminished therapeutic efficacy, solubility, unwanted side effects, and poor bioavailability necessitate the development of novel anticancer therapies. Due to their exceptional pharmacological activity, specifically their anticancer properties, heterocyclic compounds have dominated medicinal chemistry for more than a century. Currently, the available chemical galaxy includes more than 100 million organic compounds, mainly related to a limited set of classes and types. At the same time, modern drug design trends require the development of synthetic approaches to equally and diversely fill the chemical space as a source of drug-like structures. These trends have affected heterocyclic chemistry as the main "supplier" of drug-like molecules (all top 10 brand name small molecule drugs contain heterocyclic moieties).

This book, which is named **"Key Heterocyclic Cores for Smart Anticancer Drug-Design-Part II,"** offers a comprehensive analysis of several of the most interesting and contemporary hot topics in the research and development of cutting-edge cancer chemotherapeutics. This book is written with the intention of providing readers with a quick overview of the biological targets, structure-activity relationship (SAR), existing issues, and future prospects of heterocyclic-based anticancer drugs.

This book has piqued my interest tremendously, and I can't wait for it to be available in print as soon as possible. This book is useful as a resource for students, researchers, academicians, and medicinal chemists. The authors and Bentham publishers deserve praise for delivering timely and relevant information.

Roman Lesyk
Department of Pharmaceutical Organic and Bioorganic Chemistry,
Danylo Halytsky Lviv National Medical University
Pekarska, 69, Lviv, 79010,
Ukraine

PREFACE

Cancer which takes millions of lives every year, has been a curse on humans for a long time. New cancer targets are the prime need for researchers worldwide to develop effective anticancer drugs. The heterocyclic compounds and typically prevalent heterocyclic fragments present in most clinical drugs are the foundation of anticancer drug discovery.

This second volume of the book series "***Key Heterocyclic cores for Smart Anticancer Drug-Design-Part II***" focuses on various green methodologies for the synthesis of these heterocyclic cores. Furthermore, different chapters provide insight into the structure-activity relationship (SAR) of heterocyclic cores to reveal different pharmacophores accountable for anticancer activity. The volume comprises 6 scholarly written review chapters by leading researchers in the field, covering a broad range of topics.

The basic metabolism and biochemical process in the human body leading to cancer can play a decisive role in identifying and revealing new anticancer drug targets. In the first chapter of this book, Shweta *et al.* reviewed the various biochemical modes of action, biological targets and futuristic development for these heterocyclic cores for treating various types of cancer. The novel targets are also illustrated with a pictorial presentation to understand heterocyclic drug action on various cancer targets.

The concept of molecular hybridization has opened new doors towards designing and developing therapeutic candidates capable of binding to multiple targets. In this direction, several research groups have explored the therapeutic potentials of coumarin and its derivatives against cancer. In chapter two, Rohit *et al.* contributed a comprehensive review on important targets and their significance in the development of cancer. A description of reported potent anticancer coumarin hybrids inhibiting/interacting with particular targets investigated in the last five years has been provided, along with their structure-activity relationship (SAR).

Researchers and scientists have paid much attention to the drug design, and drug discovery of nitrogen (*N*) and sulphur (*S*) based heterocyclic compounds in the last decade. These *N* and *S*-based heterocyclic compounds such as pyrrole, quinazoline, thiadiazole and quinoline are widely used in the rational drug design for anticancer drugs with a favourable therapeutic index. In Chapter 3, Koli and Singh have reviewed the SAR study of recent literatures (2016-2020) in which *N* and *S* heterocyclic compounds are present as the core structure in the molecule. This chapter also emphasized the benefits of hybrid heterocyclic molecules acting *via* multiple target mechanisms.

The search for new anticancer agents to fight against cancer is not an ending process. Keeping in view, the aromatic diazole heterocyclic nucleus named imidazole proved promising health benefits. The significant therapeutic potential of the imidazole derivatives has triggered the medicinal chemist to develop a large number of novel anticancer compounds with a low toxicity profile. Chapter 4 by Dhingra *et al.* critically assessed the imidazole, demonstrating its number of anticancer analogues synthesized by various synthetic procedures. In addition, the chapter also describes the available marketed drugs having an imidazole nucleus bearing distinct substituents.

Morpholine is a highly privileged and versatile heterocyclic ring in medicinal chemistry with various biological activities due to its distinct mechanistic pathways. The talent of the morpholine ring to modulate the pharmacokinetic properties of the compounds further motivated the researchers to exploit the morpholine ring as a vital pharmacophore in developing lead compounds. Chapter 5 by Kumari and Singh outlined various synthetic strategies of morpholine ring and morpholine derivatives as potent anticancer agents. The latest data on novel anticancer morpholine derivatives with structural-activity relationship (SAR) is elaborated. The chapter also highlighted the clinical data of morpholine derivatives with anticancer activity and mechanism of action.

Natural products have played a significant role in providing novel and effective treatment inputs in anticancer research. Natural products have been a source of many anticancer agents that are being used in clinical or pre-clinical trials. Further, many compounds derived from natural products have shown the potential to be future anticancer agents. Due to their actions on numerous targets, natural products are considered ideal for anticancer drug development. In Chapter 7, Chaudhary *et al.* discuss the progress and ongoing developments in natural products and their analogues as anticancer agents. The challenges and future prospects of natural-based anticancer agents are also discussed.

The editor wishes to express their considerable appreciation to all the contributors of the chapters for their hard and scholarly work. We are also grateful to Mr. Mahmood Alam (Director Publication) and Ms. Humaira Hashmi (Manager Publication) of Bentham Science Publisher, who took over the management of the production of this book during the difficult circumstances of the COVID pandemic; their contribution is much appreciated. We are confident that this book will be a compelling guide to facilitate researchers, pharmacologists, and medicinal chemists in understanding the mechanism of heterocyclic drugs, which can help develop new anticancer agents.

Rajesh Kumar Singh
Department of Pharmaceutical Chemistry,
Shivalik College of Pharmacy, Nangal,
IKG, Punjab Technical University,
Jalandhar, Punjab, 140126,
India

List of Contributors

Akram Sidhu	UNT Health Science Center, Fort Worth, Texas, United States
Alok Sharma	Department of Pharmacognosy, ISF College of Pharmacy, Moga, G.T Road, Ghal kalan, Moga, Punjab-142001, India
Amandeep Singh	Department of Pharmaceutics, ISF College of Pharmacy, Moga, Punjab-142001, India
Anurag Chaudhary	Department of Pharmaceutical Technology, Meerut Institute of Engineering and Technology, NH-58, Baghpat Road Crossing, Bypass Road, Meerut-250005, India
Archana Kumari	School of Pharmaceutical Sciences, Lovely Professional University, Phagwara, 144001, Punjab, India
Ashish Gupta	CSIR-National Physical Laboratory, New Delhi -110012, Indiaq
Ashwani K. Dhingra	Guru Gobind Singh College of Pharmacy, Yamuna Nagar-135001, Haryana, India
Bhawna Chopra	Guru Gobind Singh College of Pharmacy, Yamuna Nagar-135001, Haryana, India
Bhupinder Kumar	Department of Pharmaceutical Chemistry, ISF College of Pharmacy, Moga, Punjab-142001, India
Kalpana Singh	HIMT College of Pharmacy, 8, Institutional Area, Knowledge Park I, Greater Noida, Uttar Pradesh-201301, India
Kumar Guarve	Guru Gobind Singh College of Pharmacy, Yamuna Nagar-135001, Haryana, India
Mymoona Akhter	Department of Pharmaceutical Chemistry, Jamia Hamdard University, New Delhi 110062, India
Nishant Verma	Panchwati College of Pharmacy, Ghat Institutional Area, NH-58, Delhi-Haridwar Bypass Road, Meerut, Uttar Pradesh-250001, India
Preet Koli	Department of Pharmaceutical Chemistry, Shivalik College of Pharmacy, Nangal, Rupnagar, Punjab, India
Rajesh Kumar Singh	Department of Pharmaceutical Chemistry, Shivalik College of Pharmacy, Nangal, Rupnagar, India
Ravindra K. Rawal	CSIR-North East Institute of Science and Technology, Formerly Regional Research Laboratory, Jorhat-785006, Assam, India
Rohit Bhatia	Department of Pharmaceutical Chemistry, ISF College of Pharmacy, Moga, Punjab-142001, India
Shweta Sharma	Department of Pharmaceutical Chemistry, Jamia Hamdard University, New Delhi 110062, India

CHAPTER 1

Understanding Promising Anticancer Targets for Heterocyclic Leads: An Introduction

Shweta Sharma[1], Mymoona Akhter[1] and **Rajesh Kumar Singh[2,*]**

[1] *Department of Pharmaceutical Chemistry, Jamia Hamdard University, New Delhi 110062, India*

[2] *Department of Pharmaceutical Chemistry, Shivalik College of Pharmacy, Nangal, Rupnagar, Punjab 140126, India*

Abstract: With the second-highest cause of mortality in the world, cancer becomes a major threat around the globe. In the last few decades, heterocyclic compounds, obtained naturally or synthetically, have been developed as a potential scaffold for developing many anticancer drugs. Heterocyclic compounds due to heteroatoms such as oxygen, nitrogen and sulphur can be employed as hydrogen bond donors as well as acceptors. Thus, they can bind suitably to pharmacological targets and receptors *via* intermolecular H-bonds more effectively, giving pharmacological effects. They can also alter liposolubility, hence the aqueous solubility of drug molecules to achieve remarkable pharmacotherapeutic properties. These heterocyclic leads exert the anticancer activity by a distinctive mechanism such as inhibiting Bcl-2, Mcl-1 proteins (induce apoptosis), inhibiting PIM proteins (hinder the cellular process and signal transduction in cells), inhibiting DNA topoisomerase, inhibiting aromatase (inhibit replication and transcription), modulating epigenetic mechanisms (inhibit histone deacetylase/HDAC) and inhibiting cellular mitosis (tubulin inhibitors).The current chapter aims to describe these promising anticancer targets. The novel targets are also illustrated with a pictorial presentation to understand heterocyclic drugs action on various cancer targets. This chapter will facilitate researchers, pharmacologists, and medicinal chemists in the understanding mechanism of heterocyclic drugs, which can help develop new anticancer agents.

Keywords: Anticancer, Apoptosis, Aromatase inhibitors, HDAC, Mitosis, Topoisomerase inhibitors, Tubulin inhibitors.

INTRODUCTION

Cancer is generally characterized by the uncontrolled growth rate of cells in any part of the body. According to recent studies presently, 9.6 million deaths out of

---

* **Corresponding author Rajesh Kumar Singh:** Department of Pharmaceutical Chemistry, Shivalik College of Pharmacy, Nangal, Dist. Rupnagar, 140126, Punjab, India; Tel: +919417513730; E-mail: rksingh244@gmail.com

Rajesh Kumar Singh (Ed.)

18.1 million new cases were reported in 2018 to publicize undivided attention to design potential leads for cancer therapy. To date, a total of 277 types of cancer have been observed, out of which small cell lung cancer leads the chart of mortality rate [1, 2].

Over the years, various heterocyclic compounds obtained either naturally or synthetically have been explored as potential scaffolds as anticancer agents. Thus, hunting for undiscovered classes of drug molecules against cancer cells captivated the attention of researchers globally. Therefore, unwrapping various cell-cycle regulators and apoptotic stimuli for cancer to dust up cancer cells seems an attractive strategy in developing potential anti-tumor agents.

In the present chapter, we aim to present an overview of different heterocyclic drugs acting on potentially known targeted proteins in a pictorial form to understand the mechanism of action better. In addition to this, novel targets have also been highlighted in the chapter.

VARIOUS HETEROCYCLIC ANTICANCER DRUG TARGETS

Heterocyclic drugs are the moieties in which one or more carbon atoms have been substituted by various hetero atoms (including oxygen, nitrogen, sulfur *etc.*) that form the backbone of the molecule [1]. Heterocycles are the basic fundamental ingredient of loads of the available anticancer agents on the market today. Almost two-thirds of anticancer agents, which were approved between 2010 and 2015, possess heterocyclic rings [3]. Therefore, we summarized various heterocyclic scaffolds reported for their anticancer potential against distinct targets pictorially to make readers understand their functioning easily.

HETEROCYCLIC DRUGS AS PROTEIN DEACETYLATION INHIBITORS

Histone Deacetylase (HDAC) Inhibitors

In the past few decades, HDAC emerged as a key drug target for the development of anticancer drugs. Histone Deacetylase inhibitors are also referred to as lysine deacetylase or deacetylase inhibitors [3]. They act exclusively not only against several types of HDACs (HDAC isoform-selective inhibitors) but also against all types of HDACs (pan-inhibitors). HDAC inhibitors can be categorized chemically into four classes of compounds: (a) hydroxamic acids; (b) short-chain fatty (aliphatic) acids; (c) benzamides; (d) cyclic tetrapeptides [4]. Various classes of HDAC inhibitors as heterocyclic drugs have been presented here in Fig. (**1**).

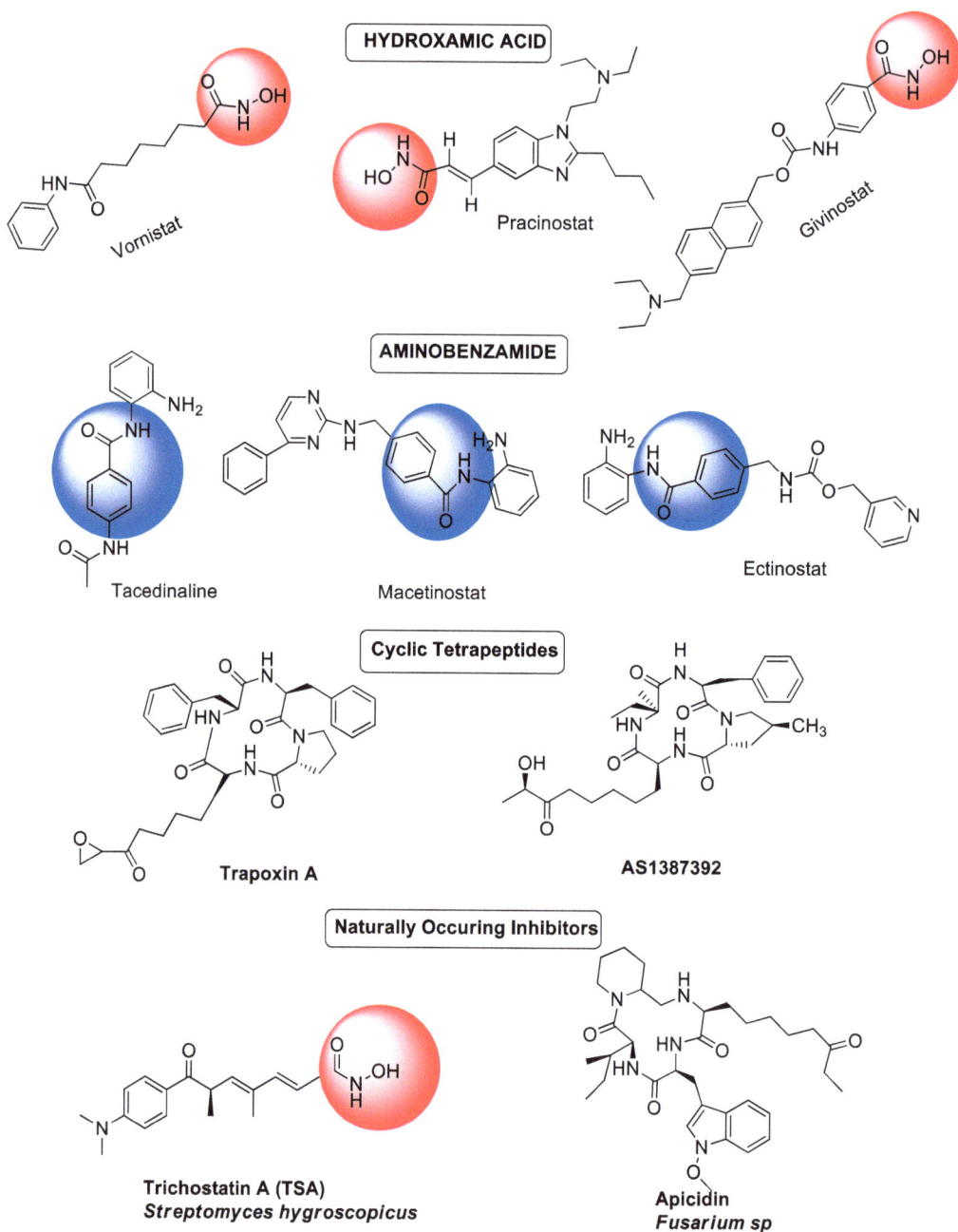

Fig. (1). Structures and name of diverse heterocyclic scaffolds as HDAC inhibitors with their chemical classes.

Mechanistically, HDAC inhibitors removed the acetyl group from lysine residue, which plays an important role in initiating and activating the cellular transcription process. Acetylation of lysine residues occurs post-transcriptionally on the NH_3 group of lysine residue entrenched in the core of N-terminal tails resulting in the emergence of transcriptionally active chromatin, which is less compact in nature. Therefore, HDAC inhibitor halts this acetylation process by deacetylating, as mentioned above, thereby preventing hyperacetylation of histones and strongly alters the gene expression process and leads to cancer [5]. The pictorial contouring of the mechanism of action of HDAC inhibitors has been shown in Fig. (**2**) for better understanding.

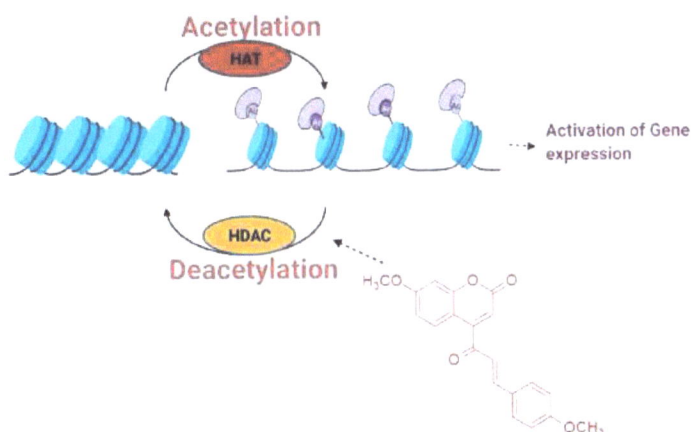

Fig. (2). Mechanism of action of HDAC inhibitors.

Till date, four drugs *viz.*, Vorniostat [6], Romidepsin [7], Belinostat [8], Panbiostat [9] have been approved as HDAC inhibitors. Vorinostat (suberanilohydroxamic acid, SAHA) is a hydroxamic acid derivative that got FDA approval in 2006, developed by Merck & Co. [6] interacts with the binding pocket of HDAC enzyme and performs a role of chelator for zinc ions which are present in the binding pocket of HDAC enzyme [10].

Vorinostat inhibits cancer in distinct ways with different combination therapy. First and foremost, it seems like a reliable option in CTCL and an efficacious radiosensitizer in human glioblastoma cell lines [11]. Moreover, in combination with temozolomide and radiotherapy, it was found effective against glioblastoma multiforme (GBM). Type I and Type II endometrial malignant cells also demonstrated their potential as a potent apoptotic and antiproliferative effect [12]. Furthermore, it inhibits cell growth, cyclin D1 and cyclin E expression, as well as p27 expression, histone acetylation, and apoptosis in both human and murine pulmonary cell lines [13]. Moreover, vorinostat, combined with capecitabine, resulted in the inhibition of *in vivo* growth of colorectal carcinoma in xenograft models [14]. Vorinostat has also shown its potential against gastrointestinal (GI) cancer [15]. Belinostat, another FDA approved hydroxamic acid derivative, is used therapeutically against relapsed or refractory PTCL [16]. It showed to be well tolerated in both groups, and it's activity was observed against Low Malignant Potential (LMP) cancer [17]. Furthermore, a phase II study in women with platinum-resistant Epithelial Ovarian Cancer (EOC) looked at the combination of belinostat and carboplatin. The three hepatocellular carcinoma cell lines (PLC/PRF/5, Hep3B, and HepG2) were also shown to inhibit cell growth and induce histone acetylation [18, 19].

Romidepsin, isolated from a culture of *Chromobacterium violaceum* by Fujisawa Pharmaceutical Company [20]. It is a prodrug, which is converted inside the cell after reduction of disulfide bond into thiol group, for the generation of an active form of the prodrug. It binds with the zinc atom located inside the Zn-dependent histone deacetylase pocket, thereupon inhibiting its activity [21, 22]. It also plays a role in preventing non-small cell lung cancer (NSCLC) cells from proliferating. When used in combination with bortezomib, it has been shown to inhibit A549 NSCLC cell growth by targeting histone acetylation and the expression of cell cycle and metalloproteinase proteins [23, 24]. It was also shown to destroy inflammatory breast cancer (IBC) emboli and improve lymphatic vascularization [25].

Sirtuin 1 Inhibitors

Sirtuin 1 (SIRT1) also emerged as a potential target for anticancer therapy. It is a nicotinamide adenosine dinucleotide (NAD)-dependent deacetylase which pulls out acetyl groups from different proteins [26]. There are seven types of sirtuins (SIRT 1 to SIRT 7), known presently in humans and found to be localized in distinct subcellular compartments. Sirtuins play a role in several biological processes, including transcriptional regulation, metabolic regulation, and cell survival [27].

Sirtuins activities can be regulated and used as a potential target in the treatment of neurodegeneration and cancer. As we are focusing on cancer so, these proteins undertake tumour-suppressing cellular activities by deacetylating proteins. It communicates with p53 and alleviates its functions by deacetylation process at the C-terminal of Lys382 residue of p53, thereby promoting tumour proliferation. Therefore, inhibition of SIRT1 leads to re-expression of Tumor Suppression Gene (TSG) and, in this way, helps in combating cancer [28]. According to some reports, it also possesses the prowess to deacetylate and nullify doubtless tumour-promoting transcription factors such as NF-κß and HIF-1α, which inhibits transcription activity, thus elevating TNF-α generated apoptosis [29]. A pictorial representation of the mechanism of action of SIRT1 inhibitors has been presented in Fig. (**3**).

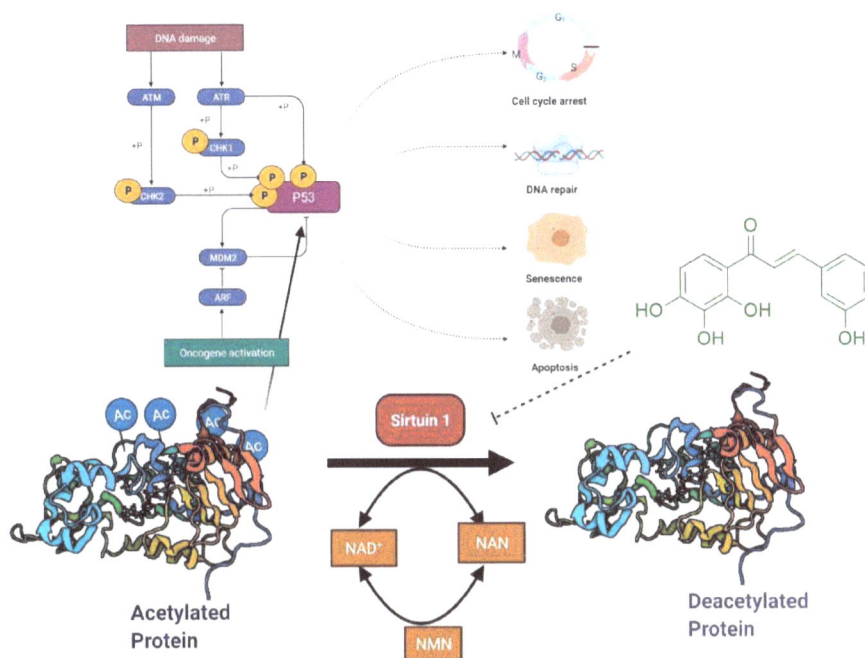

Fig. (3). Pictorial representation of mechanism of action of Sirtuin-1 inhibitors.

Sirutin-1 inhibitors are broadly classified as:

1. Nicotinamide and its analogues: Nicotinamide, acridinedione, 1,4-dihydropyridine
2. Thioacyllysine-containing compounds: Thiourea, Thioamide
3. β-napthol containing inhibitors: Sirtinol, Cambinol
4. Indole derivatives: EX-527, AC-93252
5. Suramin and its analogs
6. Atenovin and its analogs: Tenovin 1, Tenovin-6
7. Other sirtuin inhibitors: AGK2

Nicotinamide, one of the primary sirtuin inhibitors discovered. It inhibits the SIRT1 enzyme. Nicotinamide and its analogues strike as efficacious in inhibiting the growth and viability of human prostate cancer cells [30, 31]. In the cell lines, A549 lung carcinoma and MCF-7 breast carcinoma, thioacyllysine-containing compounds had an antiproliferative effect [32]. Cambinol causes hyperacetylation of tubulin, p53, KU70, and FOXO3a in cellular studies and facilitates cell cycle arrest by inhibiting SIRT1 and/or SIRT2. In a mouse xenograft model, treatment of BCL6-expressing Burkitt lymphoma cells with cambinol induces apoptosis and decreases tumour growth [33]. In N-Myc transgenic mice, a preventative treatment with cambinol reduces the formation of neuroblastoma [34]. Cambinol inhibits SIRT1-mediated deacetylation and transcription activity of the estrogen-related receptor in human breast cancer cells, resulting in a significant reduction in aromatase (CYP19A1) levels [35]. Indole derivatives EX527 induced apoptosis in leukaemia cells when combined with HDAC inhibitors [36]; protected against oculopharyngeal muscular dystrophy while AC-93253 showed cytotoxic effects in prostate DU145, pancreas MiaPaCa, lung A549 and NCI-H460 cancer cell lines [37]. Structural representation of various heterocyclic moieties as SIRT1 inhibitors is shown in Fig. (**4**).

HETEROCYCLIC DRUGS AS INHIBITORS OF CELLULAR PROLIFERATION

Tubulin Inhibitors

Tubulin, a dimeric protein, possesses two sub-units α and β, which are non-identical in nature, constitutes a key structural component to form microtubules. These microtubules are cellular components found in the eukaryotic organism and control various biological activities like mitosis, intracellular transport, and motility [38]. Tubulin inhibitors bind with tubulin protein to prevent polymerization, thereby disrupting the assembly of mitotic spindles fibres and hamper cytoskeletal function, which failed to take up successor steps [39]. The mechanism of action of tubulin inhibitors has been depicted in Fig. (**5**).

According to different binding sites present on the microtubule, inhibitors can be categorized into three different classes: (a) taxane binding domain (b) vinca binding domain. (c) Colchicine binding domain

(a)Taxane binding domain: Taxane family includes known inhibitors like Paclitaxel, Docetaxel, and Epothilones. Paclitaxel is the first inhibitor from the taxane family used for cancer chemotherapy [40]. It is used widely in a range of solid tumours as a chemotherapeutic agent. Another drug, Decetaxel, also has the same effects as Paclitaxel, which targets the M-phase of the cell cycle, which is responsible for stabilizing microtubules, thus preventing disaggregation [41]. Therapy with Docetaxel showed survival rate benefits in patients with Castration-Resistant Prostate Cancer (CRPC) [42]. Moreover, the clubbing of Histone Deacetylase Inhibitors (HDACIS) with docetaxel is observed to show

inhibition of cancer cell growth synergistically [43]. A newly developed anti-tumour drug, Epothilone, gives an added advantage over other reported taxanes as it is found effective in cells due to their ability to bind with β-tubulins I and III equally [44]. It showed potential lung cancer activity, breast cancer and prostate cancer with good therapeutic efficacy in hormone-refractory metastatic prostate cancer and taxane-refractory ovarian cancer [45].

(b)Vinca binding domain: Several heterocyclic compounds like Vinfluinine, Vincristine, Vinorelbine, Dolastatin 10 have been categorized as Vinca binding domain as all of them binds to the vinca domain in microtubules [46]. Vinflunine represents vinca alkaloid approved as second-line drug therapy against urothelial advanced transitional cell carcinoma (TCCU) [47]. Vinflunine-gemcitabine and vinflunine-carboplatin combination sound to be the most reliable preferences for first-line chemotherapy against urothelial cancer [48]. In addition, the combined therapy of oxaliplatin and vinblastine can provoke cytogenetic damage and inhibit survivin expression [49]. Another vinca alkaloid, Vincristine, when given in combination with quercetin, was found more efficacious in treatment therapy of lymphoma through a co-delivery mechanism using nanocarriers [50]. It is highly toxic and causes neuropathy, as reported in Omani study [51].

A semi-synthetic drug, Vinorelbine, blocks the polymerization of tubules, thereby inhibiting cell division in the middle stage of mitosis [52]. For stage IIIA patients with EGFR mutation-positive non-small-cell lung cancer (EVAN), a combination of Vinorelbin+Erlotinib+Cisplatin has been used as adjuvant treatment [53]. Dolastatin 10, another drug, is very effective against cytotoxic microtubules. Due to their robust *in vitro* activity and payload capacity for antibody-drug conjugates (ADC), natural synthetic analogues of dolastatin 10 have sparked a lot of interest [54]. According to studies, the 10-terminal thiazole moiety of dolastatin has functional group analogues, including amines, alcohols, and thiols, according to studies [55]. These new analogues have excellent titers in tumour cell proliferation assays. The combination of largazole and dolastatin 10 has been shown to inhibit the growth of HCT116 cancer cells, demonstrating a synergistic impact [56, 57].

A tricyclic alkaloid obtained from the colchicines binding domain possesses anti-inflammatory activity, which blocks activation of inflammatory bodies by inhibiting tubulin polymerization [58]. Furthermore, it interferes with distinct inflammatory pathways [59].

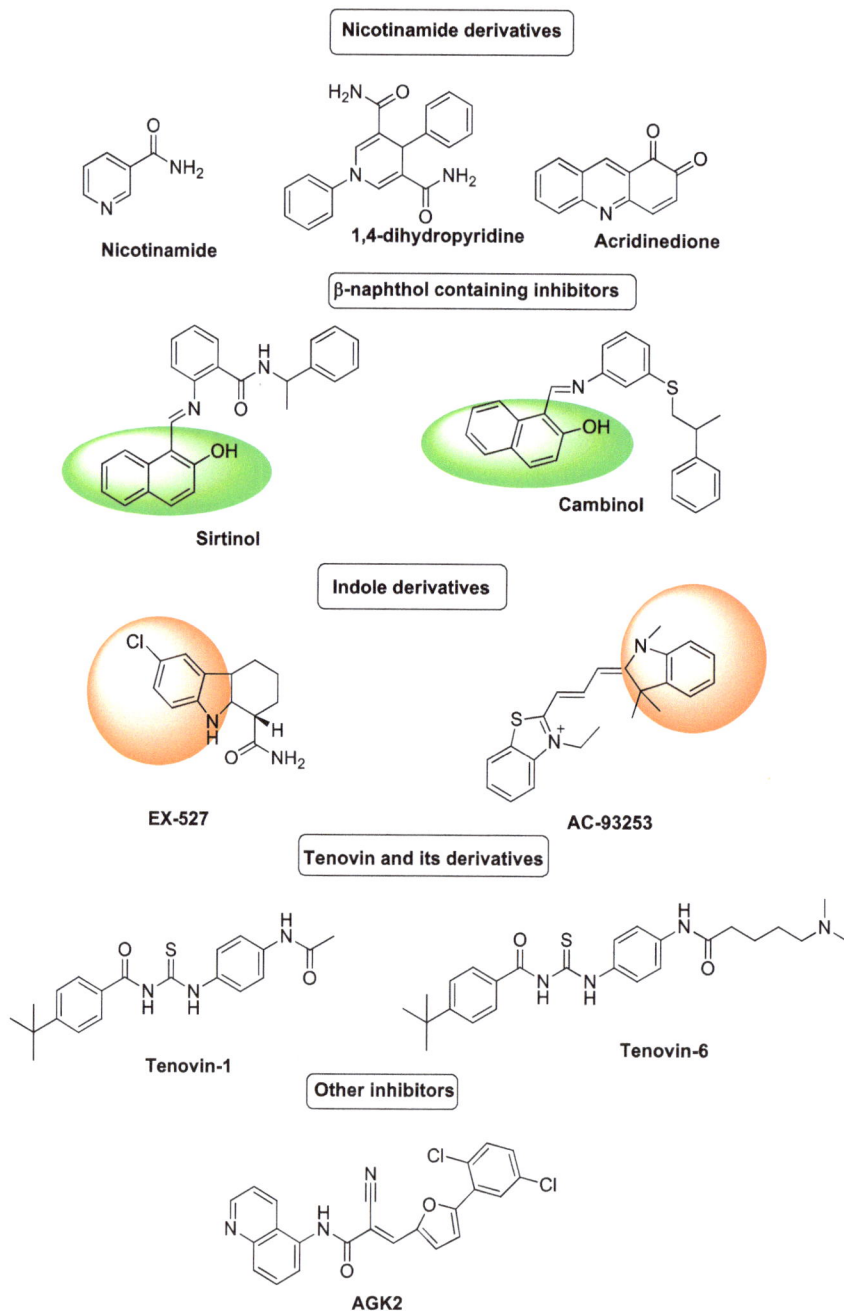

Fig. (4). Structures and name of diverse heterocyclic scaffolds as SIRT-1 inhibitors with their chemical classes.

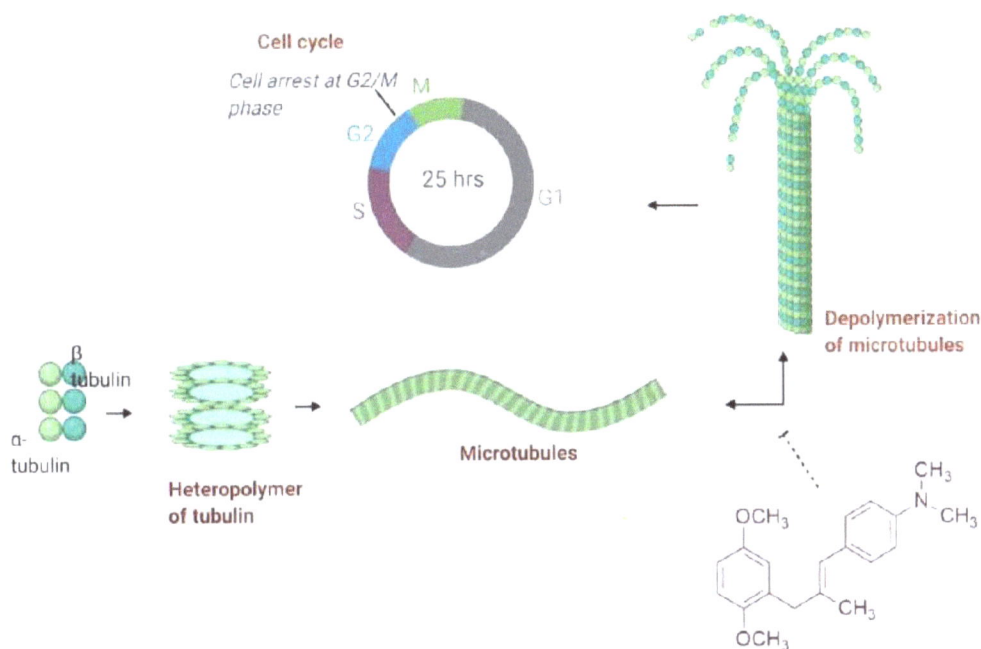

Fig. (5). Pictorial representation showing mechanism of action of Tubulin inhibitors.

(c) *Colchicine Binding Domain:*

Podophyllotoxin, another colchicine domain binding agent, is an effective cytotoxic agent [60], though its efficacy is restricted due to its resistance and side effects. In addition, Noscapine, a phthalo-isoquinoline alkaloid employed as an antitussive medicine for many years and is highly safe [61]. Noscapine capacity to force the microtubules to enhance the paused state duration, subsequently block the mitosis, and induce mitotic slip or mitotic mutation apoptosis contributed toward its anticancerous effect. Noscapine selectively blocked NF-κB, a critical transcription factor in the pathogenesis of glioblastoma; thus, it inhibits tumour growth and improves tumour chemotherapy sensitivity [62]. It has shown low toxicity as compared to colchicine and podophyllotoxin. In neurodegenerative disease and stroke mouse models, it also has shown neuroprotective properties [63]. The combination of paclitaxel and nicardipine was found to increase the proportion of apoptotic cells in human prostate cancer cell lines LNCaP and PC-3, owing to its anti-tumour effects [63]. These results established a new foundation for the treatment of prostate cancer [64]. Chemical structure of inhibitors is presented in Fig. (6).

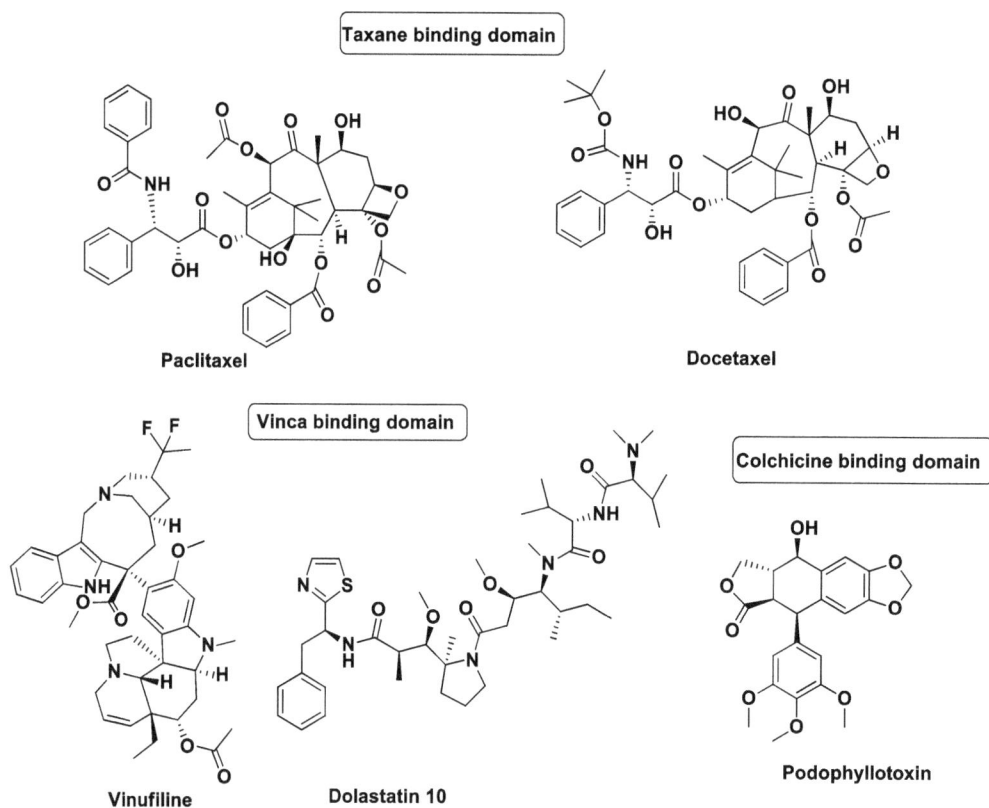

Fig. (6). Structures and name of diverse heterocyclic scaffolds as Tubulin inhibitors with their chemical classes.

Topoisomerase Expression Inhibitors

Topoisomerase II is an ATP dependent enzyme and possesses an ATP binding domain instead of the DNA binding domain. Topoisomerase II enzymes can knick/cut two DNA strands and seal the cut using ATP [65].

Mechanistically, inhibitors work by several accepted molecular mechanisms. One such theory is substrate competitive inhibition, in which the inhibitor binds to the active site of the Topoisomerase II enzyme, thus preventing DNA binding to the substrate [66]. Presently for this mechanism, no such inhibitor was reported. One more common mechanism which was more popular among the researchers is the formation of 'Topoisomerase poison', which possess a protein-DNA-drug complex that interrupts the DNA re-ligation process and locks the enzyme into 'cleavage complex'. This complex blocks enzyme turn-over and leads to the formation of a cytotoxic complex in the cell. Some compounds like aclarubicin and suramin bind to DNA and thus prevent topoisomerase binding; such compounds provide another potential inhibitory mechanism, although specificity is again an issue with such agents [67, 68]. Compound merbarone binds to the DNA protein complex and prevents cleavage and presents yet another mechanism of catalytic inhibition [69, 70]. Another mechanism that inhibits ATP-hydrolysis-driven enzymatic action is competitive inhibition of the ATP binding site, which is only observed in type II topoisomerase (discussed above). Novobiocin and Coumermycin are examples of ATP-site binders that are not used clinically due to potency, specificity, and poor pharmacokinetic properties [71, 72]. Fig. (7) depicts a pictorial representation of Topoisomerase inhibitors' mechanism of action.

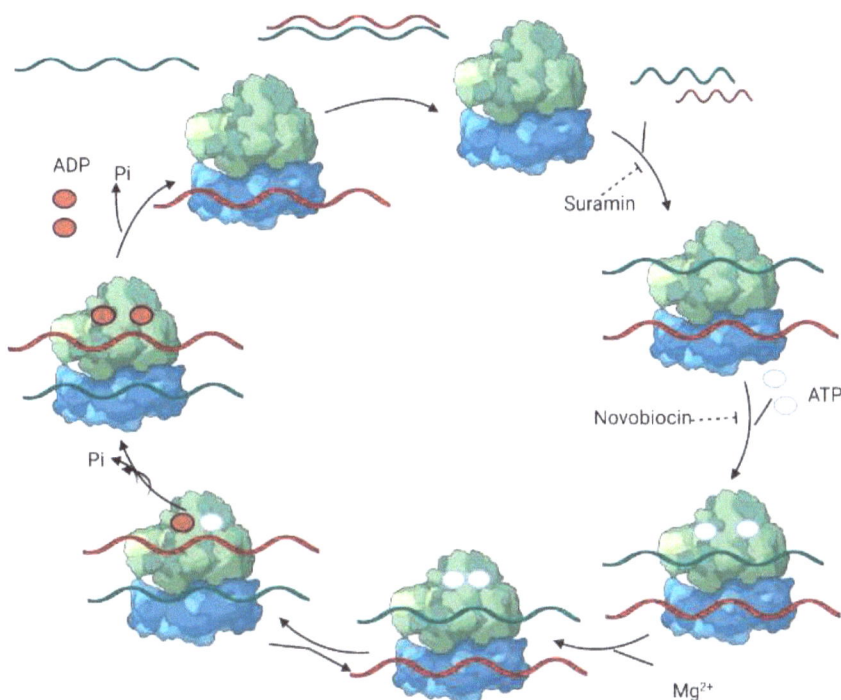

Fig. (7). Mechanism of action of various drugs as Topoisomerase inhibitors.

Topoisomerase inhibitors are categorized as:

(a) Anthracylline inhibitors: Doxorubicin, Epirubicin, Valrubicin

(b) Anthracenedione and acridine-derived topoisomerase inhibitors: Mitoxantrone, Pixantrone, Amsacrine

(c) Camptothecin-derived topoisomerase inhibitors: Camptothecin, Irinotecan, Topotecan

(d) Epipodophyllotoxin-derived topoisomerase inhibitors: Etoposide, Teniposide

The chemical structures of various Topoisomerase inhibitors are represented in Fig. (**8**). The anthracyclines were found to have antibiotic and anti-tumour activity; they were extracted from bacterial *Streptomyces* species for the first time [73]. Doxorubicin, Epirubicin, Valrubicin, Daunorubicin, and idarubicin are the clinically marketed anthracyclines derivatives. The chemical structures of some of them were shown in Fig. (**4**). Doxorubicin, an anthracyclines derivative, has been used in the treatment of breast cancer, various types of leukeamia, lymphoma, sarcomas, carcinomas, and other tumours [74]. Besides, some other derivatives are indicated for other problems, such as idarubicin for treatment of leukeamia, epirubicin for treatment of breast cancer following resection, and valrubicin to treat urinary bladder carcinoma [74]. Anthracenedione and acridine-derived topoisomerase inhibitors are the synthesized compounds known to act as anthracycline derivatives with lesser side effects [74]. Mitoxantrone, a chemotherapeutic agent used to treat leukaemia and prostate cancer, was discovered to cross the blood-brain barrier and is thus recommended for reducing the frequency and severity of multiple sclerosis relapses [75]. Pixantrone is an aza-anthracenedione that has been approved for the treatment of non-Hodgkin lymphoma. It has cytotoxic effects by intercalating into DNA like anthracyclines, but it also causes long-term cell damage and death by causing errors in mitosis and chromosome segregation [76]. Due to its inability to bind iron and contribute to free radical production in the heart, pixantrone is less toxic than doxorubicin in cardiac muscle cells. Animal models have shown that animals treated with doxorubicin have a lower heart weight than those treated with pixantrone [77, 78]. The topoisomerase poisons derived from camptothecin mainly affect type I topoisomerases. Camptotheca acuminate was the first plant from which alkaloid camptothecin was obtained (a Chinese tree). Topotecan is approved as a second-line treatment for small cell lung cancer and for patients with stage IV-B cervical carcinoma who have not had surgery or radiation [74].

Kinase Inhibitors

Receptor tyrosine kinases, ErbB participates in physiological pathways and cancer. At present, four members of the ErbB family have been known including epidermal growth factor receptor (EGFR), ErbB2, ErbB3, and ErbB4 [79]. Specifically, EGFR and ErbB2 are mutated in many epithelial tumours. The clinical studies revealed their significant roles in cancer development and progression. Therefore, considering the important role played by ErbB receptors in human cancer, efforts have been initiated in developing target-specific therapy [80].

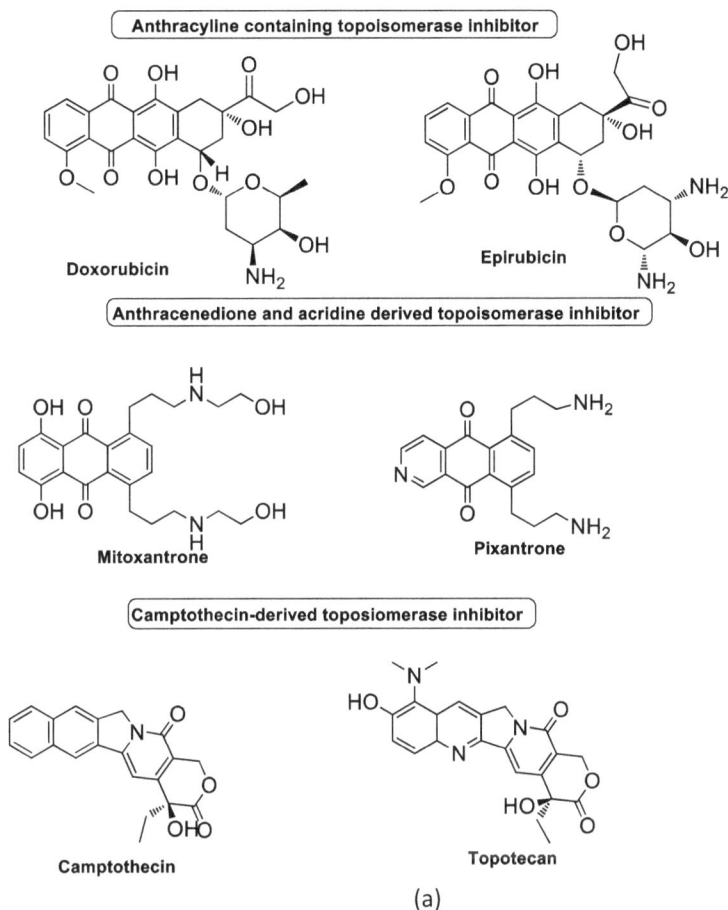

Fig. (8). Structures and name of diverse heterocyclic scaffolds as Topoisomerase inhibitors with their chemical classes.

The ErbB receptors currently constitute the primary targets of anticancer strategies. However, it was frequently observed that members of the ErbB receptor family over-expressed in several human cancers. Researchers under the leadership of Jung reported that Isoliquiritigenin (ISL) reduces cell proliferation and induces apoptosis in DU145 human prostate cancer cells and MAT-LyLu (MLL) rat prostate cancer cells [81]. Shin and colleagues synthesized 16 chromenylchalcones and used a clonogenic long-term survival assay on HCT116 human colorectal cancer cell lines to test them. The IC_{50} of one of the chromenylchalcones tested compound [82] was 93.1 nM, which is comparable to the IC_{50} values of well-known flavonoids like catechin gallate and epicatechin gallate. Fig. (**9**) shows the chemical structure of a kinase inhibitor.

Kinase Inhibitors

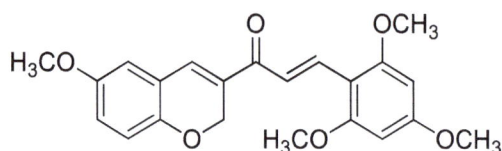

Fig. (9). Kinase Inhibitor.

mTOR Inhibitors

The mTOR (mammalian target of rapamycin) protein is serine/threonine kinase belongs to (PI3-K) phospho-inositide 3 kinase (PI3-K) family, which serve as a master switch in the regulation of cell metabolism, growth, proliferation and survival. It is clear from the published reports that the mTOR pathway got activated and deregulated, controlling various biological processes (*e.g.* tumour formation and angiogenesis, insulin resistance, adipogenesis and T-lymphocyte activation); if the patient is suffering from cancer or diabetes, the pathway is deregulated while in normal patients it got activated mTOR. Rapamycin inhibits AKT by disrupting the assembly of mTORC2, but only in certain cell types [83]. Chalcones have demonstrated mTOR inhibition in Fig. (**10**).

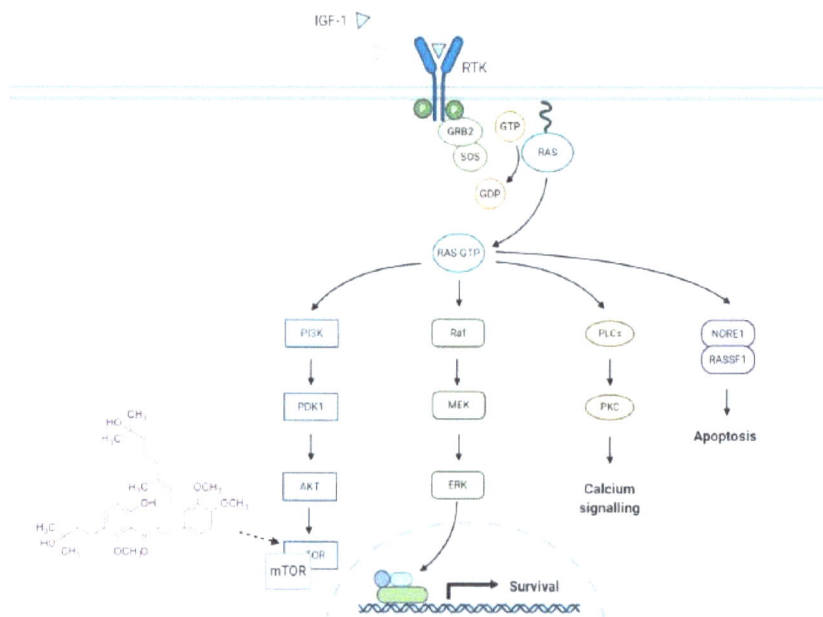

Fig. (10). Pictorial representation of the mechanism of action of mTOR inhibitors.

There are several known inhibitors as mTOR antagonists (Fig. **11**). To name a few, presently Rapamycin, Temsirolimus, Everolimus are in clinical application. Among the anticancer treatments, Rapamycin derived from the *Streptomyces hygroscopicus* bacteria found in the soil of Easter Island looks promising to slow down the tumor growth. However, some Rapamycin derivatives have been developed due to their low bioavailability and effectiveness [84]. Temsirolimus was the first rapalog approved by the FDA for the treatment of renal cell carcinoma. It is a prodrug that, when injected, converts to Rapamycin, an ester of hydroxymethyl propionic acid [85, 86].

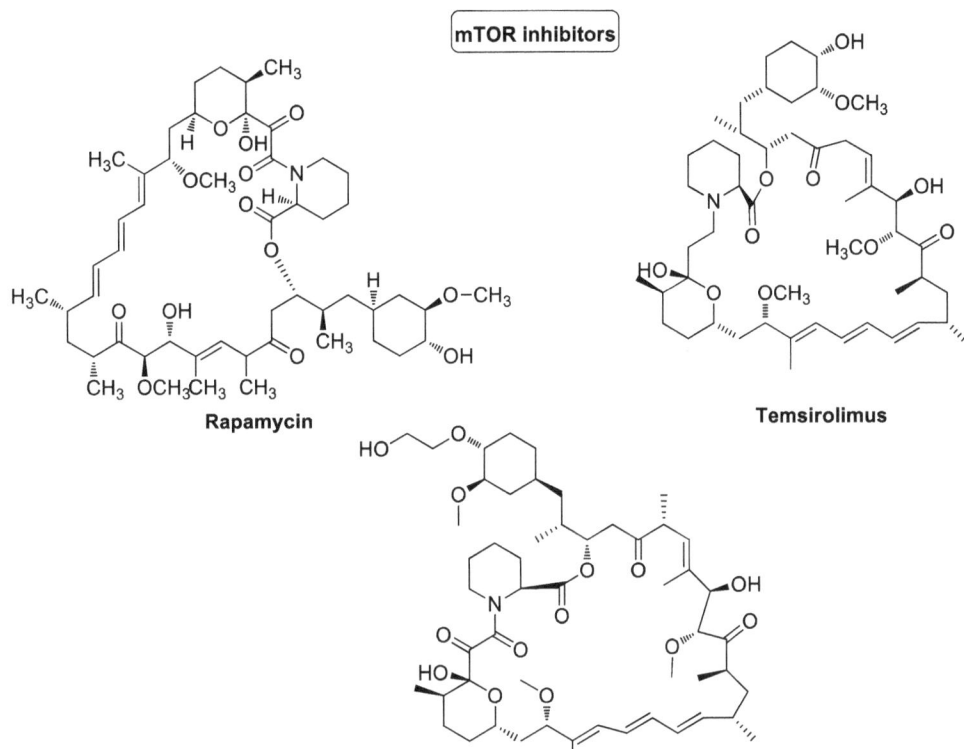

Fig. (11). Chemical structure of various mTOR inhibitors.

The FDA approved Everolimus, which has a hydroxyethyl group, for the treatment of renal cell carcinoma. Both of these rapalogs outperform rapamycin in terms of pharmacodynamic and pharmacokinetic characteristics [87].

BRAF Inhibitors

BRAF is a type of oncogene protein that directs the production of a protein that aids in transmitting chemical signals from outside the cell to the nucleus. In "RAS-RAF-MEK-ERK" pathway [also known as the mitogen-activated protein kinase (MAPK) cascade], this protein plays a significant role in the signalling pathway, which regulates the proliferation of cells, cell maturation for carrying out specific functions and apoptosis. Mutation in the BRAF gene resulted in oncogenic BRAF, which in turn leads to the generation of the overactive form of protein causing BRAFV600E mutation, thereby allowing BRAF to promote upstream cues. Therefore, these upstream cues result in overactive downstream signalling *via* MEK and ERK pathways, which causes unnecessary cell proliferation (Fig. **12**). Different types of tumours, to name a few melanoma tumours, papillary thyroid tumours, serous ovarian tumours, colorectal and prostate tumours, were generated [87].

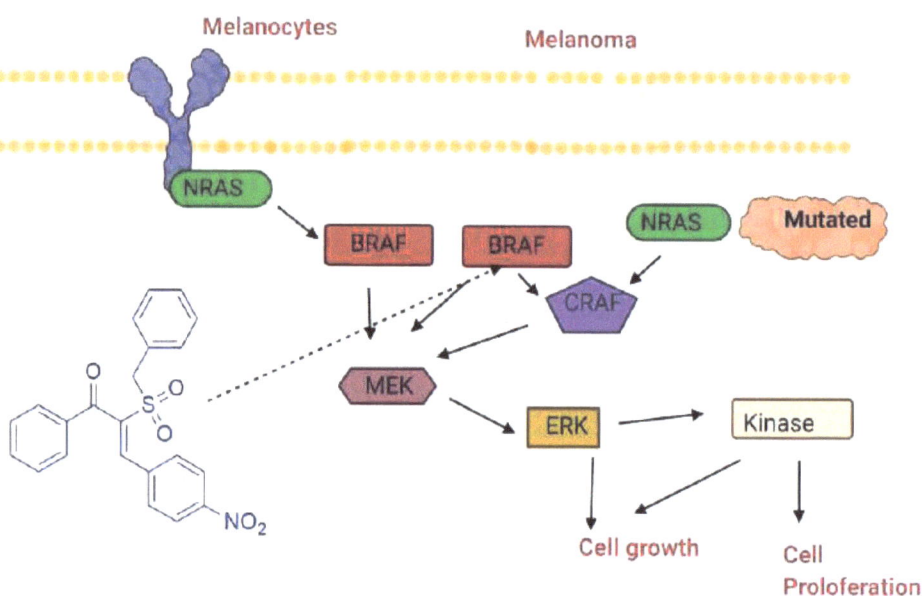

Fig. (12). Pictorial representation and mechanism of action of BRAF inhibitors.

Hence, inhibiting the BRAFV600E turns out to be successful in overcoming life-threatening cancer diseases [88]. Also, it seems like a potential therapeutic target as it helps in deactivating the tumour cell proliferation process and increases cell death.

In fact, variety of heterocyclic molecules with different scaffolds have been developed as BRAF inhibitors, including the biarylurea derivative Sorafenib, the triarylimidazole derivative SB-590885, the pyrimidine derivative Dabrafenib, the azaindole derivatives Vemurafenib and PLX4720, and the benzimidazole derivative (RAF265, compound 6).

The Food and Drug Administration (FDA) and the European Medicines Agency (EMEA) granted clinical approval for the treatment of advanced renal cell carcinoma (RCC) and unresectable hepatocellular carcinoma (HCC) in 2005 and 2007, respectively, and it is still in clinical trials for the treatment of other cancers. Its anti-angiogenic effects are mediated by inhibition of receptor tyrosine kinases VEGFR2 and PDGFR, responsible for its clinical activity [89]. Because Sorafenib is non-selective, it has failed to demonstrate therapeutic activity in malignant melanoma treatment [90], most likely due to its low BRAFV600E cell functions. The selective BRAFV600E inhibitor Vemurafenib, on the other hand, showed complete or partial tumour regression in the majority of patients with the BRAFV600E mutation, as well as a longer median survival period. The FDA approved Vemurafenib in 2011 for the treatment of BRAFV600E-mutated unresectable or metastatic melanoma [91]. In animal models, it was recently reported that combining RAF and MEK inhibitors can remove unwanted proliferative effects [91]. Patients treated with a combination of BRAF inhibitor and MEK inhibitor in phase I/II clinical trial had no cutaneous squamous cell carcinoma and had a high objective response rate [92]. Despite the promising clinical efficacy of BRAF inhibitors in cancer treatment, recent studies have shown that these inhibitors are developing substantial drug resistance. Fig. (**13**) shows BRAF inhibitors and their chemical structures.

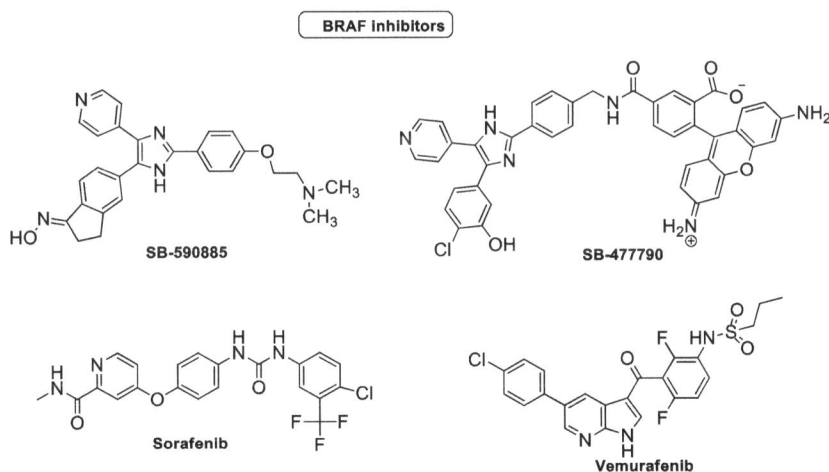

Fig. (13). Chemical structure of heterocyclic drugs as BRAF inhibitors with diverse scaffold.

NF-kβ Inhibitors

Nuclear Factor- kappa βeta (NF-kβ) is the mammalian transcription factor, which plays an important role in the regulation of over 150 genes affecting each aspect of cellular adaptation, immunity cell function activation, activation of immune cell function, apoptosis and oncogenesis [93].

In the context of cancer disease, the NF-kβ signalling pathway regulates the expression of cell death regulatory genes *via* two pathways, *i.e.* extrinsic pathway and intrinsic pathway [94]. The association of TNF-family death receptors activates the extrinsic pathway, *i.e.*, TNF receptor 1 and Fas [CD 95], while the intrinsic pathway is triggered *via* translocation of family members of pro-apoptotic BCL2 to mitochondria and later release of cytochrome-c. Other mechanisms like TNF signalling, β cell receptor, Toll receptor engagement, are also known to be responsible for activation of the NF-kβ pathway and augment the transcription of NF-kβ target genes [95]. Fig. (**14**) showed a pictorial representation of the mechanism of action of NF- *kβ* inhibitors.

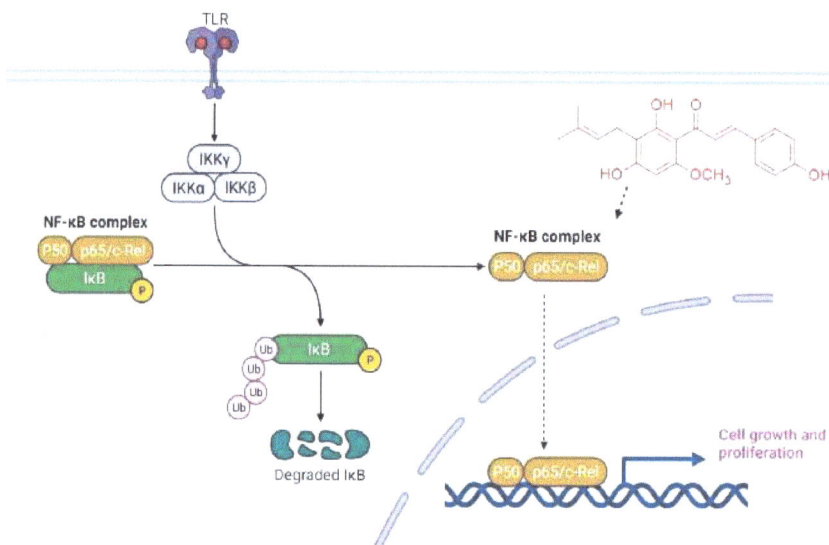

Fig. (14). Diagrammatic representation of the mechanism of action of *NF-kβ* inhibitors.

NF-kβ mediated tumorigenesis primarily occurs in the primary tumour or tumour cell lines of the cervix, ovary, breast, liver, vulva, prostate, kidney, pancreas, stomach, thyroid, *etc*. Several experiments have indicated the involvement of the NF-kb/Rel family of proteins in the growth of oncogenesis [95].

Heterocyclic drugs seem to be effective against breast cancer. Diverse scaffolds inhibitor has been reported to inhibit NF-kβ like pyrazine based inhibitor, celecoxib; (2)-S-diclofenac as thiol derivative (Fig. **15**).

Inhibition of JAK/STAT Signalling Pathway

The JAK/STAT signalling cascade controls several significant cellular functions, for instance, cell proliferation and various apoptosis as well as immune responses. Activation leads to acute neoplastic transformation and abnormal growth of cells.

An increase in STAT phosphorylation resulted in breast cancer, and the expression of STAT3 in the mitochondria seems to affect cell growth and proliferation. Furthermore, in immunocompetent mice, mitochondrial localization sequence (MLS- Stat3) affects cellular proliferation of 4T1 breast cancer [96].

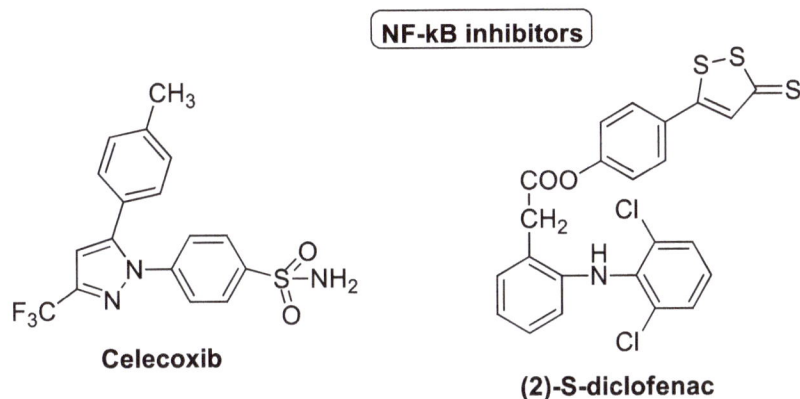

Fig. (15). Chemical structure of heterocyclic compounds as *NF-kβ* inhibitors.

Many malignancies develop slower when this pathway is inhibited by reducing aberrant phosphorylation [97] (Fig. **16**).

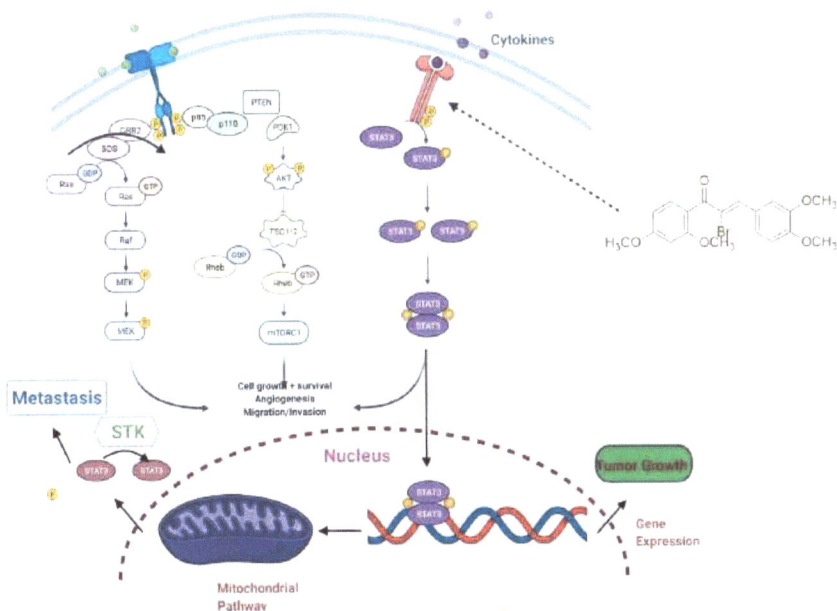

Fig. (16). Pictorial view of the mechanism of action of JAK/STAT signalling pathway inhibitors.

Pyrimethamine is used for chronic lymphocytic leukeamia, small lymphocytic leukeamia, and STA-21, an analogue of tetrangomycin (a non-peptide small molecule STAT-3 inhibitor) that was discovered using structure-based drug design and also used in various forms of cancer cell lines [97]. The chemical structure of JAK/STAT signalling pathway inhibitors has been presented in Fig. (**17**).

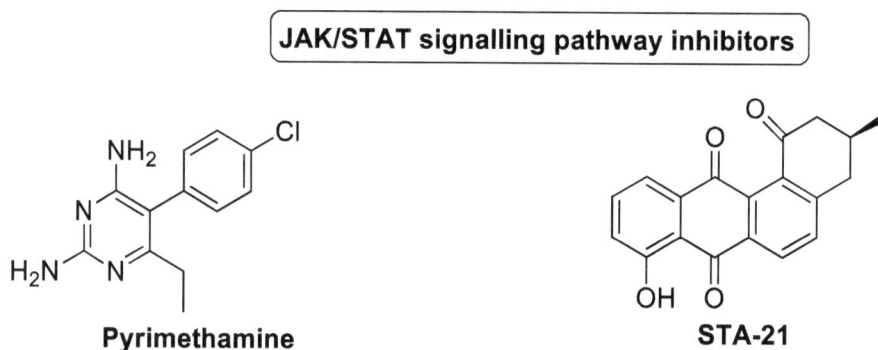

Fig. (**17**). Chemical structure of heterocyclic compounds as *JAK/STAT* signalling pathway inhibitors.

HETEROCYCLIC DRUGS AS INHIBITORS OF MULTIDRUG RESISTANCE (MDR)

ATP- Binding Cassette Transporter G2 (ABCG2) Inhibitors

ABCG2, a member of the ATP-binding cassette (ABC) transporter superfamily, has been linked to the development of multidrug resistance (MDR) in cancer patients, including those with breast cancer. ABCG2 is especially interesting among ABC transporters known to cause MDR because of its potential role in protecting cancer stem cells and its complex oligomeric structure. Small molecule compounds have also been found to modulate ABCG2 biogenesis in recent research [98]. The pictorial representation of the mechanism of action of ABCG2 inhibitors as anticancer agents has been shown in Fig. (**18**).

Recently, a drug named Febuxostat been used in cancer chemotherapy more frequently for the prophylaxis of TLS after approval in Europe and Japan [99]. TLS is a potentially fatal condition caused by the sudden release of intracellular metabolites after tumour cell lysis in chemotherapy-treated cancer patients [99]. For patients with hematologic malignancies, it is the most common emergency treatment. As a result, proper serum uric acid control is critical in the prevention of TLS. Fig. (**19**) presents the chemical structure of various ABCG2 inhibitors.

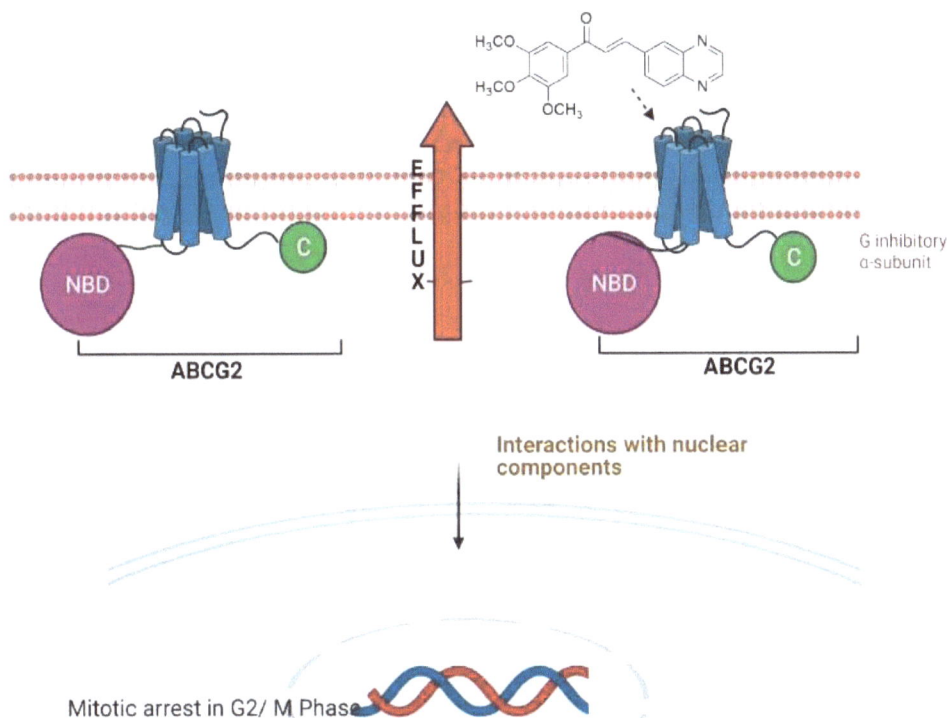

Fig. (18). Showing mechanism of action of ABCG2 inhibitors.

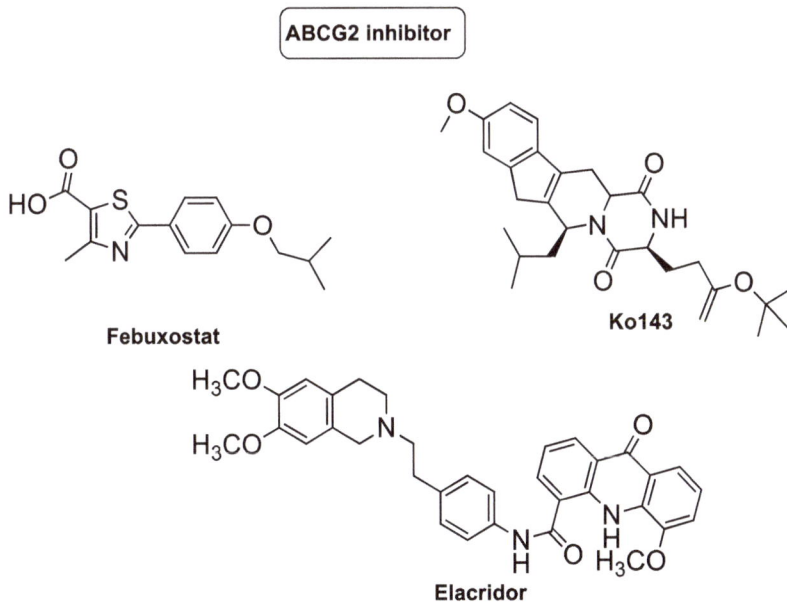

Fig. (19). Chemical structure of diverse scaffolds of heterocyclic compounds as ABCG2 inhibitors.

P-glycoprotein Inhibitors

P-glycoprotein, a protein of cell membrane, also known as multidrug resistance protein 1 (MDR1), presents in animals, fungi and bacteria and are responsible for pumping out foreign substances from the cells by an ATP-dependent efflux pump. P-gp is widely expressed and distributed in the intestinal epithelium, where it pumps xenobiotics like toxins or drugs back into the intestinal lumen. They pump drugs into bile ducts in liver cells, allowing them to be excreted quickly *via* faeces. They pump these xenobiotics back into the capillaries in the blood-brain barrier (BBB) and blood-testis barrier (BTB) [100]. P-gp is overexpressed in some cancer cells, making them resistant to a wide range of drugs (Fig. **20**). Many of the approved drugs like Verapamil, Nifedipine, Dexverapamil with diverse scaffolds have been reported as P-gp inhibitors presented in Fig. (**21**).

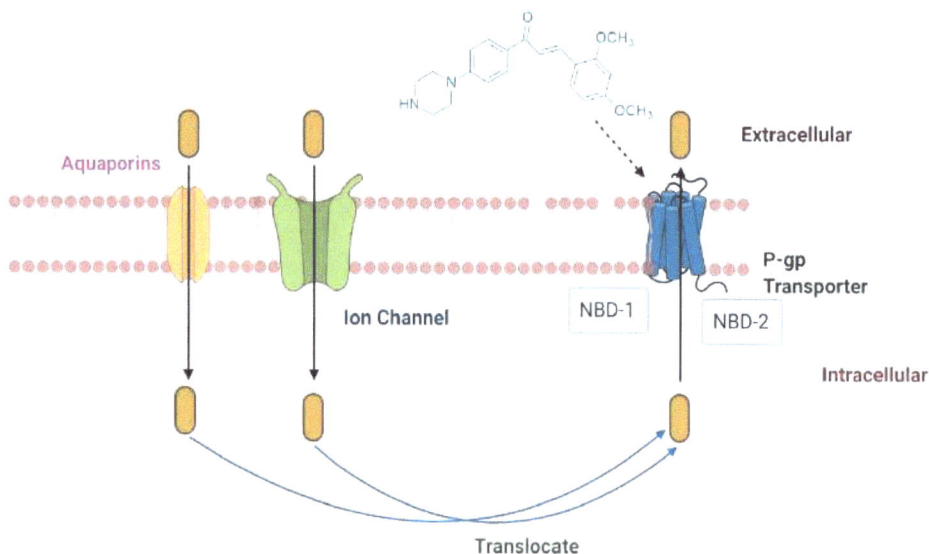

Fig. (20). The mechanism of action of P-glycoprotein inhibitors.

HETEROCYCLIC DRUGS AS P53 DEGRADATION INHIBITORS

Inhibition of Oncoprotein

Oncoprotein interaction inhibition MDM2 is a primary cellular antagonist of p53 and a p53-specific E3 ubiquitin ligase. It works by inhibiting the growth-suppressive function of p53 in unstressed cells, where MDM2 mono-ubiquitinates p53 on a regular basis and thus serves as a rate-limiting step. Multiple routes of disruption of the p53-MDM2 complex are required for p53 activation, resulting in p53 induction and biological response [101]. The figure depicting the mechanism of action has been shown in Fig. (**22**).

P-glycoprotein inhibitors

First generation P-gp Inhibitors

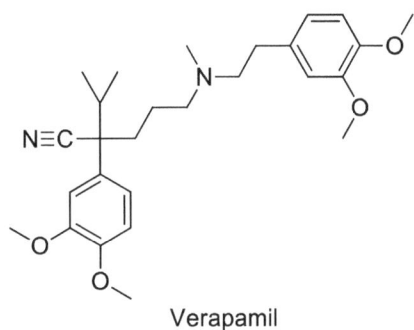

Verapamil

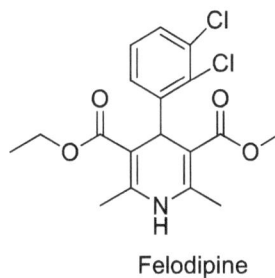

Felodipine

Second generation P-gp Inhibitors

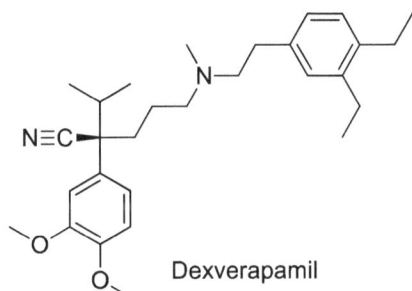

Dexverapamil

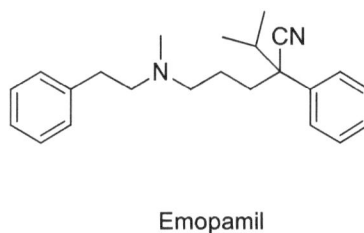

Emopamil

Third generation P-gp Inhibitors

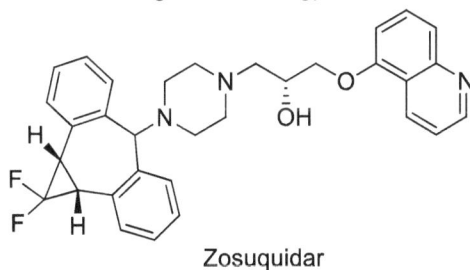

Zosuquidar

Fig. (21). Chemical structure of heterocyclic compounds as P-gp inhibitors.

PROBABLE DRUG TARGETS FOR FUTURE DEVELOPMENT

Cathepsin-k Inhibitors

Lysosomal enzyme Cathepsin-K belongs to the cysteine proteases class expressed significantly in human breast cancer cells and contributes to tumour invasiveness [102]. The published literature revealed that overexpression of Cathepsin K had been linked to metastatic cancer disease, implying that it is useful for diagnostic and prognostic purposes. Cathepsin K has been found to have different expression patterns in lung cancer cells and stromal cells, providing further support for the protease's prognostic value [103]. Cathepsin K's mechanism and role in NSCLC, on the other hand, are still unknown. In NSCLC, cathepsin K may play a role in activating the mTOR signalling pathway. Cathepsin K appears to be emerging as a potential therapeutic target for NSCLC, according to our findings [103]. Several other reports also indicated the importance of Cathepsin-k inhibitors for NSCLC. Therefore we can say that it can be an emerging target for NSCLC [104, 105].

DPP-IV Inhibitor

Several studies were published claiming for anticancer activity of DPP-IV inhibitors. Amritha *et al.* reported anticancer activity in both Sitagliptin and Vildagliptin with IC_{50} of 31.2 mcg/ml and 125 mcg/ml respectively, on colon cell lines (HT-29) using MTT assay-{3 -4, 5-dimethyl (thiazol – 2 -yl) -3, 5- dimethyl tetrazolium bromide} assay was elucidated [106]. Also, numerous other studies reported the same; hence it can be seen as a potential target for anticancer therapy [107, 108].

CONCLUSION

Globally cancer is the second-highest cause of mortality at present. Out of 277 types of cancer recognized so far, small cell lung leads the chart of mortality rate. In the last few decades, heterocyclic compounds, which may be obtained naturally or synthetically, have been developed as a potential scaffold for the development of many anticancer drugs. Heterocyclic compounds due to heteroatoms such as oxygen, nitrogen, and sulphur can be employed as hydrogen bond donors and acceptors [109 - 112]. Efforts have been made to summarize the available inform-ation regarding heterocyclic drugs *i.e.*, ABCG2/P-gp/BCRP, HDAC, Sirt-1, tubulin, topoisomerase II, kinase, mTOR, BRAF and many others. Special emphasis has been given to the diagrammatic representation of the heterocyclic drugs' mechanism inhibiting various molecular targets/pathways involved in carcinogenesis. Besides, information regarding two more drug targets, *i.e.*, DPP-IV and Cathepsin-K has also been summarized as possible anticancer drug targets, which may help researchers, medicinal chemists in designing the potential anticancer drug.

CONSENT FOR PUBLICATION

Not applicable.

CONFLICT OF INTEREST

The author declares no conflict of interest, financial or otherwise.

ACKNOWLEDGEMENTS

The author wishes to acknowledge the Management, Shivalik College of Pharmacy, Nangal and Authorities, Jamia Hamdard University, New Delhi for the constant encouragement and support.

REFERENCES

[1]   Available from: https://www.who.int/cancer/PRGlobocanFinal.pdf

[2]   Singh, R.K.; Kumar, S.; Prasad, D.N.; Bhardwaj, T.R. Therapeutic journery of nitrogen mustard as alkylating anticancer agents: Historic to future perspectives. *Eur. J. Med. Chem.*, **2018**, *151*, 401-433.
[http://dx.doi.org/10.1016/j.ejmech.2018.04.001] [PMID: 29649739]

[3]   Available   from: https://www.ddw-online.com/the-importance-of-heterocyclic-compounds--n-anti-cancer-drug-design-1106-201708/

[4]   Eckschlager, T.; Plch, J.; Stiborova, M.; Hrabeta, J. Histone deacetylase inhibitors as anticancer drugs. *Int. J. Mol. Sci.*, **2017**, *18*(7), 1414.
[http://dx.doi.org/10.3390/ijms18071414] [PMID: 28671573]

[5]   Ceccacci, E.; Minucci, S. Inhibition of histone deacetylases in cancer therapy: Lessons from leukaemia. *Br. J. Cancer*, **2016**, *114*(6), 605-611.
[http://dx.doi.org/10.1038/bjc.2016.36] [PMID: 26908329]

[6]   Grant, S.; Easley, C.; Kirkpatrick, P. Vorinostat. *Nat. Rev. Drug Discov.*, **2007**, *6*(1), 21-22.
[http://dx.doi.org/10.1038/nrd2227] [PMID: 17269160]

[7]   VanderMolen, K.M.; McCulloch, W.; Pearce, C.J.; Oberlies, N.H. Romidepsin (Istodax, NSC 630176, FR901228, FK228, depsipeptide): A natural product recently approved for cutaneous T-cell lymphoma. *J. Antibiot. (Tokyo)*, **2011**, *64*(8), 525-531.
[http://dx.doi.org/10.1038/ja.2011.35] [PMID: 21587264]

[8]   Bolden, J.E.; Peart, M.J.; Johnstone, R.W. Anticancer activities of histone deacetylase inhibitors. *Nat. Rev. Drug Discov.*, **2006**, *5*(9), 769-784.
[http://dx.doi.org/10.1038/nrd2133] [PMID: 16955068]

[9]   Atadja, P. Development of the pan-DAC inhibitor panobinostat (LBH589): Successes and challenges. *Cancer Lett.*, **2009**, *280*(2), 233-241.
[http://dx.doi.org/10.1016/j.canlet.2009.02.019] [PMID: 19344997]

[10]   Manal, M.; Chandrasekar, M.J.N.; Gomathi Priya, J.; Nanjan, M.J. Inhibitors of histone deacetylase as antitumor agents: A critical review. *Bioorg. Chem.*, **2016**, *67*, 18-42.
[http://dx.doi.org/10.1016/j.bioorg.2016.05.005] [PMID: 27239721]

[11]   Eyüpoglu, I.Y.; Hahnen, E.; Buslei, R.; Siebzehnrübl, F.A.; Savaskan, N.E.; Lüders, M.; Tränkle, C.;

Wick, W.; Weller, M.; Fahlbusch, R.; Blümcke, I. Suberoylanilide hydroxamic acid (SAHA) has potent anti-glioma properties *in vitro, ex vivo* and *in vivo. J. Neurochem.,* **2005**, *93*(4), 992-999.
[http://dx.doi.org/10.1111/j.1471-4159.2005.03098.x] [PMID: 15857402]

[12]   Stupp, R.; Mason, W.P.; van den Bent, M.J.; Weller, M.; Fisher, B.; Taphoorn, M.J.B.; Belanger, K.; Brandes, A.A.; Marosi, C.; Bogdahn, U.; Curschmann, J.; Janzer, R.C.; Ludwin, S.K.; Gorlia, T.; Allgeier, A.; Lacombe, D.; Cairncross, J.G.; Eisenhauer, E.; Mirimanoff, R.O. Radiotherapy plus concomitant and adjuvant temozolomide for glioblastoma. *N. Engl. J. Med.,* **2005**, *352*(10), 987-996.
[http://dx.doi.org/10.1056/NEJMoa043330] [PMID: 15758009]

[13]   Ma, T.; Galimberti, F.; Erkmen, C. P.; Memoli, V. Comparing histone deacetylase inhibitor responses in genetically engineered mouse lung cancer models and a window of opportunity trial in patients with lung cancer *Mol Cancer Ther.,* **2013**, *12*(8), 1545-55.
[http://dx.doi.org/10.1158/1535-7163.MCT-12-0933]

[14]   Saelen, M. G.; Ree, A. H.; Kristian, A. Radiosensitization by the histone deacetylase inhibitor vorinostat under hypoxia and with capecitabine in experimental colorectal carcinoma. *Radiat Oncol.,* **2012**, *7*, 165.
[http://dx.doi.org/10.1186/1748-717X-7-165]

[15]   Doi, T.; Hamaguchi, T.; Shirao, K.; Chin, K.; Hatake, K.; Noguchi, K.; Otsuki, T.; Mehta, A.; Ohtsu, A. Evaluation of safety, pharmacokinetics, and efficacy of vorinostat, a histone deacetylase inhibitor, in the treatment of gastrointestinal (GI) cancer in a phase I clinical trial. *Int. J. Clin. Oncol.,* **2013**, *18*(1), 87-95.
[http://dx.doi.org/10.1007/s10147-011-0348-6] [PMID: 22234637]

[16]   FDA Approves Beleodaq (belinostat) for Type of T-cell Lymphoma **2014**. Available from: http://www.cancer.org/cancer/   news/   news/fda-approves-beleodaq-belinostat-for-type-o--t-cell-lymphoma (Accessed on: Accessed August 12, 2014).

[17]   Steele, N.L.; Plumb, J.A.; Vidal, L.; Tjørnelund, J.; Knoblauch, P.; Rasmussen, A.; Ooi, C.E.; Buhl-Jensen, P.; Brown, R.; Evans, T.R.J.; DeBono, J.S. A phase 1 pharmacokinetic and pharmacodynamic study of the histone deacetylase inhibitor belinostat in patients with advanced solid tumors. *Clin. Cancer Res.,* **2008**, *14*(3), 804-810.
[http://dx.doi.org/10.1158/1078-0432.CCR-07-1786] [PMID: 18245542]

[18]   Molife, L.R.; de Bono, J.S. Belinostat: Clinical applications in solid tumors and lymphoma. *Expert Opin. Investig. Drugs,* **2011**, *20*(12), 1723-1732.
[http://dx.doi.org/10.1517/13543784.2011.629604] [PMID: 22046971]

[19]   Liu, K.Y.; Wang, L.T.; Hsu, S.H. Modification of epigenetic histone acetylation in hepatocellular carcinoma. *Cancers (Basel),* **2018**, *10*(1), 8.
[http://dx.doi.org/10.3390/cancers10010008] [PMID: 29301348]

[20]   Piekarz, R.L.; Robey, R.; Sandor, V.; Bakke, S.; Wilson, W.H.; Dahmoush, L.; Kingma, D.M.; Turner, M.L.; Altemus, R.; Bates, S.E. Inhibitor of histone deacetylation, depsipeptide (FR901228), in the treatment of peripheral and cutaneous T-cell lymphoma: A case report. *Blood,* **2001**, *98*(9), 2865-2868.
[http://dx.doi.org/10.1182/blood.V98.9.2865] [PMID: 11675364]

[21]   VanderMolen, K.M.; McCulloch, W.; Pearce, C.J.; Oberlies, N.H. Romidepsin (Istodax, NSC 630176, FR901228, FK228, depsipeptide): A natural product recently approved for cutaneous T-cell lymphoma. *J. Antibiot. (Tokyo),* **2011**, *64*(8), 525-531.
[http://dx.doi.org/10.1038/ja.2011.35] [PMID: 21587264]

[22]   Furumai, R.; Matsuyama, A.; Kobashi, N.; Lee, K.H.; Nishiyama, M.; Nakajima, H.; Tanaka, A.; Komatsu, Y.; Nishino, N.; Yoshida, M.; Horinouchi, S. FK228 (depsipeptide) as a natural prodrug that inhibits class I histone deacetylases. *Cancer Res.,* **2002**, *62*(17), 4916-4921.
[PMID: 12208741]

[23]   Denlinger, C.E.; Keller, M.D.; Mayo, M.W.; Broad, R.M.; Jones, D.R.; Jones, D.R. Combined proteasome and histone deacetylase inhibition in non–small cell lung cancer. *J. Thorac. Cardiovasc.*

Surg., **2004**, *127*(4), 1078-1086.
[http://dx.doi.org/10.1016/S0022-5223(03)01321-7] [PMID: 15052205]

[24]   Karthik, S.; Sankar, R.; Varunkumar, K.; Ravikumar, V. Romidepsin induces cell cycle arrest, apoptosis, histone hyperacetylation and reduces matrix metalloproteinases 2 and 9 expression in bortezomib sensitized non-small cell lung cancer cells. *Biomed. Pharmacother.,* **2014**, *68*(3), 327-334.
[http://dx.doi.org/10.1016/j.biopha.2014.01.002] [PMID: 24485799]

[25]   Robertson, F.R.M.; Chu, K.; Boley, Kimberly M.; Ye, Z.; Liu, H.; Wright, Moishia C.; Moraes, R.; Zhang, X.; Green, Tessa L.; Barsky, Sanford H.; Heise, C.; Cristofanilli, M. The class I HDAC inhibitor Romidepsin targets inflammatory breast cancer tumor emboli and synergizes with paclitaxel to inhibit metastasis *J. Exp. Ther. Oncol.,* **2013**, *10*(3), 219-233.
[PMID: 24416998]

[26]   Imai, S.; Armstrong, C.M.; Kaeberlein, M.; Guarente, L. Transcriptional silencing and longevity protein Sir2 is an NAD-dependent histone deacetylase. *Nature,* **2000**, *403*(6771), 795-800.
[http://dx.doi.org/10.1038/35001622] [PMID: 10693811]

[27]   Haigis, M.C.; Sinclair, D.A. Mammalian sirtuins: Biological insights and disease relevance. *Annu. Rev. Pathol.,* **2010**, *5*(1), 253-295.
[http://dx.doi.org/10.1146/annurev.pathol.4.110807.092250] [PMID: 20078221]

[28]   Luo, J.; Nikolaev, A.Y.; Imai, S.; Chen, D.; Su, F.; Shiloh, A.; Guarente, L.; Gu, W. Negative control of p53 by Sir2α promotes cell survival under stress. *Cell,* **2001**, *107*(2), 137-148.
[http://dx.doi.org/10.1016/S0092-8674(01)00524-4] [PMID: 11672522]

[29]   Jiang, H.; Khan, S.; Wang, Y.; Charron, G.; He, B.; Sebastian, C.; Du, J.; Kim, R.; Ge, E.; Mostoslavsky, R.; Hang, H.C.; Hao, Q.; Lin, H. SIRT6 regulates TNF-α secretion through hydrolysis of long-chain fatty acyl lysine. *Nature,* **2013**, *496*(7443), 110-113.
[http://dx.doi.org/10.1038/nature12038] [PMID: 23552949]

[30]   Hu, J.; Jing, H.; Lin, H. Sirtuin inhibitors as anticancer agents. *Future Med. Chem.,* **2014**, *6*(8), 945-966.
[http://dx.doi.org/10.4155/fmc.14.44] [PMID: 24962284]

[31]   Jung-Hynes, B.; Nihal, M.; Zhong, W.; Ahmad, N. Role of sirtuin histone deacetylase SIRT1 in prostate cancer. A target for prostate cancer management *via* its inhibition? *J. Biol. Chem.,* **2009**, *284*(6), 3823-3832.
[http://dx.doi.org/10.1074/jbc.M807869200] [PMID: 19075016]

[32]   Mellini, P.; Kokkola, T.; Suuronen, T.; Salo, H.S.; Tolvanen, L.; Mai, A.; Lahtela-Kakkonen, M.; Jarho, E.M. Screen of pseudopeptidic inhibitors of human sirtuins 1-3: Two lead compounds with antiproliferative effects in cancer cells. *J. Med. Chem.,* **2013**, *56*(17), 6681-6695.
[http://dx.doi.org/10.1021/jm400438k] [PMID: 23927550]

[33]   Heltweg, B.; Gatbonton, T.; Schuler, A.D.; Posakony, J.; Li, H.; Goehle, S.; Kollipara, R.; DePinho, R.A.; Gu, Y.; Simon, J.A.; Bedalov, A. Antitumor activity of a small-molecule inhibitor of human silent information regulator 2 enzymes. *Cancer Res.,* **2006**, *66*(8), 4368-4377.
[http://dx.doi.org/10.1158/0008-5472.CAN-05-3617] [PMID: 16618762]

[34]   Holloway, K.R.; Barbieri, A.; Malyarchuk, S.; Saxena, M.; Nedeljkovic-Kurepa, A.; Cameron Mehl, M.; Wang, A.; Gu, X.; Pruitt, K. SIRT1 positively regulates breast cancer associated human aromatase (CYP19A1) expression. *Mol. Endocrinol.,* **2013**, *27*(3), 480-490.
[http://dx.doi.org/10.1210/me.2012-1347] [PMID: 23340254]

[35]   Marshall, G.M.; Liu, P.Y.; Gherardi, S.; Scarlett, C.J.; Bedalov, A.; Xu, N.; Iraci, N.; Valli, E.; Ling, D.; Thomas, W.; van Bekkum, M.; Sekyere, E.; Jankowski, K.; Trahair, T.; MacKenzie, K.L.; Haber, M.; Norris, M.D.; Biankin, A.V.; Perini, G.; Liu, T. SIRT1 promotes N-Myc oncogenesis through a positive feedback loop involving the effects of MKP3 and ERK on N-Myc protein stability. *PLoS Genet.,* **2011**, *7*(6), e1002135.
[http://dx.doi.org/10.1371/journal.pgen.1002135] [PMID: 21698133]

[36]   Cea, M.; Soncini, D.; Fruscione, F.; Raffaghello, L.; Garuti, A.; Emionite, L.; Moran, E.; Magnone, M.; Zoppoli, G.; Reverberi, D.; Caffa, I.; Salis, A.; Cagnetta, A.; Bergamaschi, M.; Casciaro, S.; Pierri, I.; Damonte, G.; Ansaldi, F.; Gobbi, M.; Pistoia, V.; Ballestrero, A.; Patrone, F.; Bruzzone, S.; Nencioni, A. Synergistic interactions between HDAC and sirtuin inhibitors in human leukemia cells. *PLoS One,* **2011**, *6*(7), e22739.
        [http://dx.doi.org/10.1371/journal.pone.0022739] [PMID: 21818379]

[37]   Zhang, Y.; Au, Q.; Zhang, M.; Barber, J.R.; Ng, S.C.; Zhang, B. Identification of a small molecule SIRT2 inhibitor with selective tumor cytotoxicity. *Biochem. Biophys. Res. Commun.,* **2009**, *386*(4), 729-733.
        [http://dx.doi.org/10.1016/j.bbrc.2009.06.113] [PMID: 19559674]

[38]   Etienne-Manneville, S. Microtubules in cell migration. *Annu. Rev. Cell Dev. Biol.,* **2013**, *29*(1), 471-499.
        [http://dx.doi.org/10.1146/annurev-cellbio-101011-155711] [PMID: 23875648]

[39]   Chan, K-S.; Koh, C-G.; Li, H-Y. Mitosis-targeted anti-cancer therapies: Where they stand. *Cell Death Dis.,* **2012**, *3*(10), e411.
        [http://dx.doi.org/10.1038/cddis.2012.148] [PMID: 23076219]

[40]   Wani, M.C.; Horwitz, S.B. Nature as a remarkable chemist. *Anticancer Drugs,* **2014**, *25*(5), 482-487.
        [http://dx.doi.org/10.1097/CAD.0000000000000063] [PMID: 24413390]

[41]   Levêque, D.; Becker, G. Generic Docetaxel. *J. Clin. Pharmacol.,* **2017**, *57*(7), 935.
        [http://dx.doi.org/10.1002/jcph.893] [PMID: 28467604]

[42]   Cheetham, P.; Petrylak, D.P. Tubulin-targeted agents including docetaxel and cabazitaxel. *Cancer J.,* **2013**, *19*(1), 59-65.
        [http://dx.doi.org/10.1097/PPO.0b013e3182828d38] [PMID: 23337758]

[43]   Gross, M.E.; Dorff, T.B.; Quinn, D.I.; Diaz, P.M.; Castellanos, O.O.; Agus, D.B. Safety and efficacy of docetaxel, bevacizumab, and everolimus for Castration-resistant Prostate Cancer (CRPC). *Clin. Genitourin. Cancer,* **2018**, *16*(1), e11-e21.
        [http://dx.doi.org/10.1016/j.clgc.2017.07.003] [PMID: 28826933]

[44]   Liu, C.; Yu, F.; Liu, Q.; Bian, X.; Hu, S.; Yang, H.; Yin, Y.; Li, Y.; Shen, Y.; Xia, L.; Tu, Q.; Zhang, Y. Yield improvement of epothilones in Burkholderia strain DSM7029 *via* transporter engineering. *FEMS Microbiol. Lett.,* **2018**, *365*(9)
        [http://dx.doi.org/10.1093/femsle/fny045] [PMID: 29529178]

[45]   Marchetti, C.; Piacenti, I.; Imperiale, L.; De Felice, F.; Boccia, S.; Di Donato, V.; Perniola, G.; Monti, M.; Palaia, I.; Muzii, L.; Benedetti Panici, P. Ixabepilone for the treatment of endometrial cancer. *Expert Opin. Investig. Drugs,* **2016**, *25*(5), 613-618.
        [http://dx.doi.org/10.1517/13543784.2016.1161755] [PMID: 26949829]

[46]   Cheng, Z.; Lu, X.; Feng, B. A review of research progress of antitumor drugs based on tubulin targets. *Transl. Cancer Res.,* **2020**, *9*(6), 4020-4027.
        [http://dx.doi.org/10.21037/tcr-20-682] [PMID: 35117769]

[47]   García-Donas, J.; Font, A.; Pérez-Valderrama, B.; Virizuela, J.A.; Climent, M.Á.; Hernando-Polo, S.; Arranz, J.Á.; del Mar Llorente, M.; Lainez, N.; Villa-Guzmán, J.C.; Mellado, B.; del Alba, A.G.; Castellano, D.; Gallardo, E.; Anido, U.; del Muro, X.G.; Domènech, M.; Puente, J.; Morales-Barrera, R.; Pérez-Gracia, J.L.; Bellmunt, J. Maintenance therapy with vinflunine plus best supportive care *versus* best supportive care alone in patients with advanced urothelial carcinoma with a response after first-line chemotherapy (MAJA; SOGUG 2011/02): A multicentre, randomised, controlled, open-label, phase 2 trial. *Lancet Oncol.,* **2017**, *18*(5), 672-681a.
        [http://dx.doi.org/10.1016/S1470-2045(17)30242-5] [PMID: 28389316]

[48]   Gerullis, H.; Wawroschek, F.; Köhne, C.H.; Ecke, T.H. Vinflunine in the treatment of advanced urothelial cancer: Clinical evidence and experience. *Ther. Adv. Urol.,* **2017**, *9*(1), 28-35.
        [http://dx.doi.org/10.1177/1756287216677903] [PMID: 28042310]

[49]   Kruczynski, A.; Hill, B.T. Vinflunine, the latest Vinca alkaloid in clinical development. *Crit. Rev. Oncol. Hematol.,* **2001**, *40*(2), 159-173.
[http://dx.doi.org/10.1016/S1040-8428(01)00183-4] [PMID: 11682323]

[50]   Zhu, B.; Yu, L.; Yue, Q. Co-delivery of vincristine and quercetin by nanocarriers for lymphoma combination chemotherapy. *Biomed. Pharmacother.,* **2017**, *91*, 287-294.
[http://dx.doi.org/10.1016/j.biopha.2017.02.112] [PMID: 28463792]

[51]   Nazir, H.F.; AlFutaisi, A.; Zacharia, M.; Elshinawy, M.; Mevada, S.T.; Alrawas, A.; Khater, D.; Jaju, D.; Wali, Y. Vincristine-induced neuropathy in pediatric patients with acute lymphoblastic leukemia in Oman: Frequent autonomic and more severe cranial nerve involvement. *Pediatr. Blood Cancer,* **2017**, *64*(12), e26677.
[http://dx.doi.org/10.1002/pbc.26677] [PMID: 28623857]

[52]   Morimoto, Y.; Miyawaki, K.; Seki, R.; Watanabe, K.; Hirohara, M.; Shinohara, T. Risk factors for venous irritation in patients receiving vinorelbine: A retrospective study. *J. Pharm. Health Care Sci.,* **2018**, *4*(1), 26.
[http://dx.doi.org/10.1186/s40780-018-0122-2] [PMID: 30288295]

[53]   Yamamoto, N.; Kenmotsu, H.; Yamanaka, T.; Nakamura, S.; Tsuboi, M. Randomized Phase III study of cisplatin with pemetrexed and cisplatin with vinorelbine for completely resected nonsquamous non–small-cell lung cancer: The jipang study protocol. *Clin. Lung Cancer,* **2018**, *19*(1), e1-e3.
[http://dx.doi.org/10.1016/j.cllc.2017.05.020] [PMID: 28668204]

[54]   Dugal-Tessier, J.; Barnscher, S.D.; Kanai, A.; Mendelsohn, B.A. Synthesis and evaluation of dolastatin 10 analogues containing heteroatoms on the amino acid side chains. *J. Nat. Prod.,* **2017**, *80*(9), 2484-2491.
[http://dx.doi.org/10.1021/acs.jnatprod.7b00359] [PMID: 28885014]

[55]   Yokosaka, S.; Izawa, A.; Sakai, C.; Sakurada, E.; Morita, Y.; Nishio, Y. Synthesis and evaluation of novel dolastatin 10 derivatives for versatile conjugations. *Bioorg. Med. Chem.,* **2018**, *26*(8), 1643-1652.
[http://dx.doi.org/10.1016/j.bmc.2018.02.011] [PMID: 29454703]

[56]   Bousquet, M.S.; Ma, J.J.; Ratnayake, R.; Havre, P.A.; Yao, J.; Dang, N.H.; Paul, V.J.; Carney, T.J.; Dang, L.H.; Luesch, H. Multidimensional screening platform for simultaneously targeting oncogenic KRAS and hypoxia-inducible factors pathways in colorectal cancer. *ACS Chem. Biol.,* **2016**, *11*(5), 1322-1331.
[http://dx.doi.org/10.1021/acschembio.5b00860] [PMID: 26938486]

[57]   Salvador-Reyes, L.A.; Engene, N.; Paul, V.J.; Luesch, H. Targeted natural products discovery from marine cyanobacteria using combined phylogenetic and mass spectrometric evaluation. *J. Nat. Prod.,* **2015**, *78*(3), 486-492.
[http://dx.doi.org/10.1021/np500931q] [PMID: 25635943]

[58]   Robinson, K.P.; Chan, J.J. Colchicine in dermatology: A review. *Australas. J. Dermatol.,* **2018**, *59*(4), 278-285.
[http://dx.doi.org/10.1111/ajd.12795] [PMID: 29430631]

[59]   Angelidis, C.; Kotsialou, Z.; Kossyvakis, C.; Vrettou, A.R.; Zacharoulis, A.; Kolokathis, F.; Kekeris, V.; Giannopoulos, G. Colchicine pharmacokinetics and mechanism of action. *Curr. Pharm. Des.,* **2018**, *24*(6), 659-663.
[http://dx.doi.org/10.2174/1381612824666180123110042] [PMID: 29359661]

[60]   Zi, C.T.; Yang, L.; Xu, F.Q.; Dong, F.W.; Yang, D.; Li, Y.; Ding, Z.T.; Zhou, J.; Jiang, Z.H.; Hu, J.M. Synthesis and anticancer activity of dimeric podophyllotoxin derivatives. *Drug Des. Devel. Ther.,* **2018**, *12*, 3393-3406.
[http://dx.doi.org/10.2147/DDDT.S167382] [PMID: 30349193]

[61]   Ghaly, P.E.; Abou El-Magd, R.M.; Churchill, C.D.M.; Tuszynski, J.A.; West, F.G. A new antiproliferative noscapine analogue: Chemical synthesis and biological evaluation. *Oncotarget,* **2016**,

7(26), 40518-40530.
[http://dx.doi.org/10.18632/oncotarget.9642] [PMID: 27777381]

[62]   Altinoz, M.A.; Topcu, G.; Hacimuftuoglu, A.; Ozpinar, A.; Ozpinar, A.; Hacker, E.; Elmaci, İ. Noscapine, a Non-addictive Opioid and Microtubule-Inhibitor in Potential Treatment of Glioblastoma. *Neurochem. Res.,* **2019**, *44*(8), 1796-1806.
[http://dx.doi.org/10.1007/s11064-019-02837-x] [PMID: 31292803]

[63]   Meher, R.K.; Naik, M.R.; Bastia, B.; Naik, P.K. Comparative evaluation of anti-angiogenic effects of noscapine derivatives. *Bioinformation,* **2018**, *14*(5), 236-240.
[http://dx.doi.org/10.6026/97320630014236] [PMID: 30108421]

[64]   Eroğlu, C.; Avcı, E.; Vural, H.; Kurar, E. Anticancer mechanism of Sinapic acid in PC-3 and LNCaP human prostate cancer cell lines. *Gene,* **2018**, *671*, 127-134.
[http://dx.doi.org/10.1016/j.gene.2018.05.049] [PMID: 29792952]

[65]   Wang, J.C. Cellular roles of DNA topoisomerases: A molecular perspective. *Nat. Rev. Mol. Cell Biol.,* **2002**, *3*(6), 430-440.
[http://dx.doi.org/10.1038/nrm831] [PMID: 12042765]

[66]   Nitiss, J.L. Targeting DNA topoisomerase II in cancer chemotherapy. *Nat. Rev. Cancer,* **2009**, *9*(5), 338-350.
[http://dx.doi.org/10.1038/nrc2607] [PMID: 19377506]

[67]   Hornyak, P.; Askwith, T.; Walker, S.; Komulainen, E.; Paradowski, M.; Pennicott, L.E.; Bartlett, E.J.; Brissett, N.C.; Raoof, A.; Watson, M.; Jordan, A.M.; Ogilvie, D.J.; Ward, S.E.; Atack, J.R.; Pearl, L.H.; Caldecott, K.W.; Oliver, A.W. Mode of action of DNA-competitive small molecule inhibitors of tyrosyl DNA phosphodiesterase 2. *Biochem. J.,* **2016**, *473*(13), 1869-1879.
[http://dx.doi.org/10.1042/BCJ20160180] [PMID: 27099339]

[68]   Larsen, A.K.; Escargueil, A.E.; Skladanowski, A. Catalytic topoisomerase II inhibitors in cancer therapy. *Pharmacol. Ther.,* **2003**, *99*(2), 167-181.
[http://dx.doi.org/10.1016/S0163-7258(03)00058-5] [PMID: 12888111]

[69]   Drake, F.H.; Hofmann, G.A.; Mong, S.M.; Bartus, J.O.; Hertzberg, R.P.; Johnson, R.K.; Mattern, M.R.; Mirabelli, C.K. *In vitro* and intracellular inhibition of topoisomerase II by the antitumor agent merbarone. *Cancer Res.,* **1989**, *49*(10), 2578-2583.
[PMID: 2540903]

[70]   Fortune, J.M.; Osheroff, N. *Merbarone Inhibits the Catalytic Activity of Human Topoisomerase IIα by Blocking DNA Cleavage, Nucleic Acids, Protein Synthesis, and Molecular Genetics,* **1998**, *26*(4), P17643-P17650.

[71]   Ali, J.A.; Jackson, A.P.; Howells, A.J.; Maxwell, A. The 43-kilodalton N-terminal fragment of the DNA gyrase B protein hydrolyzes ATP and binds coumarin drugs. *Biochemistry,* **1993**, *32*(10), 2717-2724.
[http://dx.doi.org/10.1021/bi00061a033] [PMID: 8383523]

[72]   Bisacchi, G.S.; Manchester, J.I. A new-class antibacterial-almost. Lessons in drug discovery and development: A critical analysis of more than 50 years of effort toward ATPase inhibitors of DNA gyrase and topoisomerase IV. *ACS Infect. Dis.,* **2015**, *1*(1), 4-41.
[http://dx.doi.org/10.1021/id500013t] [PMID: 27620144]

[73]   Oki, T. Recent developments in the process improvement of production of antitumor anthracycline antibiotics. *Adv. Biotechnol. Processes,* **1984**, *3*, 163-196.
[PMID: 6399842]

[74]   Hevener, K.; Verstak, T.A.; Lutat, K.E.; Riggsbee, D.L.; Mooney, J.W. Recent developments in topoisomerase-targeted cancer chemotherapy. *Acta Pharm. Sin. B,* **2018**, *8*(6), 844-861.
[http://dx.doi.org/10.1016/j.apsb.2018.07.008] [PMID: 30505655]

[75]   Fox, E.J. Mechanism of action of mitoxantrone. *Neurology,* **2004**, *63*(12, Supplement 6) Suppl. 6,

S15-S18.
[http://dx.doi.org/10.1212/WNL.63.12_suppl_6.S15] [PMID: 15623664]

[76]   Beeharry, N.; Di Rora, A.G.L.; Smith, M.R.; Yen, T.J. Pixantrone induces cell death through mitotic perturbations and subsequent aberrant cell divisions. *Cancer Biol. Ther.,* **2015**, *16*(9), 1397-1406.
[http://dx.doi.org/10.1080/15384047.2015.1070979] [PMID: 26177126]

[77]   Salvatorelli, E.; Menna, P.; Paz, O.G.; Chello, M.; Covino, E.; Singer, J.W.; Minotti, G. The novel anthracenedione, pixantrone, lacks redox activity and inhibits doxorubicinol formation in human myocardium: Insight to explain the cardiac safety of pixantrone in doxorubicin-treated patients. *J. Pharmacol. Exp. Ther.,* **2013**, *344*(2), 467-478.
[http://dx.doi.org/10.1124/jpet.112.200568] [PMID: 23192654]

[78]   Longo, M.; Torre, P.D.; Allievi, C.; Morisetti, A.; Al-Fayoumi, S.; Singer, J.W. Tolerability and toxicological profile of pixantrone (Pixuvri®) in juvenile mice. Comparative study with doxorubicin. *Reprod. Toxicol.,* **2014**, *46*, 20-30.
[http://dx.doi.org/10.1016/j.reprotox.2014.02.006] [PMID: 24602559]

[79]   Wieduwilt, M.J.; Moasser, M.M. The epidermal growth factor receptor family: Biology driving targeted therapeutics. *Cell. Mol. Life Sci.,* **2008**, *65*(10), 1566-1584.
[http://dx.doi.org/10.1007/s00018-008-7440-8] [PMID: 18259690]

[80]   Available from: https://www.frontiersin.org/articles/10.3389/fphar.2015.00283/full

[81]   Jung, J.I.; Chung, E.; Seon, M.R.; Shin, H.K.; Kim, E.J.; Lim, S.S.; Chung, W.Y.; Park, K.K.; Park, J.H.Y. Isoliquiritigenin (ISL) inhibits ErbB3 signaling in prostate cancer cells. *Biofactors,* **2006**, *28*(3-4), 159-168.
[http://dx.doi.org/10.1002/biof.5520280302] [PMID: 17473376]

[82]   Shin, S.Y.; Yoon, H.; Ahn, S.; Kim, D.W.; Kim, S.H.; Koh, D.; Lee, Y.H.; Lim, Y. Chromenylchalcones showing cytotoxicity on human colon cancer cell lines and *in silico* docking with aurora kinases. *Bioorg. Med. Chem.,* **2013**, *21*(14), 4250-4258.
[http://dx.doi.org/10.1016/j.bmc.2013.04.086] [PMID: 23719279]

[83]   Sarbassov, D.D.; Ali, S.M.; Sengupta, S.; Sheen, J.H.; Hsu, P.P.; Bagley, A.F.; Markhard, A.L.; Sabatini, D.M. Prolonged rapamycin treatment inhibits mTORC2 assembly and Akt/PKB. *Mol. Cell,* **2006**, *22*(2), 159-168.
[http://dx.doi.org/10.1016/j.molcel.2006.03.029] [PMID: 16603397]

[84]   Li, J.; Kim, S.G.; Blenis, J. Rapamycin: One drug, many effects. *Cell Metab.,* **2014**, *19*(3), 373-379.
[http://dx.doi.org/10.1016/j.cmet.2014.01.001] [PMID: 24508508]

[85]   Elit, L. CCI-779 Wyeth. *Curr. Opin. Investig. Drugs,* **2002**, *3*(8), 1249-1253.
[PMID: 12211424]

[86]   Kirchner, G.I.; Meier-Wiedenbach, I.; Manns, M.P. Clinical pharmacokinetics of everolimus. *Clin. Pharmacokinet.,* **2004**, *43*(2), 83-95.
[http://dx.doi.org/10.2165/00003088-200443020-00002] [PMID: 14748618]

[87]   Holderfield, M.; Deuker, M.M.; McCormick, F.; McMahon, M. Targeting RAF kinases for cancer therapy: BRAF-mutated melanoma and beyond. *Nat. Rev. Cancer,* **2014**, *14*(7), 455-467.
[http://dx.doi.org/10.1038/nrc3760] [PMID: 24957944]

[88]   Dankort, D.; Curley, D.P.; Cartlidge, R.A.; Nelson, B.; Karnezis, A.N.; Damsky, W.E., Jr; You, M.J.; DePinho, R.A.; McMahon, M.; Bosenberg, M. BrafV600E cooperates with Pten loss to induce metastatic melanoma. *Nat. Genet.,* **2009**, *41*(5), 544-552.
[http://dx.doi.org/10.1038/ng.356] [PMID: 19282848]

[89]   Escudier, B.; Worden, F.; Kudo, M. Sorafenib: Key lessons from over 10 years of experience. *Expert Rev. Anticancer Ther.,* **2019**, *19*(2), 177-189.
[http://dx.doi.org/10.1080/14737140.2019.1559058] [PMID: 30575405]

[90]   Mousa, A.B. Sorafenib in the treatment of advanced hepatocellular carcinoma. *Saudi J.*

Gastroenterol., **2008**, *14*(1), 40-42.
[http://dx.doi.org/10.4103/1319-3767.37808] [PMID: 19568496]

[91]   Available from: http://www.fda.gov/NewsEvents/Newsroom/PressAnnouncements/ucm268241.htm

[92]   Eroglu, Z.; Ribas, A. Combination therapy with BRAF and MEK inhibitors for melanoma: Latest evidence and place in therapy. *Ther. Adv. Med. Oncol.,* **2016**, *8*(1), 48-56.
[http://dx.doi.org/10.1177/1758834015616934] [PMID: 26753005]

[93]   Oeckinghaus, A.; Ghosh, S. The NF-kappaB family of transcription factors and its regulation. *Cold Spring Harb. Perspect. Biol.,* **2009**, *1*(4), a000034.
[http://dx.doi.org/10.1101/cshperspect.a000034] [PMID: 20066092]

[94]   Zhang, H.; Sun, S.C. NF-κB in inflammation and renal diseases. *Cell Biosci.,* **2015**, *5*(1), 63.
[http://dx.doi.org/10.1186/s13578-015-0056-4] [PMID: 26579219]

[95]   Sharma, R.K.; Otsuka, M.; Gaba, G.; Mehta, S. Inhibitors of transcription factor nuclear factor-kappa beta (NF-κβ)-DNA binding. *RSC Advances,* **2013**, *3*(5), 1282-1296.
[http://dx.doi.org/10.1039/C2RA21852F]

[96]   Kiu, H.; Nicholson, S.E. Biology and significance of the JAK/STAT signalling pathways. *Growth Factors,* **2012**, *30*(2), 88-106.
[http://dx.doi.org/10.3109/08977194.2012.660936] [PMID: 22339650]

[97]   Thomas, S.J.; Snowden, J.A.; Zeidler, M.P.; Danson, S.J. The role of JAK/STAT signalling in the pathogenesis, prognosis and treatment of solid tumours. *Br. J. Cancer,* **2015**, *113*(3), 365-371.
[http://dx.doi.org/10.1038/bjc.2015.233] [PMID: 26151455]

[98]   Mo, W.; Zhang, J.T. Human ABCG2: Structure, function, and its role in multidrug resistance. *Int. J. Biochem. Mol. Biol.,* **2012**, *3*(1), 1-27.
[PMID: 22509477]

[99]   Spina, M.; Nagy, Z.; Ribera, J.M.; Federico, M.; Aurer, I.; Jordan, K.; Borsaru, G.; Pristupa, A.S.; Bosi, A.; Grosicki, S.; Glushko, N.L.; Ristic, D.; Jakucs, J.; Montesinos, P.; Mayer, J.; Rego, E.M.; Baldini, S.; Scartoni, S.; Capriati, A.; Maggi, C.A.; Simonelli, C. FLORENCE: A randomized, double-blind, phase III pivotal study of febuxostat *versus* allopurinol for the prevention of tumor lysis syndrome (TLS) in patients with hematologic malignancies at intermediate to high TLS risk. *Ann. Oncol.,* **2015**, *26*(10), 2155-2161.
[http://dx.doi.org/10.1093/annonc/mdv317] [PMID: 26216382]

[100] Chan, L.M.S.; Lowes, S.; Hirst, B.H. The ABCs of drug transport in intestine and liver: Efflux proteins limiting drug absorption and bioavailability. *Eur. J. Pharm. Sci.,* **2004**, *21*(1), 25-51.
[http://dx.doi.org/10.1016/j.ejps.2003.07.003] [PMID: 14706810]

[101] Hock, A.K.; Vousden, K.H. The role of ubiquitin modification in the regulation of p53, Biochimica et Biophysica Acta (BBA) -. *Molecular Cell Research,* **2014**, *1843*(1), 137-149.

[102] Tan, G.J.; Peng, Z.K.; Lu, J.P.; Tang, F.Q. Cathepsins mediate tumor metastasis. *World J. Biol. Chem.,* **2013**, *4*(4), 91-101.
[http://dx.doi.org/10.4331/wjbc.v4.i4.91] [PMID: 24340132]

[103] Yang, H.; Heyer, J.; Zhao, H.; Liang, S.; Guo, R.; Zhong, L. The potential role of cathepsin K in non-small cell lung cancer. *Molecules,* **2020**, *25*(18), 4136.
[http://dx.doi.org/10.3390/molecules25184136] [PMID: 32927648]

[104] Seo, S.U.; Woo, S.M.; Kim, M.W.; Lee, H.S.; Kim, S.H.; Kang, S.C.; Lee, E.W.; Min, K.; Kwon, T.K. Cathepsin K inhibition-induced mitochondrial ROS enhances sensitivity of cancer cells to anti-cancer drugs through USP27x-mediated Bim protein stabilization. *Redox Biol.,* **2020**, *30*, 101422.
[http://dx.doi.org/10.1016/j.redox.2019.101422] [PMID: 31901727]

[105] Obenauf, A.C.; Zou, Y.; Ji, A.L.; Vanharanta, S.; Shu, W.; Shi, H.; Kong, X.; Bosenberg, M.C.; Wiesner, T.; Rosen, N.; Lo, R.S.; Massagué, J. Therapy-induced tumour secretomes promote resistance and tumour progression. *Nature,* **2015**, *520*(7547), 368-372.

[http://dx.doi.org/10.1038/nature14336] [PMID: 25807485]

[106] Amritha, C.A.; Kumaravelu, P.; Chellathai, D.D. Evaluation of anti cancer effects of dpp-4 inhibitors in colon cancer- an *in vitro* study. *J. Clin. Diagn. Res.,* **2015**, *9*(12), FC14-FC16.
[PMID: 26816911]

[107] Koehler, J.A.; Kain, T.; Drucker, D.J. Glucagon-like peptide-1 receptor activation inhibits growth and augments apoptosis in murine CT26 colon cancer cells. *Endocrinology,* **2011**, *152*(9), 3362-3372.
[http://dx.doi.org/10.1210/en.2011-1201] [PMID: 21771884]

[108] De, S.; Banerjee, S.; Kumar, S.K.A.; Paira, P. Critical role of dipeptidyl peptidase IV: A therapeutic target for diabetes and cancer. *Mini Rev. Med. Chem.,* **2018**, *19*(2), 88-97.
[http://dx.doi.org/10.2174/1389557518666180423112154] [PMID: 29692250]

[109] Kumari, A.; Singh, R.K. Medicinal chemistry of indole derivatives: Current to future therapeutic prospectives. *Bioorg. Chem.,* **2019**, *89*, 103021.
[http://dx.doi.org/10.1016/j.bioorg.2019.103021] [PMID: 31176854]

[110] Kumari, A.; Singh, R.K. Morpholine as ubiquitous pharmacophore in medicinal chemistry: Deep insight into the structure-activity relationship (SAR). *Bioorg. Chem.,* **2020**, *96*, 103578.
[http://dx.doi.org/10.1016/j.bioorg.2020.103578] [PMID: 31978684]

[111] Sethi, N.S.; Prasad, D.N.; Singh, R.K. An Insight into the Synthesis and SAR of 2,4-Thiazolidinediones (2,4-TZD) as Multifunctional Scaffold: A Review. *Mini Rev. Med. Chem.,* **2020**, *20*(4), 308-330.
[http://dx.doi.org/10.2174/1389557519666191029102838] [PMID: 31660809]

[112] Kumar, S.; Singh, R.K.; Patial, B.; Goyal, S.; Bhardwaj, T.R. Recent advances in novel heterocyclic scaffolds for the treatment of drug-resistant malaria. *J. Enzyme Inhib. Med. Chem.,* **2016**, *31*(2), 173-186.
[http://dx.doi.org/10.3109/14756366.2015.1016513] [PMID: 25775094]

CHAPTER 2

Impact of Coumarin Hybrids upon Imperative Clinical Targets against Cancer

Rohit Bhatia[1], Amandeep Singh[2], Bhupinder Kumar[1] and **Ravindra K. Rawal[3,*]**

[1] *Department of Pharmaceutical Chemistry, ISF College of Pharmacy, Moga, Punjab-142001, India*

[2] *Department of Pharmaceutics, ISF College of Pharmacy, Moga, Punjab-142001, India*

[3] *CSIR-North East Institute of Science and Technology, Jorhat-785006, Assam, India*

Abstract: The severity, prevalence, and complexity of cancer do not need any introduction at present. The coumarin scaffold has been explored intermittently for its anti-cancer potential for a long time, and continuous research is further in progress. The concept of molecular hybridization has opened new doors towards the design and development of therapeutic candidates, capable of binding to multiple targets. This has been proven to be a promising approach for diseases with complex pathophysiology involving a variety of targets. In this direction, several research groups have explored the therapeutic potentials of coumarin and its derivatives against cancer. Coumarin possesses multiple sites for substitution/tethering/fusion, providing ease for constructing coumarin hybrid molecules. Coumarin and its derivatives have the ability to exert anti-cancer activity by interacting/binding with several targets, including aromatase, sulphatase, protein kinases, telomerase, carbonic anhydrase, caspases, SERD (selective estrogen receptor downregulators), tubulin, phosphoinositide 3-kinases (PI3K), topoisomerase and hormones. These targets are involved in complex pathological events during the development of cancer. Several heterocyclic moieties beyond coumarin are also capable of binding to one or more of these targets. Therefore, conjuring such a heterocycle with coumarin moiety is an ideal approach to target more than one target simultaneously. In this chapter, the authors have highlighted important targets along with their significance in the development of cancer. A description of reported potent anti-cancer coumarin hybrids (in the past five years) inhibiting/interacting with particular targets has been provided. Although there is a tremendous advancement in developing hybrid molecules against cancer, still no suitable candidate has been launched in the market for a long time. So, further clinical and toxicological investigations on reported lead molecules should be carried out on priority.

---

* **Corresponding author Ravindra K. Rawal:** CSIR-North East Institute of Science and Technology, Jorhat-785006, Assam, India; Tel: +91-8486599155; E-mails: rawal.ravindra@gmail.com and drrkrawal@neist.res.in

Rajesh Kumar Singh (Ed.)

Keywords: Aromatase, Coumarin hybrids, PI3K, Protein kinase, SERD, Sulphatase, Targets.

INTRODUCTION

Cancer is a complex, widely prevalent, and life-threatening health ailment in the modern age. It is the second leading cause of death globally, the burden is increasing day by day even after the development of advanced healthcare systems. It is a complex disease that may affect any part of the body, where the cells grow abnormally and spread to other organs through blood circulation or the lymph system [1, 2]. Cancer progresses when DNA becomes non-responsive to the normal cell growth process [3]. Reports evidence that in 2020, 1,806,590 new cancer cases and 606,520 deaths were reported in the United States, whereas in 2021, 1,898,160 new cases and 608,570 cancer deaths have been estimated in the United States [4, 5]. Cancer is the reason for 1 death/6 deaths globally. The death risk due to cancer in males is 22.05%, while in females, it is about 18.75% [6]. It is worth notable that 70% of total cancer deaths have been found in low and middle-income countries [7 - 9]. Cancer statistics in 2017 revealed that only 30% of low-income countries were able to procure treatment facilities as compared to high-income countries [10]. In a nutshell, it can be concluded that the burden of this ailment is mounting vigorously throughout the globe, striking substantial physical, mental, and economic stress on the human population. A vast population of low-income countries is still unable to get a timely diagnosis and cure for cancer, leading to a reduced survival rate.

Advancements and modernization in the healthcare sector have led to the development of several therapies against cancer. The type of treatment is dependent on the type/stage of cancer, general health of the patient, and preferences. The standard treatment strategies include chemotherapeutic agents, hormonal therapy, radiation therapy, gene therapy, immunotherapy, bone marrow transplant, and surgery [11 - 13]. Among these, chemotherapeutic agents are widely preferred as they have the potential to arrest the growth of tumor cells. These chemotherapeutic agents work through various diverse mechanisms. Although they have been proven to be significant therapeutic candidates, they are still associated with several complications and issues like lack of selectivity, toxicity, and many side effects [14, 15]. Therefore, there is an urgent need to develop newer therapeutic agents which bypass all these issues.

CONCEPT OF COUMARIN HYBRID MOLECULES AGAINST CANCER

Coumarin is a privileged motif and keeps a noteworthy place among heterocyclic compounds due to its diverse pharmacological activities, among which anti-cancer activity is the most promising. Coumarin has the potential to interact/modulate/inhibit a large number of biological targets, which are responsible for a variety of cancers [16 - 20]. Researchers have nowadays paid keen attention to exploring the potency of the coumarin nucleus to develop novel therapeutic agents in cancer treatment. Various research reports revealed that coumarin derivatives exhibit anti-cancer activity by interacting with aromatase, sulphatase, protein kinase, selective estrogen receptor modulator (SERM), selective estrogen receptor down regulator, tubulin, topoisomerase, 17β-hydroxysteroid dehydrogenase type 3 (17β-HSD3), *etc.* [21]. By focusing on these pharmacological characteristics of the coumarin scaffold, various other pharmacophores can be fused/substituted/combined with it to develop hybrid molecules with the intent to bind with multiple targets associated with cancer. The suitability of coumarin derivatives to be used as anti-cancer agents is justified by their safety as these possess very rare nephrotoxicity, neurotoxicity, epithelial toxicity, or cardiotoxicity. Coumarin scaffold exists as simple substituted compounds as well as complex hybrid forms due to its structural diversity.

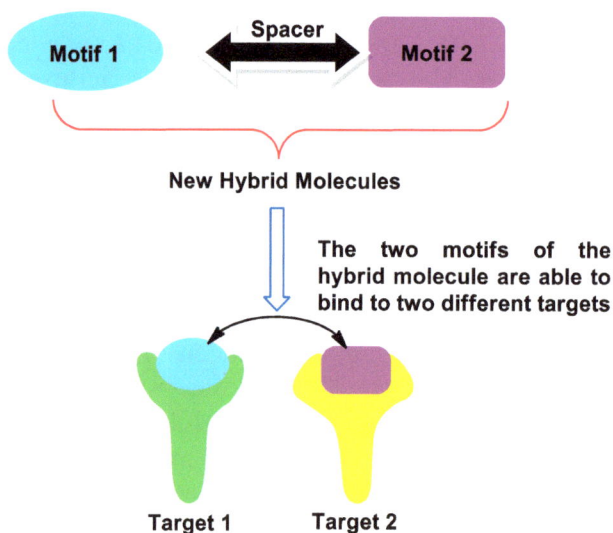

Fig. (1). Concept of molecular hybridization.

In the past few years, combination therapies have been proven to be a significant approach in developing newer anti-cancer agent drugs by utilizing the approach of molecular hybridization. Hybridization involves constructing new molecules by joining two or more existing scaffolds/sub-units through suitable ligating approaches leading to the generation of hybrid molecules [22, 23]. These newly constructed hybrids have all the properties of original scaffolds. Thus, the generated combinations can bind to two or more than two targets simultaneously and provide enhanced pharmacological activity. The different pharmacophores in the hybrid molecules may possess a similar or different mode of action to exert the activity (Fig. **1**) [24]. Coumarin hybrids can be designed through this approach by combining different bioactive motifs through suitable sites to provide excellent pharmacological activity against cancer. A few reported coumarin hybrids against cancer is depicted in Fig. (**2**). In the following sections of this chapter, the authors have summarized variously reported coumarin hybrids possessing significant anti-cancer activity by binding to the specific targets along with structural activity relationships and important clinical aspects.

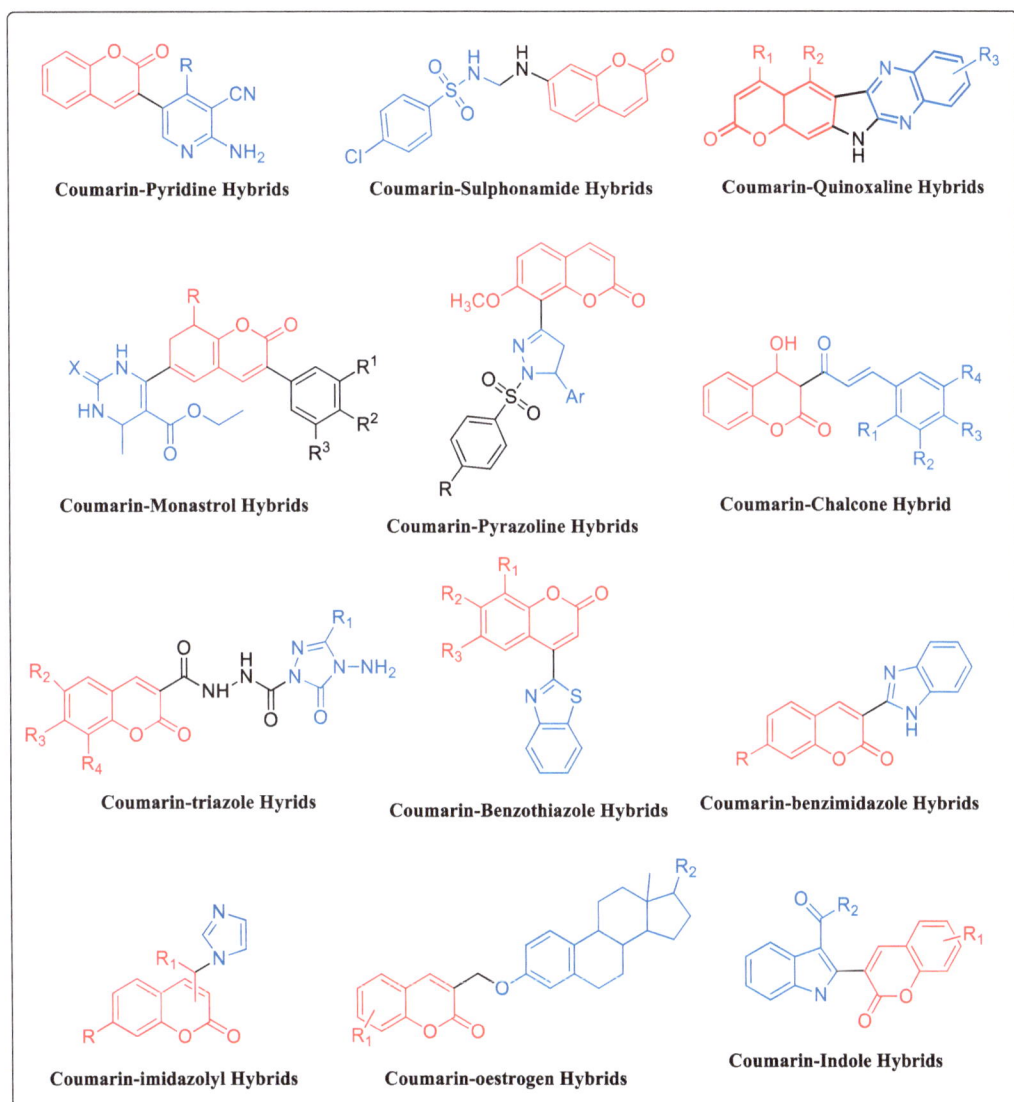

Fig. (2). Some potent coumarin hybrids against cancer.

Coumarin Hybrids as Aromatase Inhibitors

Aromatase is an enzyme belonging to the cytochrome P450 category, which is found in significant amounts in the ovaries of premenopausal, adipose tissue of postmenopausal, and the placenta of pregnant women [25]. It is well established that aromatase is exceedingly expressed in tumour sites of breasts [26]. Therefore, aromatase has been identified as a significant target for the development of therapeutic agents against breast cancer.

Aromatase is responsible for the synthesis of various estrogens, including estradiols, and estrones from substrates like androstenedione and testosterone. Coumarin derivatives inhibit aromatase expression and ultimately prevent the binding of estrogens to the estrogen receptors. Thus the proliferation of the breast cancer cells is blocked further. An underlying mechanism of inhibition has been outlined in Fig. (3). Some recent reports on aromatase inhibitory potentials of coumarin hybrids have been described in the following sections.

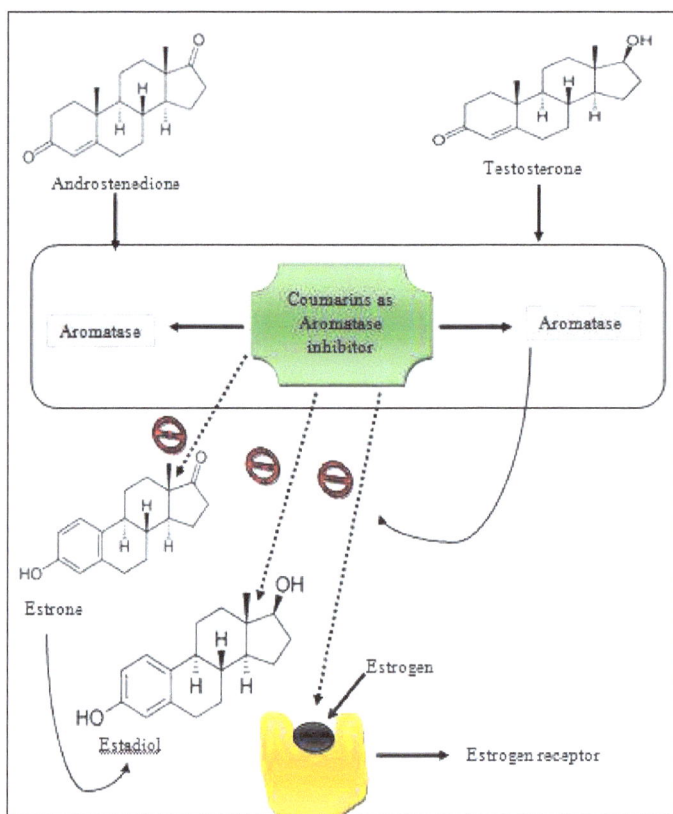

Fig. (3). Role of coumarin derivatives in aromatase inhibition.

Yamaguchi *et al.* reported a series of coumarin-pyridine and diethylamino bis-coumarin hybrids as potential aromatase inhibitors. The synthesized compounds for evaluated for the aromatase inhibitory potentials by comparing them with the well-established aromatase inhibitor exemestane. It was worth noting that substitution patterns and substituents' position presented a wide variation in inhibitory potentials. In both types of hybrid compounds, the attachment through 7th position of coumarin scaffold produced the most potent compounds. Also, the attachment pattern of pyridyl moiety varied the potency. It was found that when it was attached through its 4th position (1), the activity was maximum (IC50 = 30.3 nM) compared to the other positions. In the case of bis-coumarin hybrids, diethylamino substitution at 7th position (2) revealed maximum potency (IC$_{50}$ = 28.2 nM) as compared to other substituents (Fig. 4). The diethylamino group produced 20 times greater inhibition in comparison to methoxy substituents (3). Some derivatives revealed equivalent inhibition to exemestane ((IC$_{50}$ = 42.5 nM). These molecules may act as new substrates for aromatase with high specificity [27].

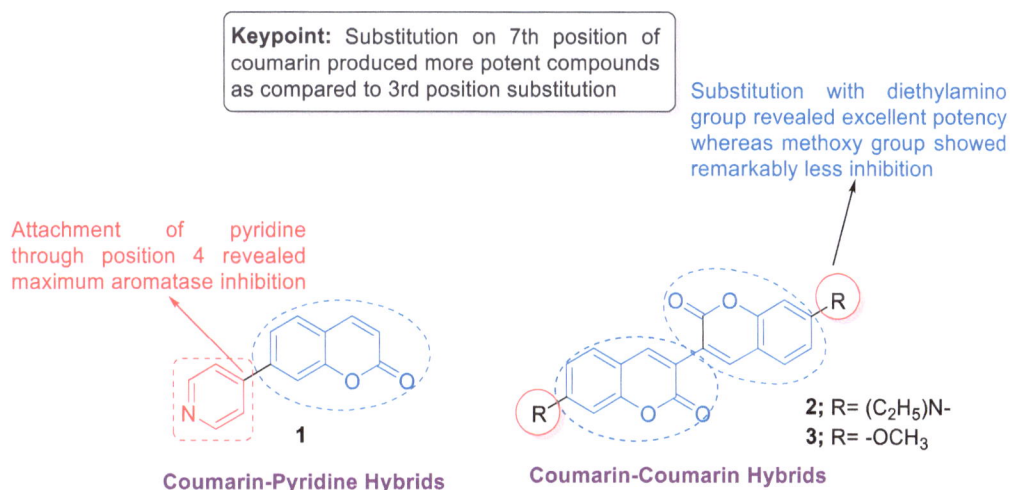

Fig. (4). SAR of Coumarin-Pyridine & Coumarin-Coumarin Hybrids.

Another series of sulphonamide-based coumarin-triazole has been reported by Pingaew *et al.* with anti-cancer and aromatase inhibitory potentials. Most of the derivatives possessing an open-chain sulphonamide group revealed good aromatase inhibition with IC$_{50}$ between 1.3 to 9.4μM. It was worth notable that dimethoxy substitution (4) on the isoquinoline ring of the hybrid molecule was found to be most potent with IC$_{50}$= 0.2μM and revealed no toxicity towards normal cells (Fig. 5). The observed biological activity was also justified by docking studies on designed hybrids against aromatase. The most potent compound with dimethoxy substituents revealed two hydrogen bonds with Met374 and Ser478, which were essential for the enzyme's significant inhibition. Additionally, the coumarin and triazole moieties showed hydrophobic interactions, which aid the inhibitory potentials. Dimethoxy substitution also enhanced the lipophilicity of the molecules [28]. Replacement of coumarin moiety and dimethoxy substitution revealed a marked reduction in the activity.

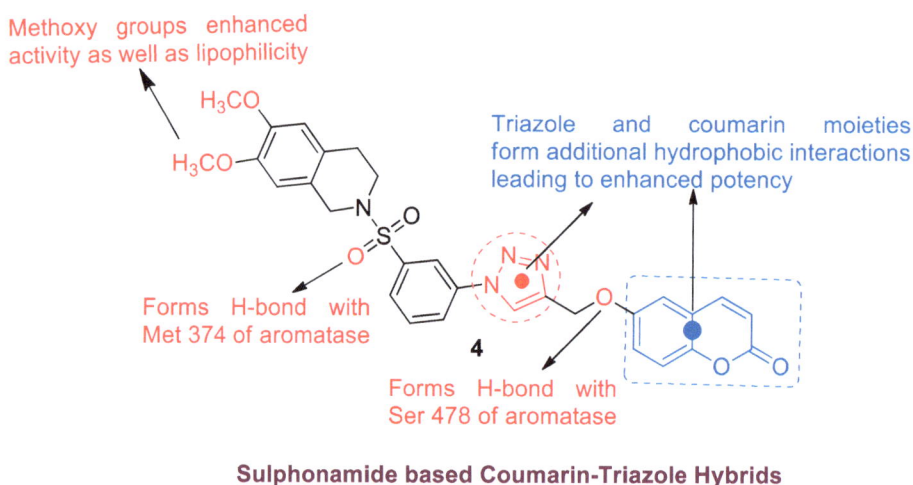

Sulphonamide based Coumarin-Triazole Hybrids

Fig. (5). Most potent sulphonamide based coumarin-triazole hybrids.

Bhatia *et al.* designed a library of coumarin-quinoxaline hybrids and carried out virtual screening against aromatase enzyme. The compound-bearing electron releasing groups like methoxy revealed excellent interactions with aromatase by forming five hydrogen bonds. The interactions and docking scores were equivalent to the standard drug exemestane. The screened best compounds were further synthesized and evaluated for anti-cancer activity. The docking outcomes were also justified by *in vitro* activity against breast cancer cell lines (MCF7), where the methoxy substituted hybrid **(5)** displayed an IC_{50} value of 7.8 µg/mL (Fig. **6**). The activity was almost comparable to the standard aromatase inhibitor exemestane. Substitution of the phenyl ring of quinoxaline with fluoro **(6)**, bromo **(7)**, trifluoromethane **(8)**, methoxy **(9)** and di-methoxy **(10)** groups produced compounds with maximum affinity [29].

With a vision to produce newer apoptosis inducers against breast cancer, Ghorab *et al.* designed and synthesized coumarin-sulphonamide hybrid molecules and evaluated them for potency against breast cancer as well as aromatase inhibition. The cytotoxic activity was evaluated against breast cancer cell lines T47D, where the compounds revealed moderate to excellent activity (IC_{50}=108.9-8.8 µM) in comparison to the reference drug doxorubicin with IC_{50}=9.8 µM. Further to investigate the mechanism of action, the compounds were also evaluated for aromatase inhibitory potentials. It was worth notable that substitution at the terminal sulphonamide group with six-membered heterocycles displayed greater inhibition as

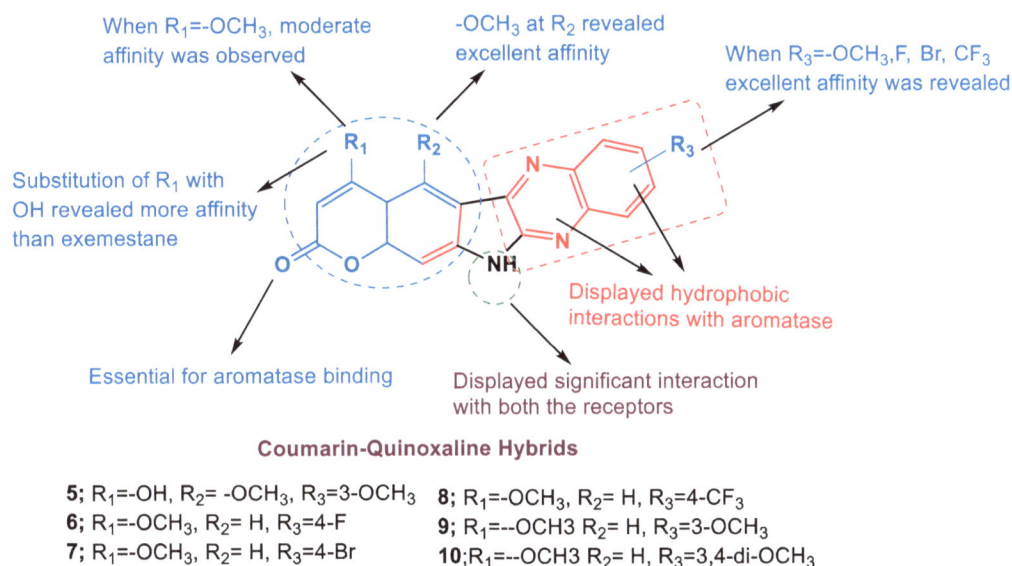

When R_1=-OCH$_3$, moderate affinity was observed

-OCH$_3$ at R_2 revealed excellent affinity

When R_3=-OCH$_3$,F, Br, CF$_3$ excellent affinity was revealed

Substitution of R_1 with OH revealed more affinity than exemestane

Essential for aromatase binding

Displayed hydrophobic interactions with aromatase

Displayed significant interaction with both the receptors

Coumarin-Quinoxaline Hybrids

5; R_1=-OH, R_2= -OCH$_3$, R_3=3-OCH$_3$ **8**; R_1=-OCH$_3$, R_2= H, R_3=4-CF$_3$
6; R_1=-OCH$_3$, R_2= H, R_3=4-F **9**; R_1=--OCH3 R_2= H, R_3=3-OCH$_3$
7; R_1=-OCH$_3$, R_2= H, R_3=4-Br **10**; R_1=--OCH3 R_2= H, R_3=3,4-di-OCH$_3$

Fig. (6). Important aspects of SAR of coumarin-quinoxaline hybrids.

compared to substitution with five-membered heterocycles. It was observed that the methoxy **(11)** and dimethoxy **(12)** substituted pyrimidinyl group displayed maximum aromatase inhibition (81%) (Fig. **7**). *In silico* investigation through molecular docking studies against aromatase also justified the *in vitro* outcomes. The synthesized molecules utterly fit into the binding pocket of aromatase and revealed good hydrogen bonds and hydrophobic interactions. Methoxy, dimethoxy substitution led to improvement in the molecules' lipophilic character and aided the potency [30].

Steroid sulphatase (STS) has been recognized as a promoter of active estrogen synthesis in the breast tissues and is responsible for breast cancer along with aromatase. It hydrolyses Estrone sulphate to Estrone and dehydroepiandrosterone sulfate (DHEAS) into dehydroepiandrosterone (DHEA). These hydrolysis products are further converted into steroids like Estradiol/androstenediol by the action of 3β-hydroxysteroid dehydrogenase (3β-HSD) or 17β-hydroxysteroid dehydrogenase (17β-HSD). These steroidal products have estrogenic properties, which may initiate breast tumour progression by stimulating estrogen-responsive elements (EREs) [31, 32]. Coumarin derivatives have been found to counteract the effect of STS by an irreversible inhibition mechanism. The mechanism of antiproliferative action of coumarin derivatives through sulphatase inhibition has been outlined in Fig. (**8**).

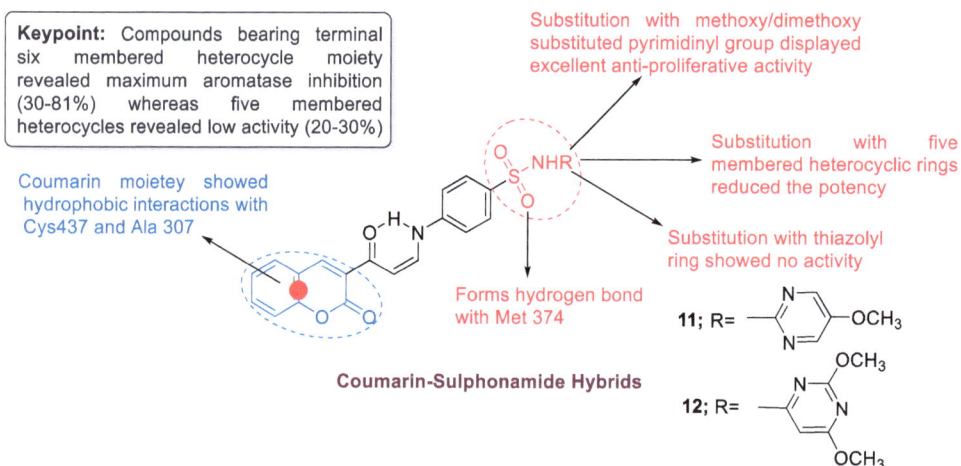

Keypoint: Compounds bearing terminal six membered heterocycle moiety revealed maximum aromatase inhibition (30-81%) whereas five membered heterocycles revealed low activity (20-30%)

Coumarin moietey showed hydrophobic interactions with Cys437 and Ala 307

Substitution with methoxy/dimethoxy substituted pyrimidinyl group displayed excellent anti-proliferative activity

Substitution with five membered heterocyclic rings reduced the potency

Substitution with thiazolyl ring showed no activity

Forms hydrogen bond with Met 374

Coumarin-Sulphonamide Hybrids

11; R=

12; R=

Fig. (7). SAR of coumarin-sulphonamide hybrids as aromatase inhibitors *Coumarin Hybrids as Sulphatase inhibitors.*

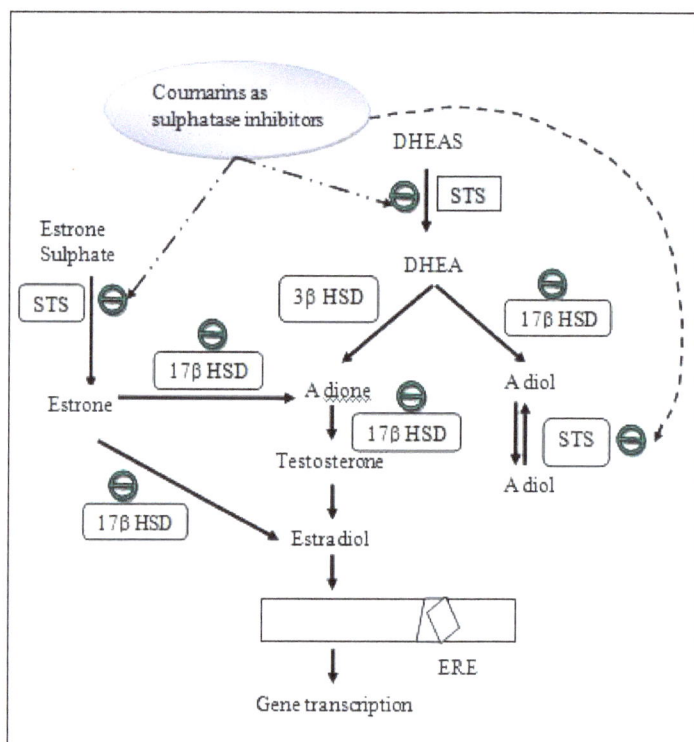

Fig. (8). Inhibition of Sulphatase action by coumarin hybrids.

Dasko *et al.* have synthesized a series of 3-(4-aminophenyl)- coumarin-7-O-sulfamate hybrids as steroid sulphatase inhibitors. The synthesized compounds were then evaluated for human placental STS inhibitory potentials for cytotoxicity against estrogen receptor-positive MCF7, T47D cell lines, and negative MDA-MB-231 SkBr3 cancer cell lines. The enzyme inhibition assay revealed that substitution on different positions of phenyl ring B remarkably influenced the inhibitory potentials. The compounds with fluoro (**13**) and trifluoro-methane (**14**) substitutions revealed excellent inhibition with IC_{50}=0.18 µM as compared to the reference compound coumarin-7-O-sulfamate (IC_{50}=1.38 µM). These outcomes were strongly justified by docking results against aromatase, where the molecules were well occupied inside the binding pocket with a good number of hydrogen bonding and hydrophobic interactions. The most potent compounds were found moderately cytotoxic against MCF7 and T47D, which was 2-3 times lower than the reference drug tamoxifen. Here, the compound with CF3 substitution on the 1st and 4th position of phenyl ring B was most potent (Fig. **9**). Also, these compounds were not selective towards estrogen-dependent cells [33].

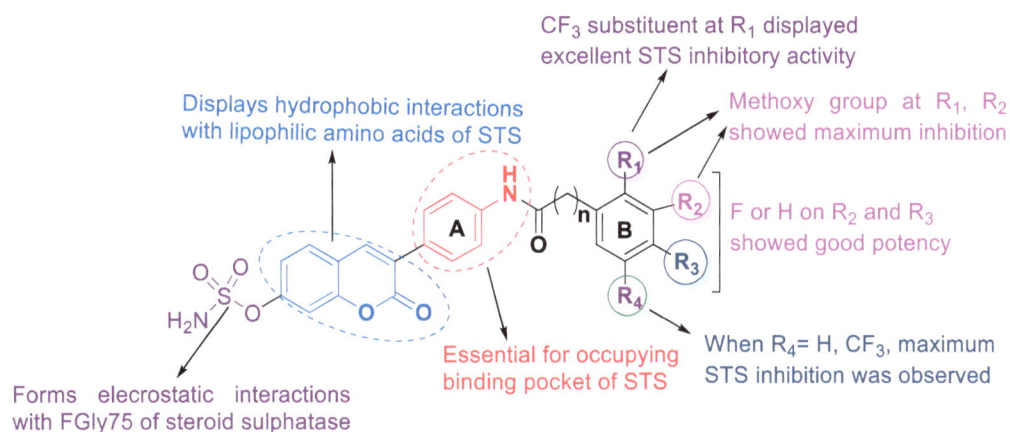

Coumarin-Amino phenyl Hybrids

13; R_1=H, R_2=F, R_3=F, R_4=H, n=1
14; R_1=-CF$_3$, R_2=H, R_3=H, R_4=-CF$_3$, n=1
15; R_1=-OCH$_3$, R_2=-OCH$_3$, R_3=H, R_4=H, n=1
(There was no carbonyl group of amide in 15)

Fig. (9). Aspects related to SAR of coumarin-aminophenyl hybrids.

Another similar kind of work was reported by Hng *et al.*, who prepared coumarin-benzylamino hybrids as potent STS inhibitors to develop therapeutic candidates against breast cancer. They replaced the carbonyl group of amide and just incorporated the methoxy substituents instead of fluoro at 1st and 2nd positions of phenyl ring B, and a significant improvement in activity was observed (IC_{50}=0.13 µM). It was also worth noting that an increase in the length of the linking alkyl chain (n) led to a remarkable decrease in inhibitory potentials. The most potent compound with dimethoxy substituent **(15)** also displayed significant cytotoxicity against MCF7 cell lines but was 13 times lower than the reference compound STX64. The methoxy substitution on the para position was not necessary for inhibition [34]. The essential aspects related to SAR have been outlined in Fig. **(9)**.

Coumarin Hybrids as Topoisomerase inhibitors

Topoisomerase enzymes play a crucial role in the development and progression of cancer. These are responsible for over/underwiding of DNA. During the phenomena of DNA replication, it becomes overwinded and leads to the development of significant torsions in its structure, leading to loss of DNA polymerase activity [35]. These deformations are corrected by topoisomerase, which binds to the DNA and cuts the phosphate backbone. This leads to the unwinding of DNA, and the backbone is sealed again at the last stage of replication [36]. Topoisomerase works on the topology of the DNA therefore, it has been proved to be a significant target for drug design against cancer. It has two subtypes: topoisomerase I (ATP independent) and topoisomerase II (ATP dependent). Topoisomerase II is targeted by several chemotherapeutic agents to induce apoptosis [37]. Topoisomerase II forms a homodimer and cleaves the double-stranded DNA, winds another DNA duplex, and re-ligates the strands [38]. It is present in sufficient concentrations in the cancer cells and is essential for proliferation. Its inhibitors, like coumarins, bind competitively to the B subunit and inhibit the ATPase activity causing cell death [39].

Konkolove *et al.* have recently reported coumarin-tacrine hybrids as potential topoisomerase inhibitors along with anti-cancer activity against lung cancer. They evaluated the potential of DNA topoisomerase I and II in the presence of designed compounds to relax supercoiled plasmid DNA through the gel electrophoresis technique. All the compounds revealed sufficient inhibition of topoisomerase I activity, whereas topoisomerase II inhibition was negligible. The anti-cancer potential was evaluated against lung cancer cell line A549, and suitable to moderate activity was observed [40]. It was worth notable that hybrids possessing longer alkyl chains with carbon lengths 6-9 **(16)** were the most potent, whereas a reduction in chain length remarkably reduced the activity (Fig. **10**).

Nikalje *et al.* also contributed to anti-cancer drug research by developing coumarin-piperazine hybrids through ultrasound-assisted synthesis as cytotoxic agents. They combined the well-established (17) anti-cancer pharmacophores by an oxy propenyl linker, contributing to anti-cancer potentials. Aromatic phenyl ring was substituted on this linker to enhance the lipophilicity of the molecules. Various substituents on this phenyl ring showed varied activities. The hybrids revealed moderate to excellent activity against breast cancer cell lines MCF7, cervical cancer cell lines HeLa, and non-small lung cancer cell lines NCI-H226 in comparison to the reference drug Adriamycin. To investigate the mode of action of developed hybrids, molecular docking studies were carried out against topoisomerase-II. The outcomes were in good agreement with the observed *in vitro* cytotoxic activity. The hybrids displayed mainly hydrogen bonding and hydrophobic interactions and were well occupied in the pocket of the enzyme. Coumarin scaffold and phenyl ring formed hydrophobic interactions, whereas piperazine nitrogen displayed hydrogen bonds with topoisomerase II's amino acids (Fig. **11**). It was notable that 4-methyl substitution at coumarin as well as at piperazine moiety was essential for activity [41]. Replacement of phenyl ring with other heterocycles remarkably decreased the activity. The compounds also displayed good *in silico* pharmacokinetic profile and drug-like properties.

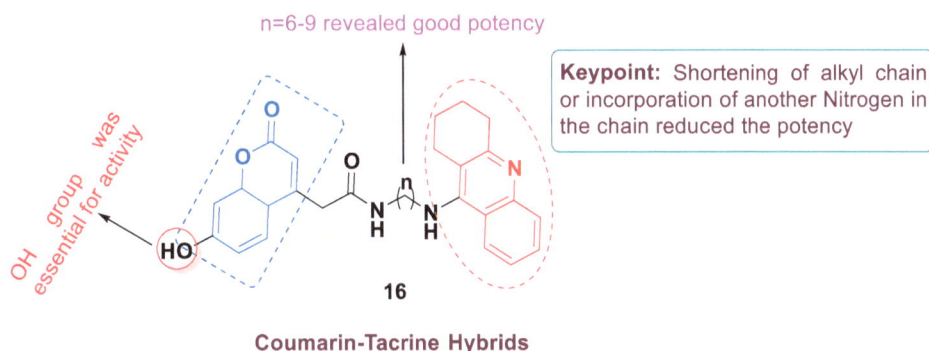

Fig. (10). SAR of coumarin-tacrine hybrids.

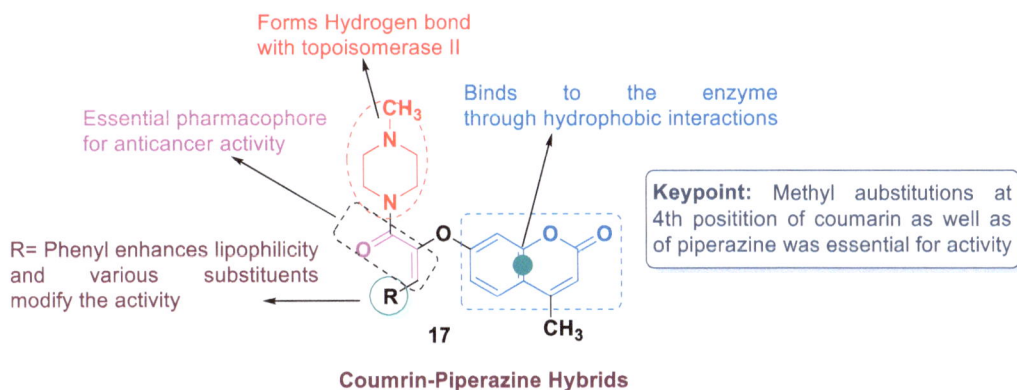

Fig. (11). SAR of potent coumarin-piperazine hybrids.

Quinone derivatives tend to cause cellular toxicity by various mechanisms like redox cycling, free radical generation, arylation of biomolecules, and DNA intercalation. Several research groups have utilized these properties to design quinine derivatives with enzyme inhibition potentials. Falcon *et al.* have prepared Coumarin-Naphthoquinone hybrids as potential topoisomerase II inhibitors. The prepared hybrid molecules were screened out for activity against human topoisomerase II, *E. coli* DNA Gyrase, and *E. coli* topoisomerase I. All the hybrids revealed excellent topoisomerase II inhibition with IC_{50} values ranging between 10-30µM in comparison to reference compounds Mebarone and Etoposide. Mechanistic studies revealed that the hybrids were catalytic type inhibitors of topoisomerase II and also inhibited the ATPase activity. It was evident that 4-nitro phenyl substituted hybrid **(18)** displayed the maximum ATPase inhibition followed by fluoro **(19)** substituents. Further, the hybrids did not reveal any DNA Gyrase and topoisomerase I inhibition. Docking studies concluded that the hybrids (S-enantiomer) fit well into the ATP-binding pocket of topoisomerase II as there was an appearance of significant pie-pie interactions between an aromatic ring of naphthoquinone and the magnesium in the binding site [42]. R-enantiomer of hybrids also displayed the pie-pie interactions between coumarin moiety and magnesium. Both the enantiomers displayed two hydrogen bond interactions but in different patterns. Important aspects related to the predicted SAR of the hybrid molecules have been summarized in Fig. **(12)**.

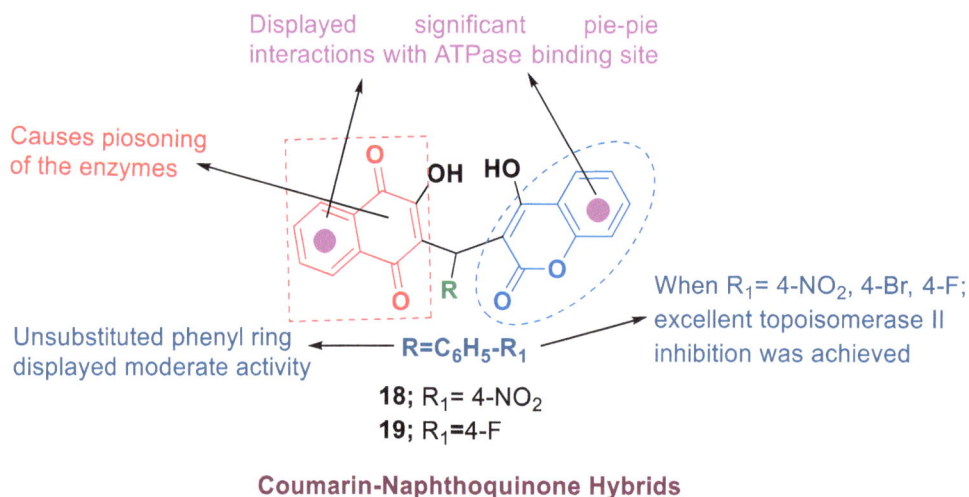

Coumarin-Naphthoquinone Hybrids

Fig. (12). SAR of coumarin-naphthoquinone hybrids.

Coumarin Hybrids as Caspase activators and Apoptosis inducers

Caspases belong to a family of aspartate-specific cysteine proteases and play a significant role in apoptosis induction and progression [43]. Based on their role, caspases have been broadly divided into two groups. Group I caspases are responsible for inflammatory responses. Group II caspases control and regulate apoptosis [44]. Coumarin derivatives have been found to induce apoptosis in cancer cells by following the caspase-dependent intrinsic mechanism. BCL2 gene is supposed to inhibit apoptosis by maintaining mitochondrial membrane integrity and preventing Bax/Bak oligomerization, which leads to the discharge of several apoptogenic molecules from the mitochondrion. Coumarins prevent the expression of BCL2 and activate p53 which leads to the activation of a pro-apoptotic protein Bax. Bax is responsible for the activation and release of cytochrome c from the mitochondrial matrix. This is followed by an apoptotic protease activating factor-1 (Apaf-1) combined with cytochrome to form a complex apoptosome. The apoptosome then activates dormant pro-caspase-9 into active caspase-9 that further activates caspase-3 leading to caspase cascade and induction of apoptosis [45, 46]. The apoptotic mechanism induced by Caspase activation has been outlined in Fig. (**13**).

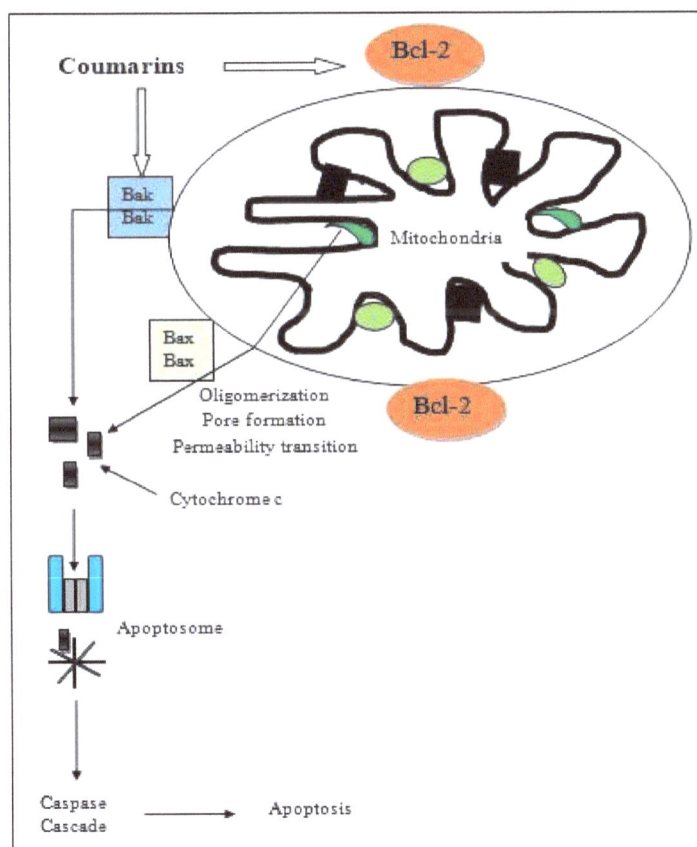

Fig. (13). Coumarin derivatives as Caspase activators.

Fayed *et al.* recently reported coumarin-pyridine hybrids as promising anti-cancer agents. The cytotoxic activity of the hybrids was evaluated against breast (MCF7), colon (HCT116), hepatocellular (HepG2) and lung cancer (A549) cell lines. All the hybrids displayed moderate to excellent activity against all the cell lines. Compounds bearing amide group, cyano group and fusion of pyrimidinone moiety on pyridine **(20, 21)** displayed excellent cytotoxic potentials with IC_{50} =1.1-2.4 µM in comparison to the reference drug fluoro-uracil (IC_{50} =7.1-8.2 µM). The fusion of pyrimidinone moiety remarkably increased the caspase-3 activity and apoptosis rate, whereas the fusion of pyridine with five-membered heterocycles reduced the activity. The outcomes were further evidenced by docking studies carried out against caspase-3. The potent compounds were well fitted inside the binding pocket with high docking scores. The significant interactions were arene-arene, arene-cation and hydrogen bonding (Fig. **14**). Coumarin moiety displayed arene-arene type interactions, whereas phenyl ring substituted on pyridine showed arene-cation type interactions. In the case of the pyrimidinone fused hybrid, additional two hydrogen bonds were observed corresponding to the oxygen atom and nitrogen atom [47].

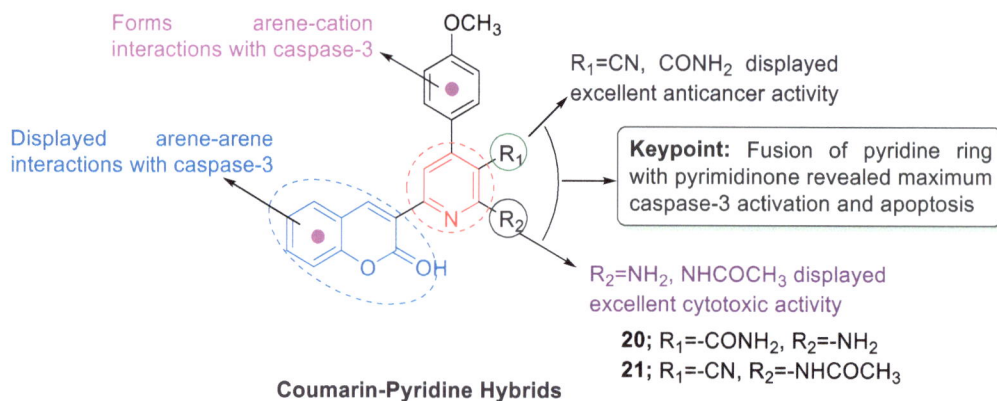

Fig. (14). SAR of coumarin-pyridine hybrids.

In another work carried out by Mohamed *et al.*, coumarin-thiazole-pyrazole hybrids were prepared and evaluated for cytotoxic and apoptosis induction potentials. The prepared hybrids were assessed against various cancer cell lines, including breast MCF7, lung A549, prostate PC3, liver HepG2 and normal melanocyte HFB4. 4-chlorophenyl **(22)** and 4-methyl phenyl diazenyl derivative **(23)** was found to be the most potent compound among the series, with an IC_{50} value of 5.41-6.1 µM against MCF7 cell lines in comparison to the reference drug doxorubicin (IC_{50}= 6.73 µM). The 5-methylthiazolidinone derivatives of coumarin revealed comparatively low cytotoxicity (Fig. **15**). The most potent compound was further evaluated for caspase activation potentials. The apoptosis induction in

MCF7 cell lines occurs due to activation of caspase-7 due to a lack of caspase-3. The treatment of MCF7 cell lines with the most potent hybrid resulted in 4.4 fold elevation in the concentration of active caspase-7 and 11 fold increase in the level of inducer caspase-9 [48]. Further QSAR studies and *in silico* ADMET studies suggested that the developed hybrids can be promising therapeutic candidates against cancer.

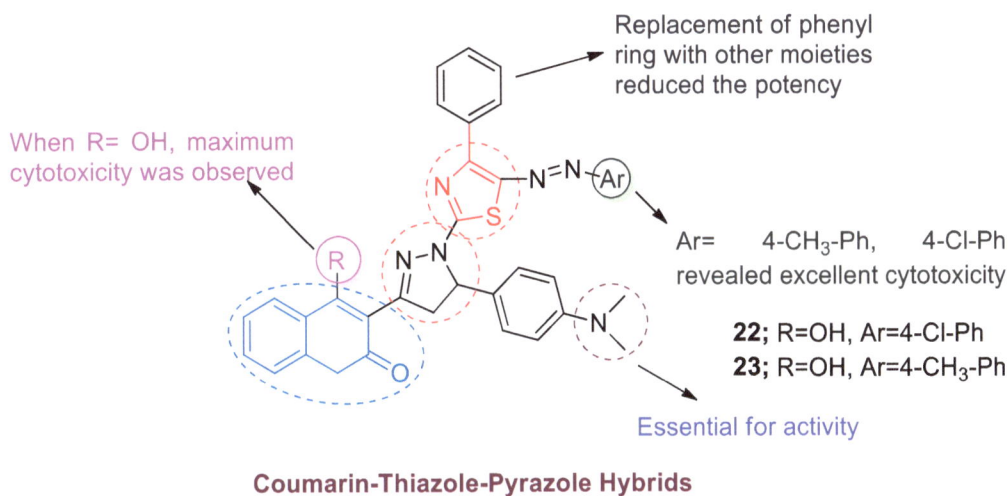

Coumarin-Thiazole-Pyrazole Hybrids

Fig. (15). SAR of coumarin-thiazole-pyrazole hybrids.

Zhang *et al.* synthesized a series of coumarin-piperazine hybrids as antiproliferative agents and apoptosis inducers. The synthesized compounds were further evaluated for cytotoxic activity against a variety of cancer cell lines (A549, H157, HepG2, MCF7 and MG63). The results revealed that the 2-cyanoacryloyl component was essential for significant activity. It was also evident that compounds having electron-donating groups like -Me, -NMe₂, -OEt, *etc.*, displayed inferior activity against all the cell lines. But it was notable that halogen substituents showed significant antiproliferative activity, suggesting that halogen substitution has a promising effect on activity. The compounds having 3,4-dichloro **(24)** and 3-bromo **(25)** substitution was found most potent among the series with IC_{50} values of 6.26 and 7.28 µM, respectively, which was slightly lower than the reference drug doxorubicin (Fig. **16**). Further, the most potent compound was evaluated for its apoptosis potentials in MG63 cell lines. The results indicated that the compound had produced significant apoptosis marked by nuclear fragmentation, chromatin damage, cell shrinkage, *etc.* Further, the mechanism of apoptosis in MG63 cell lines was studied through PCR and western blot, which revealed that the expression of the Bcl-2 gene was decreased, which suppresses apoptosis, whereas the expression of Bax was increased. Also, the levels of caspase 3, 8, and 9 were found to be elevated, which were the clear indicators of apoptosis [49].

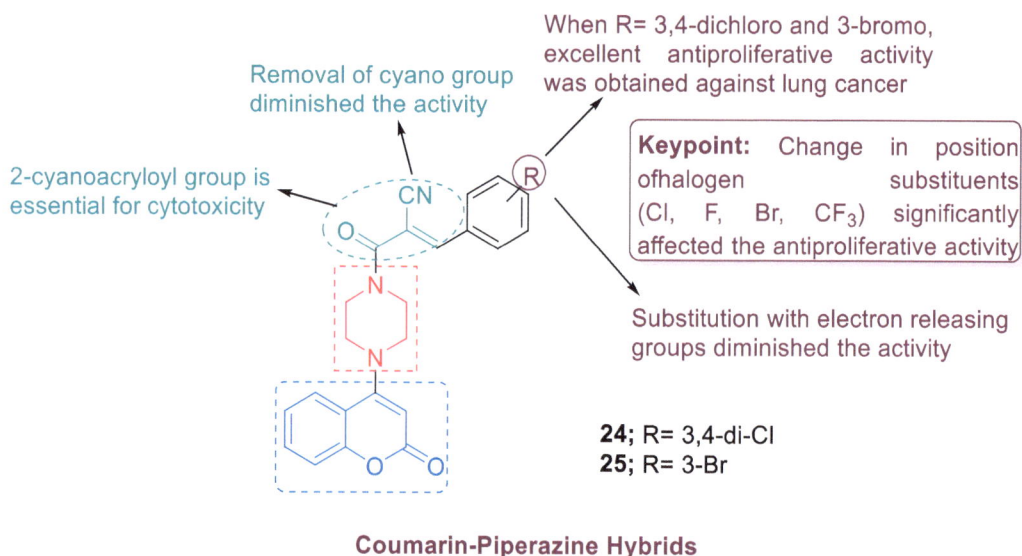

Coumarin-Piperazine Hybrids

Fig. (16). SAR of coumarin-piperazine hybrids.

Elshemy *et al.* have reported three series of coumarin hybrids by combining coumarin moiety with chalcones **(26)**, acrylohydrazides **(27)** and pyridine **(28)** scaffolds. All the prepared compounds were further evaluated for their cytotoxic activity against liver cancer cell lines HepG2 and leukemia cell lines K562. All the hybrids displayed excellent activity against both the cell lines, with IC_{50} ranging between 0.49-3.96μM. Interestingly, the hybrids bearing methoxy substituted phenyl group were the most potent among all the three series and showed better activity than the reference drugs cisplatin, combretastatin and doxorubicin. It was also worth noting that the 8-methoxy group on coumarin and substituted phenyl ring was essential for potency in all three series (Fig. **17**). Further, the potent compounds were also investigated for Caspase-3 and Caspase-9 activation to understand apoptosis's mechanism. Results revealed significant overexpression of Caspase-3 and Caspase-9 proteins suggesting in the cells treated with coumarin hybrids compared to the untreated cells, which evidenced that apoptosis was induced by increased levels of these caspases. The normal cell cytotoxicity study against fibroblast cells (WI-38) showed very low selectivity towards the normal cells in comparison to the cancer cells suggesting the low toxicity of designed coumarin hybrids [50].

Fig. (17). SAR of coumarin-chalcone/acrylohydrazide/pyridine Hybrids.

Coumarin Hybrids as Selective Estrogen Receptor Degraders (SERDs)

Selective estrogen receptor degraders bind to the estrogen receptors and cause its degradation and downregulation [51]. These agents are used to treat estrogen receptor (ER) sensitive breast cancer. The coumarin derivatives bind to the AF1/AF2 domain of the estrogen receptor and prevent estrogen from binding to it. Coumarins cause accelerated degradation of the AF1 domain and prevent its dimerization. Due to the prevention of dimerization, both the domains remain inactive, and there is no nuclear localization of these domains. The degraded receptor is now not able to recruit the coactivators for transcription. Due to all these consequences, no transcription occurs, and no further tumor growth exists. The mechanism of antitumor activity of coumarin mediated by SERD inhibition has been presented in Fig. (**18**) [52]. Hence SERDs have been proven to be a significant target to design antitumor drugs.

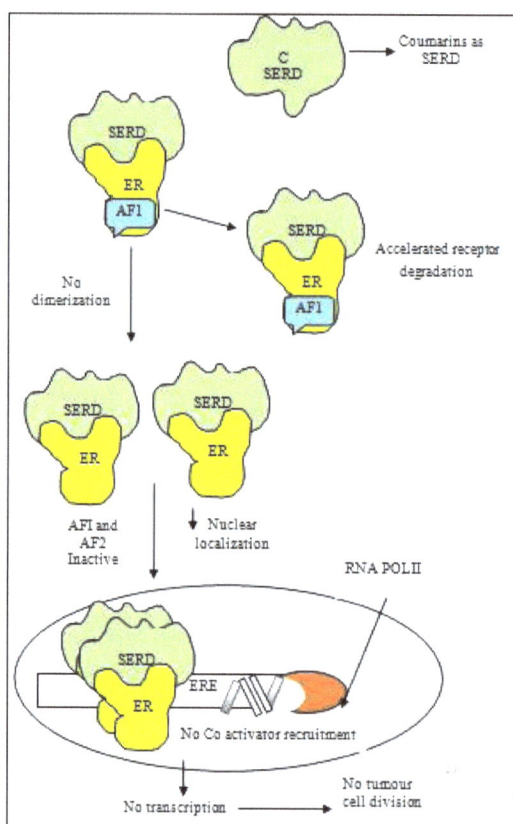

Fig. (18). Coumarin derivatives as selective estrogen receptor degraders.

Degorce *et al.* synthesized coumarin-oxyphenyl acrylic acid hybrids as potential oral selective estrogen receptor downregulation. They have investigated several aspects such as sown regulating potentials, pharmacokinetics, bioavailability, and lipophilicity. It was worth noting that the critical factors affecting all these properties were the type of linker between phenyl and coumarin moiety, substitution on the 7th position of coumarin, and substitution on the phenyl ring attached to the 3rd position of coumarin. Compounds with trifluoromethane (29) and fluorine (30) substituents on the phenyl ring displayed excellent estrogen downregulation with IC_{50}=0.0004-0.0005µM. Similarly, an oxy linker and hydroxyl substitution on the 7th position of coumarin produced maximum downregulation. Although these compounds showed excellent potency, the bioavailability was found poor (Fig. **19**). Removal of 7-hydroxy groups remarkably improved the pharmacokinetics of the compounds but reduced the potency [53].

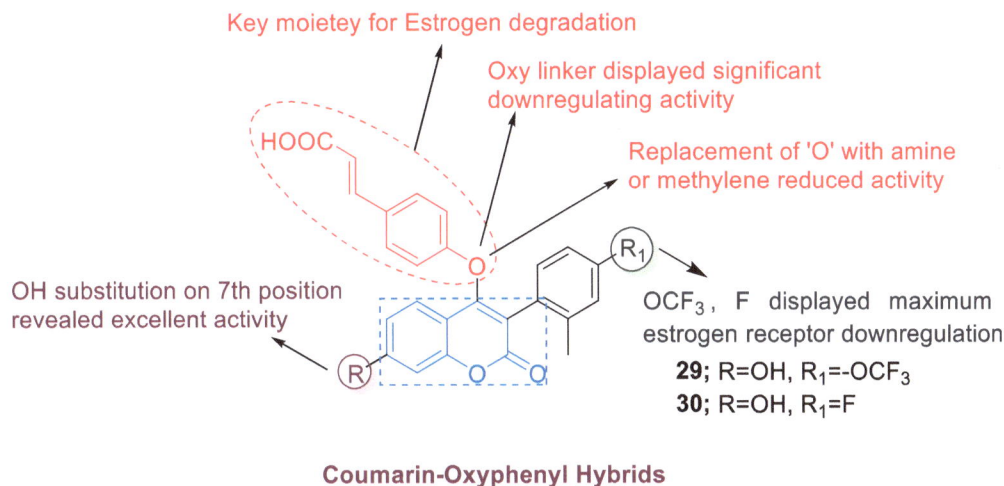

Coumarin-Oxyphenyl Hybrids

Fig. (19). SAR of coumarin-oxyphenyl acrylic acid hybrids.

Lu *et al.* also discovered chromene-oxyphenyl hybrids as potent SERDs by hopping of coumarin scaffold. They also evaluated the pharmacokinetic profiles and antiestrogen potentials against MCF7 cell lines. Ki67 is a marker of proliferation in tumour cells. The synthesized hybrid with methoxy substitution on phenyl ring (**31**) showed remarkable suppression in levels of Ki67. It also displayed excellent estrogen receptor deregulation with $IC_{50}= 0.8$ μM (Fig. **20**). The same compound revealed a good human pharmacokinetic profile and a lower log D value than fulvestrant. Further molecular docking studies against estrogen receptors justified the observations as the hybrids showed prominent fitting in the binding pocket with a good number of interactions. All these aspects evidenced that proposed scaffolds may act as a suitable skeleton for the design of ERα antagonists [54].

Coumarin Hybrids As Tubulin Targeting Agents

Microtubules, formed of α and β tubulin heterodimers, are cytoskeletal and play a key role in various cellular functions such as signalling, division (spindle formation) and cellular movements [55]. It plays a crucial role in cell development and helps in maintaining the cell shape [56]. Tubulin and microtubules exist in dynamic equilibrium, which is a key factor in cell division [57]. Any disruption in this dynamic equilibrium blocks the cell division at the metaphase–anaphase transition, leading to mitochondrial apoptosis [58, 59]. Thus, tubulins are well-explored targets to develop anti-cancer agents.

Keypoint: Scaffold hopping improved the antiestrogen activity, pharmacokinetic profile as well as as better volume of distribution

Methoxy substitutent displayed maximum estrogen binding capacity

OCH_3

HOOC

Scaffold Hopping

7-hydroxy substitution is essential for SERD potential

31

Chromene-Oxyphenyl Hybrids

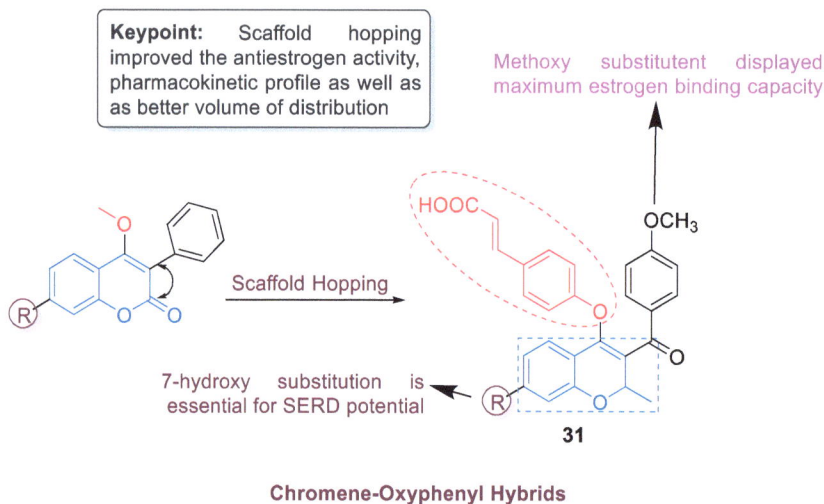

Fig. (20). SAR of chromene-oxyphenyl hybrids.

Mutai *et al.* reported the design and synthesis of pyridyl substituted coumarin derivatives **32** (Fig. **21**) as tubulin targeting agents as 4-arylcoumarins share colchicine binding sites [60]. Against CA-4 resistant parental HT29 cells, the pattern of activity from highest to lowest observed was $Cl > H > OCH_3 > F > CH_3$. On activity against A549 cells, cytotoxicity order changed to $CH_3 > Cl > F > H > OCH_3$. Further, SAR studies revealed that the presence of electron-donating group methoxy can enhance the activity to some extent in 4-arylcoumarins while electron-withdrawing group fluoro causes the loss of activity. Thus, compounds with methoxy or no substitution ($R_1 = OCH_3$, H) inhibited the *in vitro* microtubule formation similar to Combretastatin A-4 and led to microtubule framework disruption significantly.

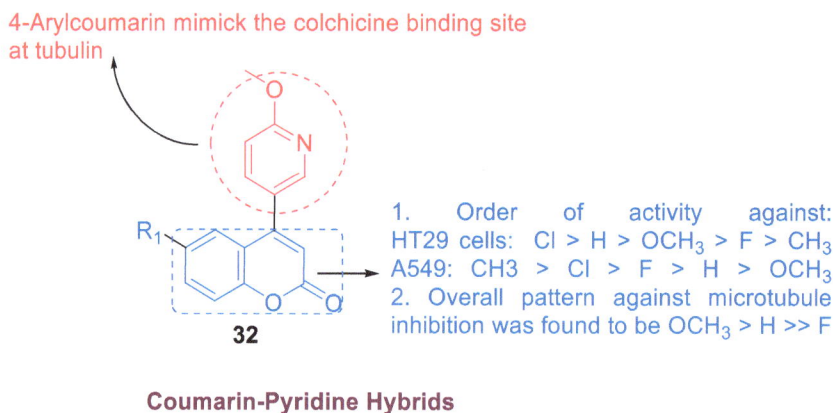

4-Arylcoumarin mimick the colchicine binding site at tubulin

R_1

1. Order of activity against: HT29 cells: $Cl > H > OCH_3 > F > CH_3$ A549: $CH3 > Cl > F > H > OCH_3$
2. Overall pattern against microtubule inhibition was found to be $OCH_3 > H >> F$

32

Coumarin-Pyridine Hybrids

Fig. (21). SAR studies of 4-pyridylcoumarins hybrids as tubulin disrupting agents.

Fu *et al.* reported trimethoxyphenyl-1,2,3-triazole and coumarin hybrids (Fig. **22**) as potential tubulin targeting agents [61]. This study demonstrated that trimethoxyphenyl-1,2,3-triazole containing coumarin hybrids possess potent antiproliferative activity having IC_{50} values from 0.13 µM to 1.74 µM against PC3, MGC803 and HepG2 cancer cells, which was found to be better than colchicine. The results of the MTT assay revealed that compounds with C4 substitution at coumarin (**33**) possess less activity in comparison to C7 substituted coumarin compounds (**34**) (Fig. **22**). The methyl group at the C4 position of the coumarin ring showed increased antiproliferative activity against PC3 and MGC803 cancer cells but decreased potency against HepG2 cancer cells. Coumarin moiety was found to play a key role in antiproliferative activity as a replacement of coumarin with indole, thiazole, oxazole or other results in significant loss of activity. These results demonstrate that coumarin moiety plays a crucial role in cytotoxicity. The synthesized hybrids were found to inhibit the tubulin polymerization by binding at the colchicine binding site of tubulins and causing G2/M phase arrest in apoptosis.

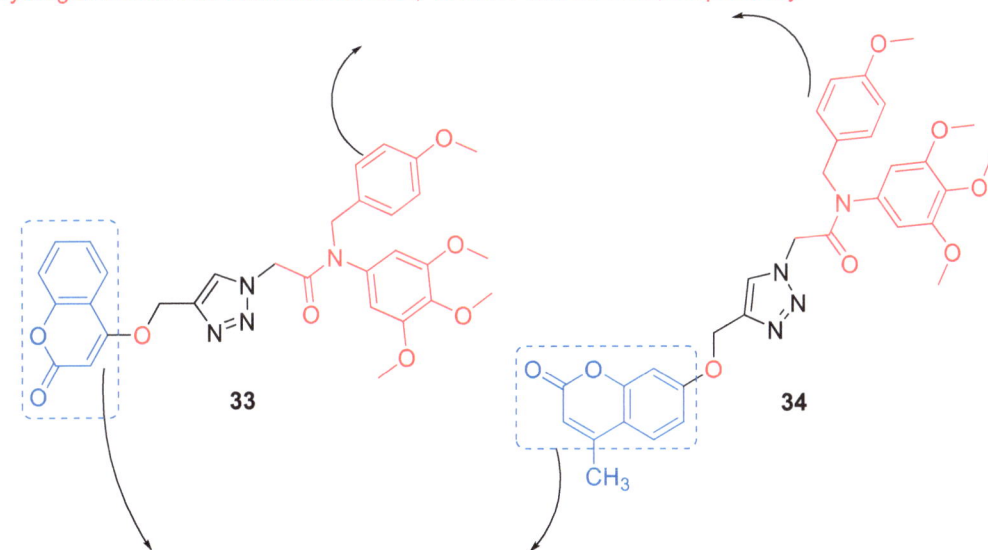

3,4,5-trimethoxyphenyl ring, 4-methoxyphenyl ring, and amide group formed three hydrogen bonds with residues ASN329, TYR224 and LYS352, respectively

33

34

CH₃

1. C4 subtituted coumrin derivatives possess less anti-proliferative activity than C7 coumarin derivatives.
2. Methyl subtitution at C4 (**34**) leads to increase in anti-proliferative activity.
3. Replacement of coumarin with other rings decreases the activity.

Coumarn-trimethoxy Triazole Hybrids

Fig. (22). SAR of coumarin-trimethoxyphenyl-1,2,3-triazole hybrids as tubulin disrupting agents.

Pilli *et al.* evaluated coumarin-hydrazone derivatives **35** (Fig. **23**) as tubulin-targeted antiproliferative agents [62]. The MTT studies against A549, HeLa, SK-N-SH, MCF-7 and NRK-49F cancer cells revealed potent antiproliferative activity with IC_{50} values ranging from 6.07 to 60.45 µM. Coumarin derivative with hydroxy substitution at C7 showed the most potent antiproliferative activity. These compounds attack cancerous cells at the primary and metastatic phase and also possess antimitotic properties. The compounds were found to bind at β-tubulin protein in the mitotic spindle and help in apoptosis. Among these 4,7-dihydroxycoumarin and 4-hydroxylcoumarin derivatives with benzoyl, toulenesulphonyl and pyridinoyl aromatic rings, the benzoyl derivatives were found to possess the most potent anti-cancer activity.

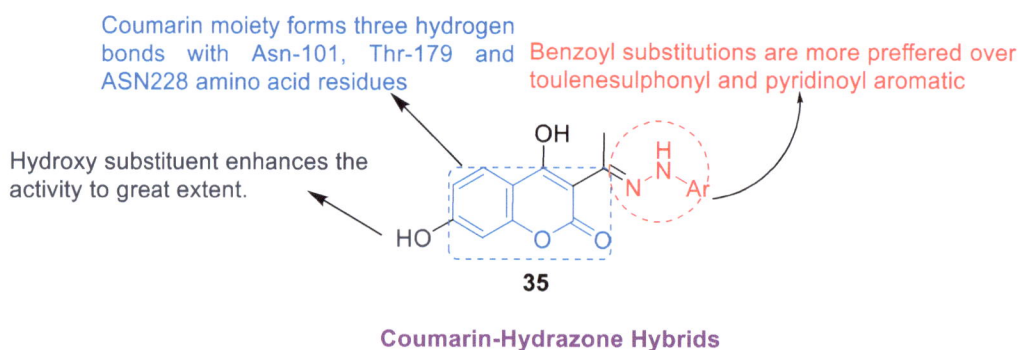

Coumarin-Hydrazone Hybrids

Fig. (23). SAR studies of coumarin-hydrazone hybrids as tubulin disrupting agents.

Coumarin hybrids as Protein Kinase Inhibitors (PKI)

Protein kinases regulate the various cellular functions such as transcription, translation, cell growth, proliferation, *etc* [63]. Phosphatidylinositol 3-kinases (PI3Ks) are a large family of kinases belonging to the lipid kinase family from these kinases. PI3Ks generally phosphorylate the hydroxyl group present at 3rd position phosphatidylinositol bisphosphate (PIP2) and produce phosphatidylinositol trisphosphate (PIP3) [64, 65]. In almost all types of cancer cells, PI3Ks and their components are dysregulated, which describes their importance as a target for cancer treatment [66]. Various studies describe the role of coumarins in PI3K/AKT (protein kinase B)/mTOR/MAPK (mitogen-activated protein kinase) inhibition for the treatment of cancer along with their mechanism [67 - 70]. Jiang *et al.* [71] and Sumorek-Wiadro *et al.* [72] described the role of coumarins extracted from natural sources in PI3K inhibition and cancer treatment. The role of coumarin derivatives as protein kinase inhibitors has been depicted in Fig. (**24**).

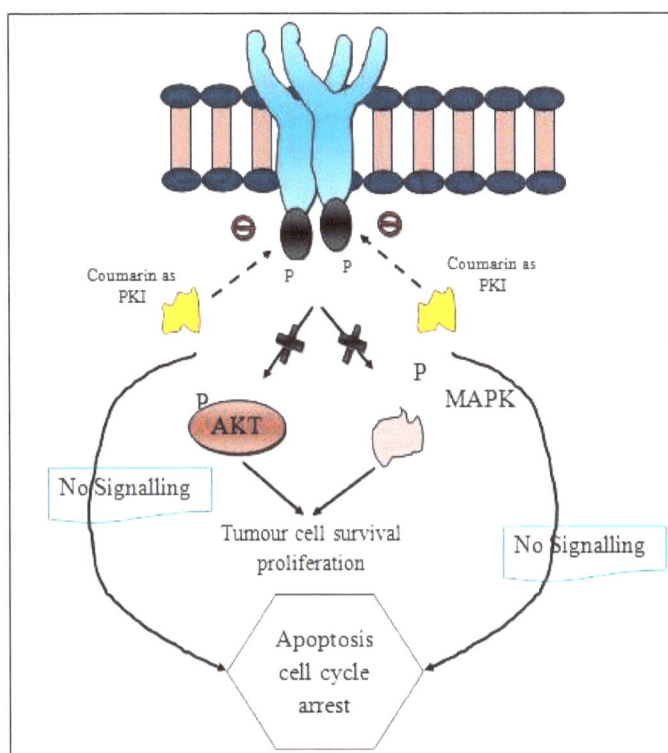

Fig. (24). Coumarin derivatives as protein kinase inhibitors.

Ma *et al.* reported multi-substituted coumarin derivatives (Fig. **25**) having pyridine scaffold in structure as potential PI3K inhibitors [73]. The synthesized coumarin derivatives showed good *in vitro* inhibitory activities in MTT assay against K562, Hela, A549 and MCF-7 cancer cells, with some of them possessing potency better than BENC-511. Compounds with halogen substituents such as chloro **(36)** and bromo groups **(37)** were found to have more potent PI3K inhibitory activity with an affinity toward PI3Kα/β/δ. Further SAR studies revealed that di-substitution at phenyl ring is more preferred over mono substitution.

Liu *et al.* reported coumarin-benzimidazole hybrids (Fig. **26**) as potential PI3K inhibitors for the treatment of cancer [74]. The synthesized compounds showed promising antiproliferative profile against stomach cancer cell lines such as AGS, KATO-III, and SNU-1 cells, ovarian cancer cell lines such as SKOV3 and OVCAR-8 cells, pancreatic cancer cell lines such as BXPC-3 and PANC-1, T24, WiDr, HepG2, SN12C, and K562 cells with GI_{50} values ranging from 0.07 μM to 3.57 μM. Interestingly, these compounds were found inactive against breast cancer cell line MCF-7. SAR studies revealed that N, N-diethyl substitution at C7 position of coumarin **(38)** moiety is most favoured for anti-cancer profile against all above-mentioned cancer cells except MCF-7. The mechanistic studies revealed that compounds cause the caspase-induced cell apoptosis and inhibit the PI3K-AKT-mTOR pathway, which is a key intracellular pathway in cell proliferation and cell death. Mohareb *et al.* proved that introduction of thiourea moiety at the N1 position of benzimidazole **(39)** gives a more potent compound against MCF-7, NCI-H460, and SF-268 cancer cells, which were found 1.5 to 2 times more potent (GI$_{50}$: 0.05 μM to 0.08 μM, SRB assay) than Doxorubicin [75]. Another study showed that N-sulfonated benzimidazole-coumarin hybrids are More potent anti-cancer agents against HeLa cells with methyl and methoxy substitutions at the C6 position of coumarin [76].

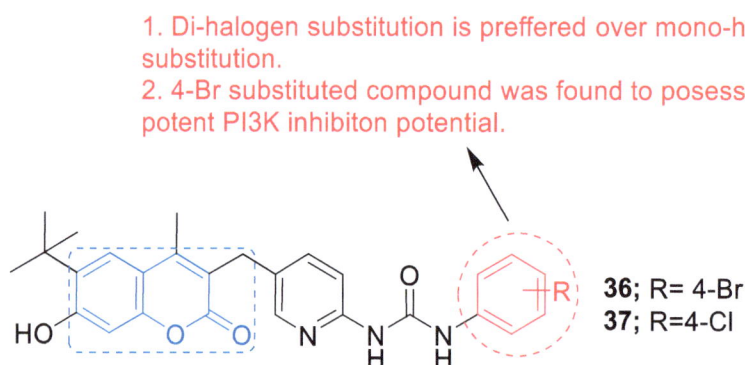

Coumarin-Pyridine Hybrids

Fig. (25). SAR studies of pyridine-coumarin hybrids as PI3K inhibitors.

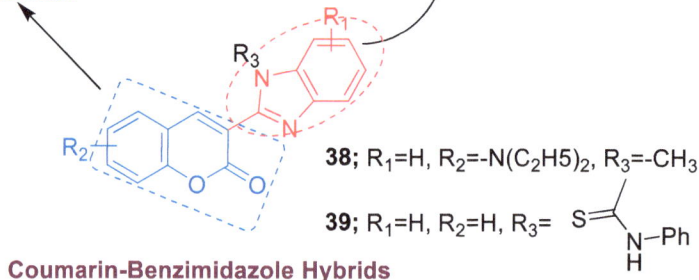

Coumarin-Benzimidazole Hybrids

Fig. (26). SAR studies of benzimidazole-coumarin hybrids as PI3K inhibitors.

Wang *et al.* introduced benzylsulfone coumarin derivatives (Fig. **27**) as promising PI3K inhibitors [77]. The synthesized compounds showed significant cytotoxicity against Hela, HepG2, H1299, HCT-116, and MCF-7 cancer cells. Compound with 4-fluorobenzyl sulfonyl and nitro substituent at the C6 position of coumarin (40) was most potent against all these cell lines with IC_{50} values from 18.12 to 32.60 µM. It also inhibited PI3K by 50.3% at 20 µM concentration, according to *in vitro* cell line studies. The nature of the substituent at coumarin was sought to play a key role in the activity and the pattern observed was found to be nitro group > bromine atom > hydrogen atom. At benzylsufonyl, moiety para-substitution was most preferred, followed by ortho-substitution and meta-substitution. In summary, para-fluorine at benzylsulfonyl and nitro group at coumarin moiety showed the best antitumor activity.

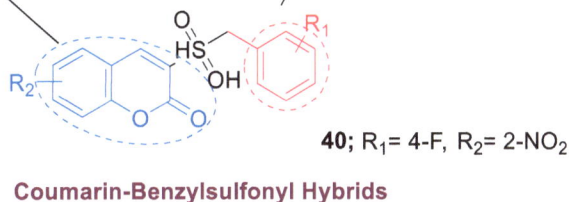

Coumarin-Benzylsulfonyl Hybrids

Fig. (27). SAR studies of benzylsulfonyl-coumarin hybrids as PI3K inhibitors.

Coumarin Hybrids as CDK Inhibitor

Cyclin-dependent kinases (CDKs), serine/threonine kinase proteins, are key enzymes in the cell cycle process [78]. These CDKs act to regulate the cell cycle process via a protein called "cyclins" which are key regulator proteins to control the cell cycle process throughout its different phases [79]. Since the 1980s, after establishing the role of kinases in tumour growth [80], the CDKs have been sought as a potential target for the treatment of cancer. The CDKs inhibitors are used as promising chemotherapeutic agents [81, 82]. Flavopiridol and Eupatilin arc two examples of coumarin derivatives having CDK inhibitory potential.

Lu *et al.* reported C4 (Fig. **28**) pyrimidine substituted coumarin derivatives with potent anticancer activities against various cell lines [83]. The 6-methyl-4-substituted coumarin-pyrimidine hybrids **41** were found to possess promising anticancer activity against HepG2 and MCF-7 cell lines. The presence of hydrogen bond donors such as hydrazyl or piperazinyl groups at the R position of pyrimidine is favoured, while its replacement with an aniline group reduced activity. The docking studies revealed the binding mode of ligands in which the carbonyl group of coumarin was found to favour hydrogen binding with Leu83 amino acid residue of cyclin-dependent kinase 2 (CDK2). This is key interaction for CDK2 inhibition in anti-cancer activity.

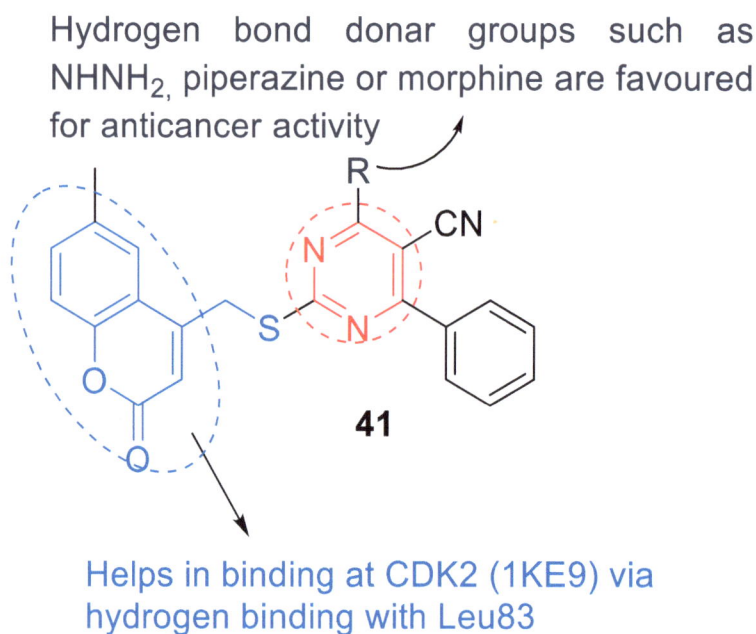

Coumarin-Pyrimidine Hybrids

Fig. (28). SAR studies of C4 substituted coumarin derivatives as CDK inhibitor.

El-Karim *et al.* synthesized thiazol-hydrazono-coumarin hybrids as CDK2 inhibitors for the treatment of cervical cancer [84]. These new thiazol-2--l-hydrazono-chromen-2-one analogs were found to possess significant CDK2 inhibitory activity with an IC_{50} range of 0.022–1.629 nM. The most potent compound (**42**) with methyl and ethyl acetate substitution was found to increase the level of CDK2 regulators, *i.e.*, P21 and P27, by 2.30 and 5.7 folds, respectively, which further establishes the mechanistic pathway behind the cytotoxic effect of these coumarin hybrids (Fig. **29**). The QSAR analysis revealed that the molecular charge distribution is a key structural feature to regulate the cytotoxic profile of compounds. This feature affects the ability of the molecule to cause electrostatics-dependent interactions along with its hydrophilicity. These two features are inversely proportional to the cytotoxic potential of compounds.

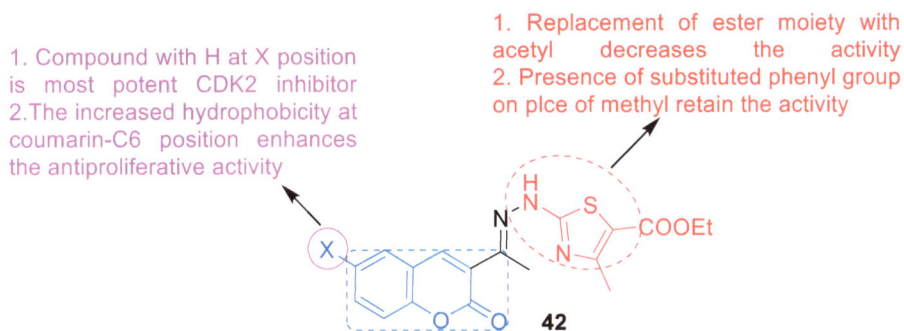

Coumarin-Hydrazone-Thiazol Hybrids

Fig. (29). SAR studies of thiazol-hydrazono-coumarin hybrids as CDK2 inhibitor.

Xu *et al.* reported coumarin-pyrimidine hybrids **43** as potent CDK9 inhibitors with high selectivity (160- to 8300-fold) over CDK1/2/3/4/5/6/7/8/19 [85]. In these molecules, substituted coumarin moiety was found to bind at the flexible hinge/αD region of CDK9, *i.e.*, a key target site for this kinase inhibition. SAR studies revealed that the di-substitution is preferred over the phenyl ring attached to pyrimidine moiety. On replacement of halogen atom with electron donation or a less electronegative atom, the CDK9 inhibition activity was lost. This effect was thought to be due to the alteration of electron density which ultimately disrupts the hydrogen-bond interaction with Cys106 in the hinge region. Replacement of morpholino moiety with 4-methylpiperazin-1-yl, 4-ethylpiperazin-1-yl or piperidin-1-yl does not affect the cytotoxic and CDK9 inhibitory potential significantly. Similarly, the replacement of acetyl moiety with a 3-propionyl also gives the same inhibitory activity (Fig. **30**).

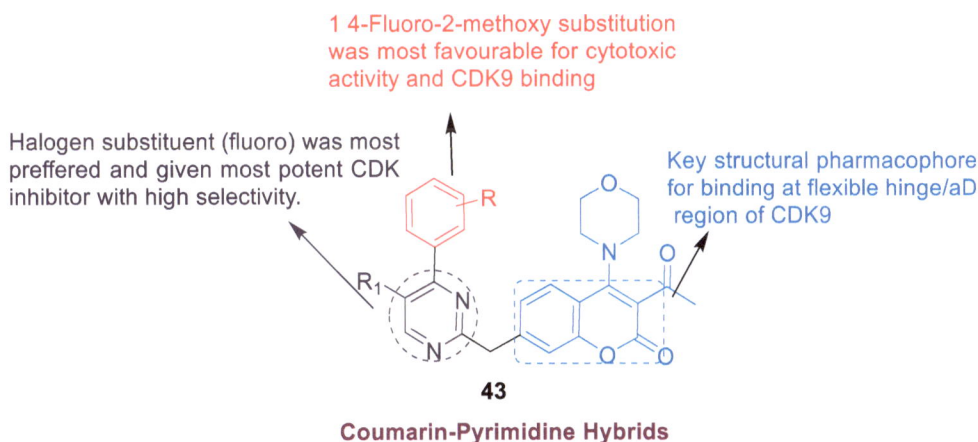

Coumarin-Pyrimidine Hybrids

Fig. (30). SAR studies of coumarin-pyrimidine hybrids as CDK9 inhibitor.

Coumarin Hybrids as Histone Deacetylase Inhibitors (HDI)

Histone deacetylases (HDACs) group of enzymes is responsible for the regulation and expression of activities of several proteins associated with the development and progression of tumours. HDACs remove the acetyl group from histone and generate an unusual chromatin conformation, leading to the inhibition of transcription of genes encoded for proteins involved in tumour formation. Beyond histones, HDACs deacetylate several other targets, such as transcription mediators, and cellular proteins associated with growth, differentiation and apoptosis [86]. Therefore inhibition of HDACs is a promising approach in drug design against cancer. Coumarin derivatives have been found to inhibit the activity of HDACs, resulting in hyperacetylation of substrates. This leads to the generation of oxidative stress, protein deactivation/degradation and finally causes apoptosis. The events involved in the induction of apoptosis have been depicted in Fig. (**31**).

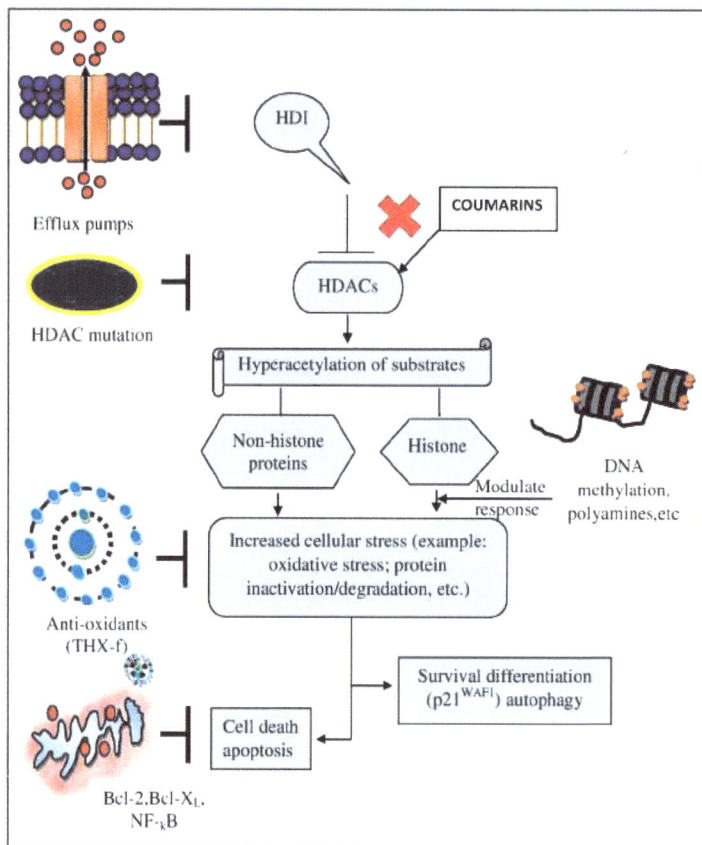

Fig. (31). Coumarin derivatives as HDAC activators.

Working towards the development of newer anti-cancer agents, Ding *et al.* have prepared coumarin-N-hydroxycinnamide hybrids as potential histone deacetylase inhibitors. The prepared compounds were also investigated for antiproliferative activity against MCF-7, HepG2, HeLa and HCT-116 cell lines. The synthesized compounds moderate to excellent antiproliferative activity and HDAC inhibition. It was worth notable that various substitutions on the $6^{th}, 7^{th}$ and 8th positions of coumarin moiety produced great diversity in the activity. Compounds with methoxy substitution at 7th position (**44**) showed excellent HDAC inhibition with $IC_{50} = 0.32\mu M$ in comparison to the reference drug suberanilohydroxamic acid (SAHA) with $IC_{50} = 0.48\mu M$. The compounds bearing ethoxy (**45**) and propyloxy (**46**) substituents at the same position also displayed good HDAC inhibition as well as antiproliferative activity. The substitution of halogens on 6th and 8th positions of coumarin remarkably reduced the activity up to many folds. Further, the potent compounds were subjected to molecular docking against HDAC and were completely fit inside the binding pocket. Aryl ring linker displayed hydrophobic interactions, whereas –NH and –OH groups of hydroxycinnamide segment displayed hydrogen bondings (Fig. **32**). The coumarin scaffold showed arene-cation type interactions [87].

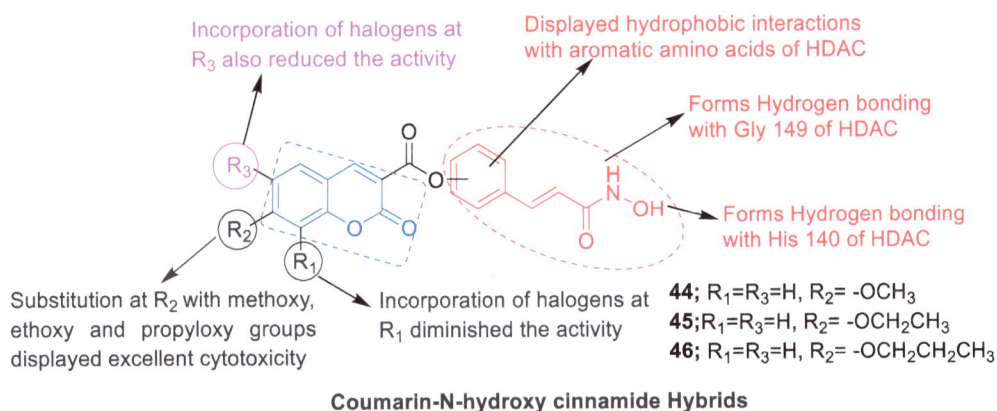

Keypoint: Antiproliferative activity was found maximum in case of electron donating groups as compared to electron withdrawing groups

Incorporation of halogens at R_3 also reduced the activity

Displayed hydrophobic interactions with aromatic amino acids of HDAC

Forms Hydrogen bonding with Gly 149 of HDAC

Forms Hydrogen bonding with His 140 of HDAC

Substitution at R_2 with methoxy, ethoxy and propyloxy groups displayed excellent cytotoxicity

Incorporation of halogens at R_1 diminished the activity

44; $R_1 = R_3 = H$, $R_2 = -OCH_3$
45; $R_1 = R_3 = H$, $R_2 = -OCH_2CH_3$
46; $R_1 = R_3 = H$, $R_2 = -OCH_2CH_2CH_3$

Coumarin-N-hydroxy cinnamide Hybrids

Fig. (32). SAR of Coumarin-n-hydroxy cinnamide hybrids.

Lagunes *et al.* reported novel coumarin-selenourea hybrids as multitargeted antiproliferative agents by hybridization of coumarin with organoselenium motif. The cytotoxicity of the compounds was evaluated against breast, lung, cervix, colon cancer and normal fibroblast cell lines. The compounds displayed good to excellent activity with a GI_{50} range between 3-28µM. The compound bearing p-bromo phenyl substituent (47) on the terminal urea nitrogen displayed maximum activity against all the cell lines (GI_{50}=2.7-3.5 µM) in comparison to the reference drug cisplatin with GI_{50}=1.8-14 µM. Simple phenyl and methoxyphenyl substituents displayed reduced activity, whereas the aliphatic butyl group (48) on the same position displayed excellent activity. The compounds also displayed promising potential for increasing the levels of reactive oxygen species, which is also an effective cancer therapy approach. The potent hybrids were further subjected to molecular docking studies against human HDAC8. The coumarin moiety displayed significant arene-arene interactions, whereas electrostatic interactions were observed between the keto group of coumarin and zinc cofactor. The amino group of urea displayed significant hydrogen bond interactions (Fig. 33). These docking outcomes were further justified by *in vitro* HDAC8 inhibitory assay [88]. The compounds revealed good to moderate HDAC8 inhibition, but the designed hybrids' dimeric form displayed maximum HDAC8 inhibition.

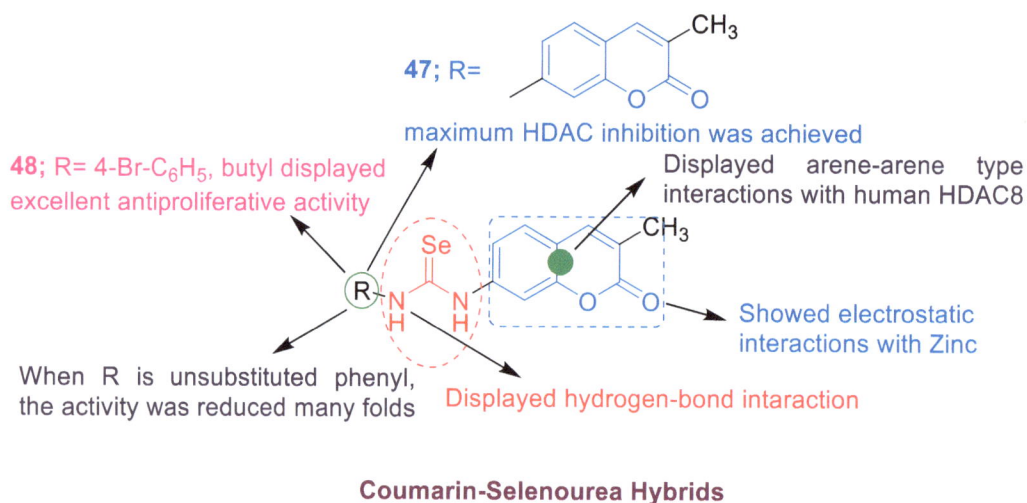

Coumarin-Selenourea Hybrids

Fig. (33). SAR of coumarin-selenourea hybrids.

Abdizadeh *et al.* also prepared a series of coumarin-benzamide hybrids and evaluated them for anti-cancer and histone deacetylase inhibitory potentials. The antiproliferative activity of the synthesized hybrids was evaluated against HCT116, A2780, MCF7, A549, PC3 and HL60 cell lines. The title compounds revealed promising cytotoxic activity with the IC_{50} values in the range of 0.27-80 µM against all cell lines. The compound with 4-methyl-benzyloxy substitution on the 7th position of coumarin (49) was found to be the most potent compound among the series displaying IC_{50} values of 0.2--6.0 µM. It showed higher potency against HCT116, A549 and HL60 cells as compared to the reference drug

Entinostat. Further HDAC inhibition assay was carried out, suggesting that the substitutions on the coumarin moiety are responsible for diverse activity variety. It was observed that methoxy or ethoxy groups on the 7th position of coumarin revealed more cytotoxicity than their 8-alkoxy isomers. The compound having a p-tolyloxy group showed maximum HDAC inhibition with an IC_{50} value of 0.25 and 2.06 μM, in HCT116 and A2780 cell lines, respectively. The incorporation of 6-bromo substituent on the coumarin ring increased the HDAC inhibition. A similar kind of inhibition was also observed in compounds with 8-methoxy and 8-ethoxy substitutions. Inhibitory activity in the hybrids was further improved by the incorporation of electron-donating or electron-withdrawing groups on the benzyl ring of the coumarin. The order of activity here was observed as methyl > methoxy > Bromo > Chloro > Fluoro > H [89]. The potent compounds were found to be least toxic towards the normal Huvec cell lines. Further docking studies against HDAC revealed that the Zinc ion was in Penta-coordinated form with amino acid residues and the carbonyl and aniline of benzamide. Aniline protons revealed hydrogen bond interaction with Gly 149, and the carbonyl oxygen of the benzamide showed hydrogen bonding with Tyr 303 (Fig. **34**). Pie-Pie stacking interactions were also observed with Phe150, which improved the binding affinity of hybrids to HDAC.

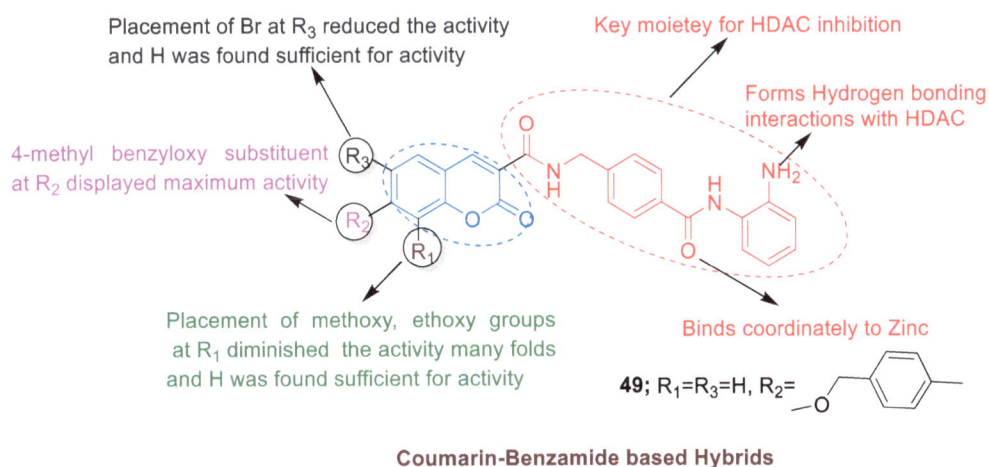

Keypoint: 1. The substitutions on the 7th position of coumarin moietey played a crucial role in activity.
2. Various substituted aryl derivatives' incorporation on 7th postion showed good HDAC inhibition

Placement of Br at R_3 reduced the activity and H was found sufficient for activity

Key moietey for HDAC inhibition

Forms Hydrogen bonding interactions with HDAC

4-methyl benzyloxy substituent at R_2 displayed maximum activity

Placement of methoxy, ethoxy groups at R_1 diminished the activity many folds and H was found sufficient for activity

Binds coordinately to Zinc

49; $R_1=R_3=H$, $R_2=$

Coumarin-Benzamide based Hybrids

Fig. (34). SAR of coumarin-benzamide based hybrids.

Miscellaneous

Pyrimidine scaffold has been reported as a key structural feature in various bioactive molecules [90 - 92] and is sought as a key pharmacophore in anti-cancer drug designing. Lv *et al.* reported 2-phenyl pyrimidine coumarin derivatives (Fig. **35**) as a key structural framework for possessing telomerase-inhibiting activity [93]. The synthesized compounds were found to possess potent anti-cancer activity (MTT assay) against the CNE2 and Cal27 cell lines while weak anti-cancer activity against the KB cells. The structure-activity relationship studies demonstrated that compounds bearing aromatic substitution possess better antiproliferative activity against resisting tumour cell proliferation as compared to compounds having thiophene and alkyl substituents. At aromatic moiety, a compound with *N,N*-dimethyl substituent **(50)** (IC_{50} against CNE2, KB, and Cal27 cell lines were 1.92 ± 0.13, 3.72 ± 0.54, and 1.97 ± 0.51 µM, respectively) is much more potent as compared to compounds with halogen substituents. The mechanistic studies against CNE2 cells proved the antiproliferative activity of 2-phenylpyrimidines via telomerase inhibition which further extends the importance of the coumarin-pyrimidine framework in anti-cancer drug designing.

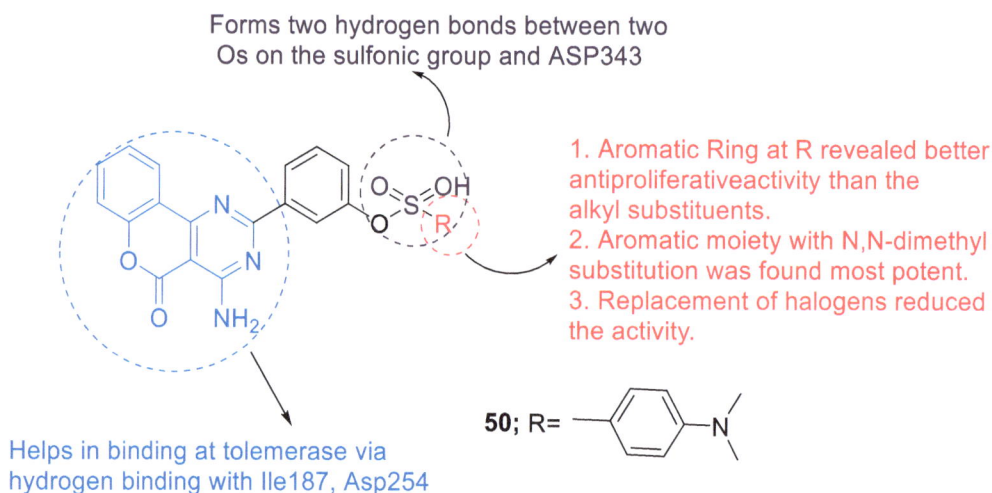

Coumarin fused Pyrimidine Hybrids

Fig. (35). SAR studies of 2-phenylpyrimidine coumarin derivatives as telomerase inhibitors.

Morsy *et al.* [94] reported C3 (Fig. **36**) pyrimidine substituted coumarin derivatives **(51),** respectively having potent anti-cancer activities against various cell lines. C3 substituted coumarins showed good inhibitory potential against A549 and MDA-MB-231 cancer cells. The SAR studies revealed that the para substitution on phenyl rings is more favourable for anti-cancer activity. Shifting the substituents to meta and ortho positions led to a decrease in anti-cancer activity significantly. This pyrimidine substituted coumarin scaffold caused the destruction of DNA, which also signify that it can play a key role in killing microorganism via destroying their genome.

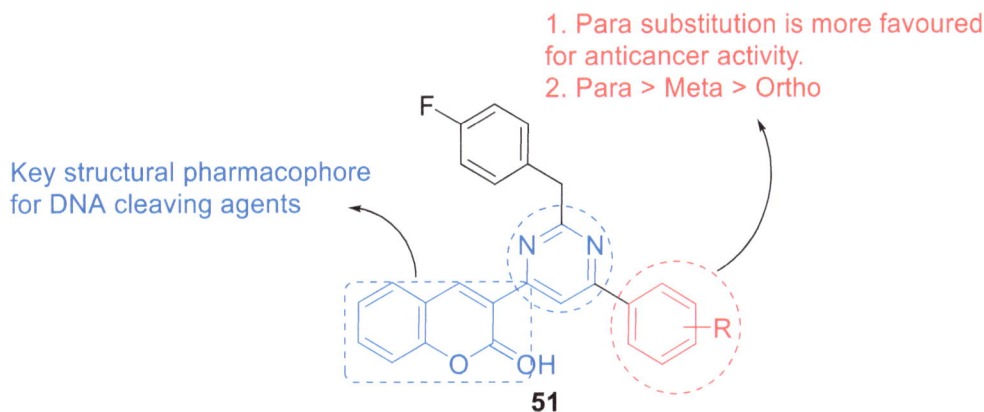

C3 Substituted Coumarin-Pyrimidine Hybrids

Fig. (36). SAR studies of C3 and C4 substituted coumarin derivatives as DNA cleaving agents.

Lingaraju *et al.* reported isoxazole tethered coumarin derivatives (**52**) (Fig. **37**) as promising anti-cancer agents [95]. The synthesized compounds were evaluated for their cytotoxicity against human melanoma (UACC 903) and fibroblast (FF2441) cancer and normal cells, respectively. The synthesized compounds showed promising activity against cancer cells with IC_{50} values ranging from 4.5 µM to 10.5 µM. SAR studies revealed that the substitution pattern at phenyl ring substituted with isoxazoline plays an important role in cytotoxicity against UACC 903 cancer cells. Electron withdrawing halogen substituents at ortho while electron releasing (methoxy) substituents at meta and para positions are favourable for good cytotoxic activity. These compounds were also found to possess little toxicity to normal cells. On change of substitution pattern to 3,4-dimethoxy at phenyl ring removed the toxicity to normal cells and increased selectivity toward cancer cells. This most active compound was also found to possess good *in vitro* activity and increased the life span in treated mice significantly.

Narella *et al.* [96] and Dhawan *et al.* [97] reported coumarin-1,3,4-oxadiazole hybrids **53** and **54,** respectively, as potential anti-cancer agents. The SAR studies against MCF-7 and MDA-MB-231 hybrids **30** (IC_{50}: <5 - >100 µM) and **31** (IC_{50}:

7.07 - >100 µM) with aromatic rings possess much potent antiproliferative activity in comparison to hybrids with alkyl group against carbonic anhdrase. Similarly, conversion of sulfur to sulfone moiety could improve the carbonic anhydarse inhibitory activity. Pattern for subtitution agianst hCA XII was observed as benzoyl > benzyl > phenacyl > isobutyl group (Fig. **38**).

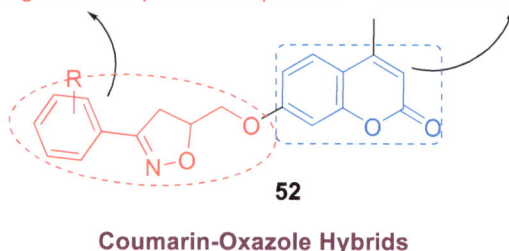

Coumarin-Oxazole Hybrids

Fig. (37). SAR studies of isoxazole thetred coumarin derivatives as anti-cancer agents.

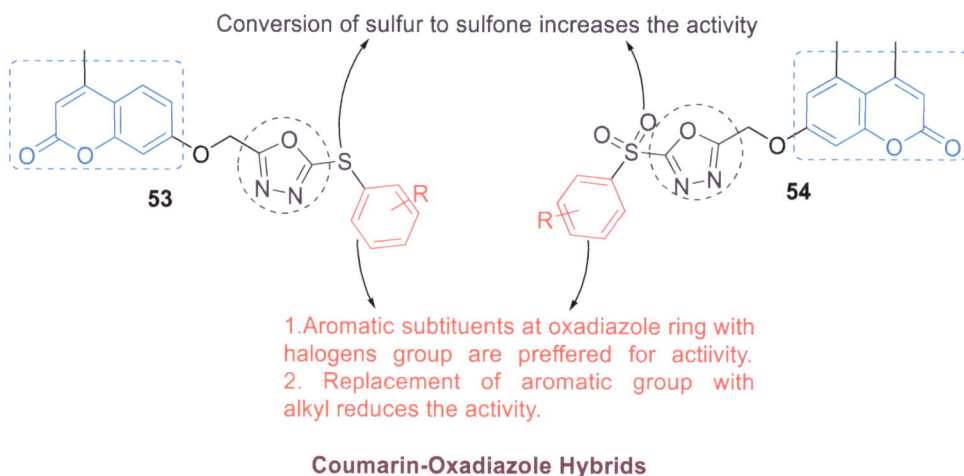

Coumarin-Oxadiazole Hybrids

Fig. (38). SAR studies of coumarin-1,3,4-oxadiazole hybrids as carbonic anhydarse inhibitors.

Chalcone hybrids of coumarins are another class of potential anti-cancer agents [98, 99]. Mokale *et al.* reported potent chalcone-coumarin hybrids as potent anti-cancer agents [100]. The SAR studies of coumarin-chalcone hybrids (**55**) (Fig. **39**) against MCF-7 and MDA-MB-435 cell lines (MTT assay) revealed that hybrids with para substituents are more potent than hybrids with ortho substituents. The introduction of methoxy substituents at the meta position along with para substituents reduced the activity significantly. At R position pattern for activity was observed as piperidyl > pyrrolidinyl > dimethylamino. This data reveals that cycloamine hybrids are more potent anti-cancer agents than alkylamine hybrids, with piperidyl hybrids possessing the most potent activity. These compounds were found to increase the latency time and reduce tumor volume and weight in treated mice compared to the untreated group.

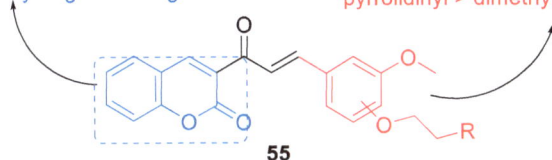

Coumarin-Chalcone Hybrids

Fig. (39). SAR studies of coumarin-chalcone hybrids as carbonic anhydrase inhibitors.

CONCLUSION

The cancer burden is increasing consistently throughout the globe, and medicinal chemists, researchers as well as drug developers are working continuously in the direction of developing more potent and safer therapeutic candidates. The concept of molecular hybridization has been widely adopted these days by researchers as it has the advantages of utilizing the therapeutic properties of two different scaffolds/groups into one molecule. Coumarin hybrids have been proven to be promising anti-cancer agents as they tend to work against several types of cancer, and their action is mediated through interaction/modulating/inhibiting several biological targets. In the presented chapter, the authors have presented the anti-cancer potentials of coumarin hybrids reported recently in the past 5-6 years. Various targets through which these hybrids mediate their action have been discussed briefly, along with important aspects of the structure-activity relationships of the potent compounds. Various outcomes related to antiproliferative activities and enzyme inhibition/activation were also highlighted. Docking outcomes revealing significant interactions of coumarin hybrids with various target enzymes were also discussed. Therefore, it can be concluded that the coumarin hybrids have significant potential to defeat a variety of cancers, and they can provide new leads to the scientists for launching and formulating new therapeutic candidates for the market.

CONSENT FOR PUBLICATION

Not applicable.

CONFLICT OF INTEREST

The author declares no conflict of interest, financial or otherwise.

ACKNOWLEDGEMENTS

Declared None.

REFERENCES

[1]   Weir, H.K.; Anderson, R.N.; Coleman King, S.M.; Soman, A.; Thompson, T.D.; Hong, Y.; Moller, B.; Leadbetter, S. Heart disease and cancer deaths — trends and projections in the United States, 1969–2020. *Prev. Chronic Dis.,* **2016,** *13,* 160211.
[http://dx.doi.org/10.5888/pcd13.160211] [PMID: 27854420]

[2]   Bray, F.; Ferlay, J.; Soerjomataram, I.; Siegel, R.L.; Torre, L.A.; Jemal, A. Global cancer statistics 2018: GLOBOCAN estimates of incidence and mortality worldwide for 36 cancers in 185 countries. *CA Cancer J. Clin.,* **2018,** *68*(6), 394-424.
[http://dx.doi.org/10.3322/caac.21492] [PMID: 30207593]

[3]   Chow, A.Y. Cell cycle control by oncogenes and tumor suppressors: Driving the transformation of normal cells into cancerous cells. *Nature Education,* **2010,** *3*(9), 7.

[4]   Siegel, R.L.; Miller, K.D.; Fuchs, H.E.; Jemal, A. Cancer statistics, 2021. *CA Cancer J. Clin.,* **2021,** *71*(1), 7-33.
[http://dx.doi.org/10.3322/caac.21654] [PMID: 33433946]

[5]   Siegel, R.L.; Miller, K.D.; Jemal, A. Cancer statistics, 2020. *CA Cancer J. Clin.,* **2020,** *70*(1), 7-30.
[http://dx.doi.org/10.3322/caac.21590] [PMID: 31912902]

[6]   Ferlay, J.; Soerjomataram, I.; Ervik, M.; Dikshit, R.; Eser, S.; Mathers, C. GLOBOCAN 2012 v1.0, Cancer Incidence and Mortality Worldwide: IARC Cancer Base No. 11 Lyon, France. Int. Agency for Res. *Int. Agency for Res. Cancer,* **2013.**

[7]   World Health Organization (WHO). *Global Health Estimates 2020: Deaths by Cause, Age, Sex, by Country and by Region, 2000 2019*; WHO, **2020.**

[8]   Shah, S.C.; Kayamba, V.; Peek, R.M., Jr; Heimburger, D. Cancer control in low- and middle-income countries: Is it time to consider screening? *J. Glob. Oncol.,* **2019,** *5*(5), 1-8.
[http://dx.doi.org/10.1200/JGO.18.00200] [PMID: 30908147]

[9]   Ferlay, J.; Colombet, M.; Soerjomataram, I.; Mathers, C.; Parkin, D.M.; Piñeros, M.; Znaor, A.; Bray, F. Estimating the global cancer incidence and mortality in 2018: GLOBOCAN sources and methods. *Int. J. Cancer,* **2019,** *144*(8), 1941-1953.
[http://dx.doi.org/10.1002/ijc.31937] [PMID: 30350310]

[10]   LaVigne, A.W.; Triedman, S.A.; Randall, T.C.; Trimble, E.L.; Viswanathan, A.N. Cervical cancer in low and middle income countries: Addressing barriers to radiotherapy delivery. *Gynecol. Oncol. Rep.,* **2017,** *22,* 16-20.
[http://dx.doi.org/10.1016/j.gore.2017.08.004] [PMID: 28948205]

[11]   Arruebo, M.; Vilaboa, N.; Sáez-Gutierrez, B.; Lambea, J.; Tres, A.; Valladares, M.; González-Fernández, Á. Assessment of the evolution of cancer treatment therapies. *Cancers (Basel),* **2011,** *3*(3), 3279-3330.
[http://dx.doi.org/10.3390/cancers3033279] [PMID: 24212956]

[12]   Charmsaz, S.; Collins, D.; Perry, A.; Prencipe, M. Novel strategies for cancer treatment: Highlights from the 55th IACR annual conference. *Cancers (Basel),* **2019,** *11*(8), 1125.
[http://dx.doi.org/10.3390/cancers11081125] [PMID: 31394729]

[13]   Cross, D.; Burmester, J.K. Gene therapy for cancer treatment: Past, present and future. *Clin. Med. Res.,* **2006**, *4*(3), 218-227.
       [http://dx.doi.org/10.3121/cmr.4.3.218] [PMID: 16988102]

[14]   Schirrmacher, V. From chemotherapy to biological therapy: A review of novel concepts to reduce the side effects of systemic cancer treatment (Review). *Int. J. Oncol.,* **2019**, *54*(2), 407-419.
       [PMID: 30570109]

[15]   Nurgali, K.; Jagoe, R.T.; Abalo, R. Editorial: Adverse effects of cancer chemotherapy: Anything new to improve tolerance and reduce sequelae? *Front. Pharmacol.,* **2018**, *9*(9), 245.
       [http://dx.doi.org/10.3389/fphar.2018.00245] [PMID: 29623040]

[16]   Stefanachi, A.; Leonetti, F.; Pisani, L.; Catto, M.; Carotti, A. Coumarin: A natural, privileged and versatile scaffold for bioactive compounds. *Molecules,* **2018**, *23*(2), 250.
       [http://dx.doi.org/10.3390/molecules23020250] [PMID: 29382051]

[17]   Küpeli Akkol, E.; Genç, Y.; Karpuz, B.; Sobarzo-Sánchez, E.; Capasso, R. Coumarins and coumarin-related compounds in pharmacotherapy of cancer. *Cancers (Basel),* **2020**, *12*(7), 1959.
       [http://dx.doi.org/10.3390/cancers12071959] [PMID: 32707666]

[18]   Bhatia, R.; Rawal, R.K. Coumarin hybrids: Promising scaffolds in the treatment of breast cancer. *Mini Rev. Med. Chem.,* **2019**, *19*(17), 1443-1458.
       [http://dx.doi.org/10.2174/1389557519666190308122509] [PMID: 30854961]

[19]   Chen, S.; Cho, M.; Karlsberg, K.; Zhou, D.; Yuan, Y.C. Biochemical and biological characterization of a novel anti-aromatase coumarin derivative. *J. Biol. Chem.,* **2004**, *279*(46), 48071-48078.
       [http://dx.doi.org/10.1074/jbc.M406847200] [PMID: 15358790]

[20]   Hao, S.Y.; Feng, S.L.; Wang, X.R.; Wang, Z.; Chen, S.W.; Hui, L. Novel conjugates of podophyllotoxin and coumarin: Synthesis, cytotoxicities, cell cycle arrest, binding CT DNA and inhibition of Topo IIβ. *Bioorg. Med. Chem. Lett.,* **2019**, *29*(16), 2129-2135.
       [http://dx.doi.org/10.1016/j.bmcl.2019.06.063] [PMID: 31278032]

[21]   Dandriyal, J.; Singla, R.; Kumar, M.; Jaitak, V. Recent developments of C-4 substituted coumarin derivatives as anticancer agents. *Eur. J. Med. Chem.,* **2016**, *119*, 141-168.
       [http://dx.doi.org/10.1016/j.ejmech.2016.03.087] [PMID: 27155469]

[22]   Andricopulo, A.; Salum, L.; Abraham, D. Structure-based drug design strategies in medicinal chemistry. *Curr. Top. Med. Chem.,* **2009**, *9*(9), 771-790.
       [http://dx.doi.org/10.2174/156802609789207127] [PMID: 19754394]

[23]   Shaveta, ; Mishra, S.; Singh, P. Hybrid molecules: The privileged scaffolds for various pharmaceuticals. *Eur. J. Med. Chem.,* **2016**, *124*, 500-536.
       [http://dx.doi.org/10.1016/j.ejmech.2016.08.039] [PMID: 27598238]

[24]   Ballazhi, L.; Popovski, E.; Jashari, A.; Imeri, F.; Ibrahimi, I.; Mikhova, B.; Mladenovska, K. Potential antiproliferative effect of isoxazolo- and thiazolo coumarin derivatives on breast cancer mediated bone and lung metastases. *Acta Pharm.,* **2015**, *65*(1), 53-63.
       [http://dx.doi.org/10.1515/acph-2015-0002] [PMID: 25781704]

[25]   Brueggemeier, R.W.; Hackett, J.C.; Diaz-Cruz, E.S. Aromatase inhibitors in the treatment of breast cancer. *Endocr. Rev.,* **2005**, *26*(3), 331-345.
       [http://dx.doi.org/10.1210/er.2004-0015] [PMID: 15814851]

[26]   Bulun, S.E.; Price, T.M.; Aitken, J.; Mahendroo, M.S.; Simpson, E.R. A link between breast cancer and local estrogen biosynthesis suggested by quantification of breast adipose tissue aromatase cytochrome P450 transcripts using competitive polymerase chain reaction after reverse transcription. *J. Clin. Endocrinol. Metab.,* **1993**, *77*(6), 1622-1628.
       [http://dx.doi.org/10.1210/jcem.77.6.8117355] [PMID: 8117355]

[27]   Yamaguchi, Y.; Nishizono, N.; Kobayashi, D.; Yoshimura, T.; Wada, K.; Oda, K. Evaluation of synthesized coumarin derivatives on aromatase inhibitory activity. *Bioorg. Med. Chem. Lett.,* **2017**,

27(12), 2645-2649.
[http://dx.doi.org/10.1016/j.bmcl.2017.01.062] [PMID: 28512028]

[28]   Pingaew, R.; Prachayasittikul, V.; Mandi, P.; Nantasenamat, C.; Prachayasittikul, S.; Ruchirawat, S.; Prachayasittikul, V. Synthesis and molecular docking of 1,2,3-triazole-based sulfonamides as aromatase inhibitors. *Bioorg. Med. Chem.*, **2015**, *23*(13), 3472-3480.
[http://dx.doi.org/10.1016/j.bmc.2015.04.036] [PMID: 25934226]

[29]   Bhatia, R.; Narang, R.K; Rawal, R.K *In silico* investigation of therapeutic potentials of coumarin-quinoxaline hybrids against Breast Cancer, synthesis and *in vitro* activity. *Ind. J. Het. Chem.*, **2020**, *30*(4), 489-502.

[30]   Ghorab, M.M.; Alsaid, M.S.; Al-Ansary, G.H.; Abdel-Latif, G.A.; Abou El Ella, D.A. Analogue based drug design, synthesis, molecular docking and anticancer evaluation of novel chromene sulfonamide hybrids as aromatase inhibitors and apoptosis enhancers. *Eur. J. Med. Chem.*, **2016**, *124*, 946-958.
[http://dx.doi.org/10.1016/j.ejmech.2016.10.020] [PMID: 27770735]

[31]   Malini, B.; Purohit, A.; Ganeshapillai, D.; Woo, L.W.L.; Potter, B.V.L.; Reed, M.J. Inhibition of steroid sulphatase activity by tricyclic coumarin sulphamates. *J. Steroid Biochem. Mol. Biol.*, **2000**, *75*(4-5), 253-258.
[http://dx.doi.org/10.1016/S0960-0760(00)00178-3] [PMID: 11282279]

[32]   Woo, L.W.L.; Purohit, A.; Malini, B.; Reed, M.J.; Potter, B.V.L. Potent active site-directed inhibition of steroid sulphatase by tricyclic coumarin-based sulphamates. *Chem. Biol.*, **2000**, *7*(10), 773-791.
[http://dx.doi.org/10.1016/S1074-5521(00)00023-5] [PMID: 11033081]

[33]   Daśko, M.; Demkowicz, S.; Biernacki, K.; Ciupak, O.; Kozak, W.; Masłyk, M.; Rachon, J. Recent progress in the development of steroid sulphatase inhibitors – examples of the novel and most promising compounds from the last decade. *J. Enzyme Inhib. Med. Chem.*, **2020**, *35*(1), 1163-1184.
[http://dx.doi.org/10.1080/14756366.2020.1758692] [PMID: 32363947]

[34]   Hng, Y.; Lin, M.H.; Lin, T.S.; Liu, I.C.; Lin, I.C.; Lu, Y.L.; Chang, C.N.; Chiu, P.F.; Tsai, K.C.; Chen, M.J.; Liang, P.H. Design and synthesis of 3-benzylaminocoumarin-7-O-sulfamate derivatives as steroid sulfatase inhibitors. *Bioorg. Chem.*, **2020**, *96*, 103618.
[http://dx.doi.org/10.1016/j.bioorg.2020.103618] [PMID: 32059152]

[35]   Champoux, J.J. DNA topoisomerases: structure, function, and mechanism. *Annu. Rev. Biochem.*, **2001**, *70*(1), 369-413.
[http://dx.doi.org/10.1146/annurev.biochem.70.1.369] [PMID: 11395412]

[36]   Champoux, J.J. DNA TOPOISOMERASES: Structure, function, and mechanism. *Ann. Rev. Biochem.*, **2001**, *70*, 369-413.

[37]   Vologodskii, A. Unlinking of supercoiled DNA catenanes by type IIA topoisomerases. *Biophys. J.*, **2011**, *101*(6), 1403-1411.
[http://dx.doi.org/10.1016/j.bpj.2011.08.011] [PMID: 21943421]

[38]   Seol, Y.; Neuman, K.C. The dynamic interplay between DNA topoisomerases and DNA topology. *Biophys. Rev.*, **2016**, *8*(S1) Suppl. 1, 101-111.
[http://dx.doi.org/10.1007/s12551-016-0240-8] [PMID: 28510219]

[39]   Pommier, Y.; Leo, E.; Zhang, H.; Marchand, C. DNA topoisomerases and their poisoning by anticancer and antibacterial drugs. *Chem. Biol.*, **2010**, *17*(5), 421-433.
[http://dx.doi.org/10.1016/j.chembiol.2010.04.012] [PMID: 20534341]

[40]   Konkoľová, E.; Hudáčová, M.; Hamuľaková, S.; Jendželovský, R.; Vargová, J.; Ševc, J.; Fedoročko, P.; Kožurková, M. Tacrine-coumarin derivatives as topoisomerase inhibitors with antitumor effects on A549 human lung carcinoma cancer cell lines. *Molecules*, **2021**, *26*(4), 1133.
[http://dx.doi.org/10.3390/molecules26041133]

[41]   Nikalje, A.P.G.; Tiwari, S.V.; Tupe, J.G.; Vyas, V.K.; Qureshi, G. Ultrasound Assisted-synthesis and Biological Evaluation of Piperazinylprop- 1-en-2-yloxy-2H-chromen-2-ones as Cytotoxic Agents.

Lett. Drug Des. Discov., **2017**, *14*(10), 1195-1205.
[http://dx.doi.org/10.2174/1570180814666170322154750]

[42]   Hueso-Falcón, I.; Amesty, Á.; Anaissi-Afonso, L.; Lorenzo-Castrillejo, I.; Machín, F.; Estévez-Braun, A. Synthesis and biological evaluation of naphthoquinone-coumarin conjugates as topoisomerase II inhibitors. *Bioorg. Med. Chem. Lett.,* **2017**, *27*(3), 484-489.
[http://dx.doi.org/10.1016/j.bmcl.2016.12.040] [PMID: 28040393]

[43]   Adams, J.M.; Cory, S. Life-or-death decisions by the Bcl-2 protein family. *Trends Biochem. Sci.,* **2001**, *26*(1), 61-66.
[http://dx.doi.org/10.1016/S0968-0004(00)01740-0] [PMID: 11165519]

[44]   Zimmermann, K.C.; Green, D.R. How cells die: Apoptosis pathways. *J. Allergy Clin. Immunol.,* **2001**, *108*(4) Suppl., S99-S103.
[http://dx.doi.org/10.1067/mai.2001.117819] [PMID: 11586274]

[45]   Salvesen, G.S. Caspases and apoptosis. *Essays Biochem.,* **2002**, *38*, 9-19.
[http://dx.doi.org/10.1042/bse0380009] [PMID: 12463158]

[46]   Brentnall, M.; Rodriguez-Menocal, L.; De Guevara, R.L.; Cepero, E.; Boise, L.H. Caspase-9, caspase-3 and caspase-7 have distinct roles during intrinsic apoptosis. *BMC Cell Biol.,* **2013**, *14*(1), 32.
[http://dx.doi.org/10.1186/1471-2121-14-32] [PMID: 23834359]

[47]   Fayed, E.A.; Sabour, R.; Harras, M.F.; Mehany, A.B.M. Design, synthesis, biological evaluation and molecular modeling of new coumarin derivatives as potent anticancer agents. *Med. Chem. Res.,* **2019**, *28*(8), 1284-1297.
[http://dx.doi.org/10.1007/s00044-019-02373-x]

[48]   Mohamed, T.K.; Batran, R.Z.; Elseginy, S.A.; Ali, M.M.; Mahmoud, A.E. Synthesis, anticancer effect and molecular modeling of new thiazolylpyrazolyl coumarin derivatives targeting VEGFR-2 kinase and inducing cell cycle arrest and apoptosis. *Bioorg. Chem.,* **2019**, *85*, 253-273.
[http://dx.doi.org/10.1016/j.bioorg.2018.12.040] [PMID: 30641320]

[49]   Zhang, Y.Y.; Zhang, Q.Q.; Song, J.L.; Zhang, L.; Jiang, C.S.; Zhang, H. Design, Synthesis, and Antiproliferative Evaluation of Novel Coumarin/2-Cyanoacryloyl Hybrids as Apoptosis Inducing Agents by Activation of Caspase-Dependent Pathway. *Molecules,* **2018**, *23*(8), 1972.
[http://dx.doi.org/10.3390/molecules23081972] [PMID: 30087276]

[50]   Elshemy, H.A.H.; Zaki, M.A. Design and synthesis of new coumarin hybrids and insight into their mode of antiproliferative action. *Bioorg. Med. Chem.,* **2017**, *25*(3), 1066-1075.
[http://dx.doi.org/10.1016/j.bmc.2016.12.019] [PMID: 28038941]

[51]   Wang, L.; Guillen, V.S.; Sharma, N.; Flessa, K.; Min, J.; Carlson, K.E.; Toy, W.; Braqi, S.; Katzenellenbogen, B.S.; Katzenellenbogen, J.A.; Chandarlapaty, S.; Sharma, A. New Class of Selective Estrogen Receptor Degraders (SERDs): Expanding the Toolbox of PROTAC Degrons. *ACS Med. Chem. Lett.,* **2018**, *9*(8), 803-808.
[http://dx.doi.org/10.1021/acsmedchemlett.8b00106] [PMID: 30128071]

[52]   Xiong, R.; Zhao, J.; Gutgesell, L.M.; Wang, Y.; Lee, S.; Karumudi, B.; Zhao, H.; Lu, Y.; Tonetti, D.A.; Thatcher, G.R.J. Novel Selective Estrogen Receptor Downregulators (SERDs) Developed against Treatment-Resistant Breast Cancer. *J. Med. Chem.,* **2017**, *60*(4), 1325-1342.
[http://dx.doi.org/10.1021/acs.jmedchem.6b01355] [PMID: 28117994]

[53]   Degorce, S.L.; Bailey, A.; Callis, R.; De Savi, C.; Ducray, R.; Lamont, G.; MacFaul, P.; Maudet, M.; Martin, S.; Morgentin, R.; Norman, R.A.; Peru, A.; Pink, J.H.; Plé, P.A.; Roberts, B.; Scott, J.S. Investigation of (*E*)-3-[4-(2-Oxo-3-aryl-chromen-4-yl)oxyphenyl]acrylic Acids as Oral Selective Estrogen Receptor Down-Regulators. *J. Med. Chem.,* **2015**, *58*(8), 3522-3533.
[http://dx.doi.org/10.1021/acs.jmedchem.5b00066] [PMID: 25790336]

[54]   Luo, G.; Chen, M.; Lyu, W.; Zhao, R.; Xu, Q.; You, Q.; Xiang, H. Design, synthesis, biological evaluation and molecular docking studies of novel 3-aryl-4-anilino-2 H -chromen-2-one derivatives targeting ERα as anti-breast cancer agents. *Bioorg. Med. Chem. Lett.,* **2017**, *27*(12), 2668-2673.

[http://dx.doi.org/10.1016/j.bmcl.2017.04.029] [PMID: 28460819]

[55]   Kumar, B.; Kumar, R.; Skvortsova, I.; Kumar, V. Mechanisms of tubulin binding ligands to target cancer cells: Updates on their therapeutic potential and clinical trials. *Curr. Cancer Drug Targets,* **2017**, *17*(4), 357-375.
[http://dx.doi.org/10.2174/1568009616666160928110818] [PMID: 27697026]

[56]   Dustin, P. *Microtubules*; Springer Verlag: Berlin, Heidelberg, New York, **1978**, 452, .
[http://dx.doi.org/10.1007/978-3-642-96436-7]

[57]   Cao, D.; Liu, Y.; Yan, W.; Wang, C.; Bai, P.; Wang, T.; Tang, M.; Wang, X.; Yang, Z.; Ma, B.; Ma, L.; Lei, L.; Wang, F.; Xu, B.; Zhou, Y.; Yang, T.; Chen, L. Design, synthesis, and evaluation of *in vitro* and *in vivo* anti-cancer activity of 4-substituted coumarins: A novel class of potent tubulin polymerization inhibitors. *J. Med. Chem.,* **2016**, *59*(12), 5721-5739.
[http://dx.doi.org/10.1021/acs.jmedchem.6b00158] [PMID: 27213819]

[58]   Pasquier, E.; Kavallaris, M. Microtubules: A dynamic target in cancer therapy. *IUBMB Life,* **2008**, *60*(3), 165-170.
[http://dx.doi.org/10.1002/iub.25] [PMID: 18380008]

[59]   Kumar, B.; Sharma, P.; Gupta, V.P.; Khullar, M.; Singh, S.; Dogra, N.; Kumar, V. Synthesis and biological evaluation of pyrimidine bridged combretastatin derivatives as potential anticancer agents and mechanistic studies. *Bioorg. Chem.,* **2018**, *78*, 130-140.
[http://dx.doi.org/10.1016/j.bioorg.2018.02.027] [PMID: 29554587]

[60]   Mutai, P.; Breuzard, G.; Pagano, A.; Allegro, D.; Peyrot, V.; Chibale, K. Synthesis and biological evaluation of 4 arylcoumarin analogues as tubulin-targeting antitumor agents. *Bioorg. Med. Chem.,* **2017**, *25*(5), 1652-1665.
[http://dx.doi.org/10.1016/j.bmc.2017.01.035] [PMID: 28174064]

[61]   Fu, D.J.; Li, P.; Wu, B.W.; Cui, X.X.; Zhao, C.B.; Zhang, S.Y. Molecular diversity of trimethoxyphenyl-1,2,3-triazole hybrids as novel colchicine site tubulin polymerization inhibitors. *Eur. J. Med. Chem.,* **2019**, *165*, 309-322.
[http://dx.doi.org/10.1016/j.ejmech.2019.01.033] [PMID: 30690300]

[62]   Govindaiah, P.; Dumala, N.; Mattan, I.; Grover, P.; Jaya Prakash, M. Design, synthesis, biological and *in silico* evaluation of coumarin-hydrazone derivatives as tubulin targeted antiproliferative agents. *Bioorg. Chem.,* **2019**, *91*, 103143.
[http://dx.doi.org/10.1016/j.bioorg.2019.103143] [PMID: 31374528]

[63]   Asati, V.; Mahapatra, D.K.; Bharti, S.K. PI3K/Akt/mTOR and Ras/Raf/MEK/ERK signaling pathways inhibitors as anticancer agents: Structural and pharmacological perspectives. *Eur. J. Med. Chem.,* **2016**, *109*, 314-341.
[http://dx.doi.org/10.1016/j.ejmech.2016.01.012] [PMID: 26807863]

[64]   McMullen, J.R.; Jay, P.Y. PI3K(p110α) inhibitors as anti-cancer agents: Minding the heart. *Cell Cycle,* **2007**, *6*(8), 910-913.
[http://dx.doi.org/10.4161/cc.6.8.4124] [PMID: 17404510]

[65]   Vanhaesebroeck, B.; Leevers, S.J.; Panayotou, G.; Waterfield, M.D. Phosphoinositide 3-kinases: A conserved family of signal transducers. *Trends Biochem. Sci.,* **1997**, *22*(7), 267-272.
[http://dx.doi.org/10.1016/S0968-0004(97)01061-X] [PMID: 9255069]

[66]   Yang, J.; Nie, J.; Ma, X.; Wei, Y.; Peng, Y.; Wei, X. Targeting PI3K in cancer: Mechanisms and advances in clinical trials. *Mol. Cancer,* **2019**, *18*(1), 26.
[http://dx.doi.org/10.1186/s12943-019-0954-x] [PMID: 30782187]

[67]   Thakur, A.; Singla, R.; Jaitak, V. Coumarins as anticancer agents: A review on synthetic strategies, mechanism of action and SAR studies. *Eur. J. Med. Chem.,* **2015**, *101*, 476-495.
[http://dx.doi.org/10.1016/j.ejmech.2015.07.010] [PMID: 26188907]

[68]   Wu, Y.; Xu, J.; Liu, Y.; Zeng, Y.; Wu, G. A review on anti-tumor mechanisms of coumarins. *Front.*

Oncol., **2020**, *10*, 592853.
[http://dx.doi.org/10.3389/fonc.2020.592853] [PMID: 33344242]

[69]   Wu, L.; Wang, X.; Xu, W.; Farzaneh, F.; Xu, R. The structure and pharmacological functions of coumarins and their derivatives. *Curr. Med. Chem.,* **2009**, *16*(32), 4236-4260.
[http://dx.doi.org/10.2174/092986709789578187] [PMID: 19754420]

[70]   Riveiro, M.; De Kimpe, N.; Moglioni, A.; Vázquez, R.; Monczor, F.; Shayo, C.; Davio, C. Coumarins: Old compounds with novel promising therapeutic perspectives. *Curr. Med. Chem.,* **2010**, *17*(13), 1325-1338.
[http://dx.doi.org/10.2174/092986710790936284] [PMID: 20166938]

[71]   Jiang, J.; Wang, B.; Li, J.; Ye, B.; Lin, S.; Qian, W.; Shan, L.; Efferth, T. Total coumarins of Hedyotis diffusa induces apoptosis of myelodysplastic syndrome SKM-1 cells by activation of caspases and inhibition of PI3K/Akt pathway proteins. *J. Ethnopharmacol.,* **2017**, *196*, 253-260.
[http://dx.doi.org/10.1016/j.jep.2016.12.012] [PMID: 27988397]

[72]   Sumorek-Wiadro, J.; Zając, A.; Langner, E.; Skalicka-Woźniak, K.; Maciejczyk, A.; Rzeski, W.; Jakubowicz-Gil, J. Antiglioma potential of coumarins combined with sorafenib. *Molecules,* **2020**, *25*(21), 5192.
[http://dx.doi.org/10.3390/molecules25215192] [PMID: 33171577]

[73]   Ma, C.C.; Liu, Z.P. Design and synthesis of coumarin derivatives as novel PI3K inhibitors. Anti-Canc. *Anticancer. Agents Med. Chem.,* **2017**, *17*(3), 395-403.
[http://dx.doi.org/10.2174/1871520616666160223120207] [PMID: 26902599]

[74]   Liu, H.; Wang, Y.; Sharma, A.; Mao, R.; Jiang, N.; Dun, B.; She, J.X. Derivatives containing both coumarin and benzimidazole potently induce caspase-dependent apoptosis of cancer cells through inhibition of PI3K-AKT-mTOR signaling. *Anticancer Drugs,* **2015**, *26*(6), 667-677.
[http://dx.doi.org/10.1097/CAD.0000000000000232] [PMID: 25811964]

[75]   Mohareb, R.M.; Gamaan, M.S. The uses of ethyl 2-(1H-benzo [D] imidazol-2-yl) acetate to synthesis pyrazole, thiophene, pyridine and coumarin derivatives with antitumor activities. *Bull. Chem. Soc. Ethiop.,* **2018**, *32*(3), 541-557.
[http://dx.doi.org/10.4314/bcse.v32i3.13]

[76]   Holiyachi, M.; Shastri, S.L.; Chougala, B.M.; Shastri, L.A.; Joshi, S.D.; Dixit, S.R.; Nagarajaiah, H.; Sunagar, V.A. Design, Synthesis and structure-activity relationship study of coumarin benzimidazole hybrid as potent antibacterial and anticancer agents. *ChemistrySelect,* **2016**, *1*(15), 4638-4644.
[http://dx.doi.org/10.1002/slct.201600665]

[77]   Wang, T.; Peng, T.; Wen, X.; Wang, G.; Sun, Y.; Liu, S.; Zhang, S.; Wang, L. Design, synthesis and preliminary biological evaluation of benzylsulfone coumarin derivatives as anti-cancer agents. *Molecules,* **2019**, *24*(22), 4034.
[http://dx.doi.org/10.3390/molecules24224034] [PMID: 31703373]

[78]   Al-Warhi, T.; El Kerdawy, A.M.; Aljaeed, N.; Ismael, O.E.; Ayyad, R.R.; Eldehna, W.M.; Abdel-Aziz, H.A.; Al-Ansary, G.H. Synthesis, biological evaluation and *in silico* studies of certain oxindole–indole conjugates as anti-cancer CDK inhibitors. *Molecules,* **2020**, *25*(9), 2031.
[http://dx.doi.org/10.3390/molecules25092031] [PMID: 32349307]

[79]   Lim, S.; Kaldis, P. Cdks, cyclins and CKIs: Roles beyond cell cycle regulation. *Development,* **2013**, *140*(15), 3079-3093.
[http://dx.doi.org/10.1242/dev.091744] [PMID: 23861057]

[80]   Matthews, D.J.; Gerritsen, M.E. *Targeting protein kinases for cancer therapy*; John Wiley & Sons, **2011**.

[81]   Mariaule, G.; Belmont, P. Cyclin-dependent kinase inhibitors as marketed anticancer drugs: Where are we now? A short survey. *Molecules,* **2014**, *19*(9), 14366-14382.
[http://dx.doi.org/10.3390/molecules190914366] [PMID: 25215591]

[82] Kalra, S.; Joshi, G.; Munshi, A.; Kumar, R. Structural insights of cyclin dependent kinases: Implications in design of selective inhibitors. *Eur. J. Med. Chem.,* **2017**, *142*, 424-458.
[http://dx.doi.org/10.1016/j.ejmech.2017.08.071] [PMID: 28911822]

[83] Lu, X.Y.; Wang, Z.C.; Ren, S.Z.; Shen, F.Q.; Man, R.J.; Zhu, H.L. Coumarin sulfonamides derivatives as potent and selective COX-2 inhibitors with efficacy in suppressing cancer proliferation and metastasis. *Bioorg. Med. Chem. Lett.,* **2016**, *26*(15), 3491-3498.
[http://dx.doi.org/10.1016/j.bmcl.2016.06.037] [PMID: 27349331]

[84] Abd El-Karim, S.S.; Syam, Y.M.; El Kerdawy, A.M.; Abdelghany, T.M. New thiazol-hydrazon--coumarin hybrids targeting human cervical cancer cells: Synthesis, CDK2 inhibition, QSAR and molecular docking studies. *Bioorg. Chem.,* **2019**, *86*, 80-96.
[http://dx.doi.org/10.1016/j.bioorg.2019.01.026] [PMID: 30685646]

[85] Xu, J.; Li, H.; Wang, X.; Huang, J.; Li, S.; Liu, C.; Dong, R.; Zhu, G.; Duan, C.; Jiang, F.; Zhang, Y.; Zhu, Y.; Zhang, T.; Chen, Y.; Tang, W.; Lu, T. Discovery of coumarin derivatives as potent and selective cyclin-dependent kinase 9 (CDK9) inhibitors with high antitumour activity. *Eur. J. Med. Chem.,* **2020**, *200*, 112424.
[http://dx.doi.org/10.1016/j.ejmech.2020.112424] [PMID: 32447197]

[86] Glozak, M.A.; Seto, E. Histone deacetylases and cancer. *Oncogene,* **2007**, *26*(37), 5420-5432.
[http://dx.doi.org/10.1038/sj.onc.1210610] [PMID: 17694083]

[87] Ding, J.; Liu, J.; Zhang, Z.; Guo, J.; Cheng, M.; Wan, Y.; Wang, R.; Fang, Y.; Guan, Z.; Jin, Y.; Xie, S.S. Design, synthesis and biological evaluation of coumarin-based N-hydroxycinnamamide derivatives as novel histone deacetylase inhibitors with anticancer activities. *Bioorg. Chem.,* **2020**, *101*, 104023.
[http://dx.doi.org/10.1016/j.bioorg.2020.104023] [PMID: 32650178]

[88] Lagunes, I.; Begines, P.; Silva, A.; Galán, A.R.; Puerta, A.; Fernandes, M.X.; Maya, I.; Fernández-Bolaños, J.G.; López, Ó.; Padrón, J.M. Selenocoumarins as new multitarget antiproliferative agents: Synthesis, biological evaluation and *in silico* calculations. *Eur. J. Med. Chem.,* **2019**, *179*, 493-501.
[http://dx.doi.org/10.1016/j.ejmech.2019.06.073] [PMID: 31271961]

[89] Abdizadeh, T.; Kalani, M.R.; Abnous, K.; Tayarani-Najaran, Z.; Khashyarmanesh, B.Z.; Abdizadeh, R.; Ghodsi, R.; Hadizadeh, F. Design, synthesis and biological evaluation of novel coumarin-based benzamides as potent histone deacetylase inhibitors and anticancer agents. *Eur. J. Med. Chem.,* **2017**, *132*, 42-62.
[http://dx.doi.org/10.1016/j.ejmech.2017.03.024] [PMID: 28340413]

[90] Wang, S.; Meades, C.; Wood, G.; Osnowski, A.; Anderson, S.; Yuill, R.; Thomas, M.; Mezna, M.; Jackson, W.; Midgley, C.; Griffiths, G.; Fleming, I.; Green, S.; McNae, I.; Wu, S.Y.; McInnes, C.; Zheleva, D.; Walkinshaw, M.D.; Fischer, P.M. 2-Anilino-4-(thiazol-5-yl)pyrimidine CDK inhibitors: Synthesis, SAR analysis, X-ray crystallography, and biological activity. *J. Med. Chem.,* **2004**, *47*(7), 1662-1675.
[http://dx.doi.org/10.1021/jm0309957] [PMID: 15027857]

[91] Ahmed, N.M.; Youns, M.; Soltan, M.K.; Said, A.M. Design, synthesis, molecular modelling, and biological evaluation of novel substituted pyrimidine derivatives as potential anticancer agents for hepatocellular carcinoma. *J. Enzyme Inhib. Med. Chem.,* **2019**, *34*(1), 1110-1120.
[http://dx.doi.org/10.1080/14756366.2019.1612889] [PMID: 31117890]

[92] Prachayasittikul, S.; Pingaew, R.; Worachartcheewan, A.; Sinthupoom, N.; Prachayasittikul, V.; Ruchirawat, S.; Prachayasittikul, V. Roles of pyridine and pyrimidine derivatives as privileged scaffolds in anticancer agents. *Mini Rev. Med. Chem.,* **2017**, *17*(10), 869-901.
[http://dx.doi.org/10.2174/1389557516666160923125801] [PMID: 27670581]

[93] Lv, N.; Sun, M.; Liu, C.; Li, J. Design and synthesis of 2-phenylpyrimidine coumarin derivatives as anticancer agents. *Bioorg. Med. Chem. Lett.,* **2017**, *27*(19), 4578-4581.
[http://dx.doi.org/10.1016/j.bmcl.2017.08.044] [PMID: 28888820]

[94]   Hosamani, K.M.; Reddy, D.S.; Devarajegowda, H.C. Microwave-assisted synthesis of new fluorinated coumarin–pyrimidine hybrids as potent anticancer agents, their DNA cleavage and X-ray crystal studies. *RSC Advances,* **2015**, *5*(15), 11261-11271.
[http://dx.doi.org/10.1039/C4RA12222D]

[95]   Lingaraju, G.S.; Balaji, K.S.; Jayarama, S.; Anil, S.M.; Kiran, K.R.; Sadashiva, M.P. Synthesis of new coumarin tethered isoxazolines as potential anticancer agents. *Bioorg. Med. Chem. Lett.,* **2018**, *28*(23-24), 3606-3612.
[http://dx.doi.org/10.1016/j.bmcl.2018.10.046] [PMID: 30396758]

[96]   Narella, S.G.; Shaik, M.G.; Mohammed, A.; Alvala, M.; Angeli, A.; Supuran, C.T. Synthesis and biological evaluation of coumarin-1,3,4-oxadiazole hybrids as selective carbonic anhydrase IX and XII inhibitors. *Bioorg. Chem.,* **2019**, *87*, 765-772.
[http://dx.doi.org/10.1016/j.bioorg.2019.04.004] [PMID: 30974299]

[97]   Dhawan, S.; Kerru, N.; Awolade, P.; Singh-Pillay, A.; Saha, S.T.; Kaur, M.; Jonnalagadda, S.B.; Singh, P. Synthesis, computational studies and antiproliferative activities of coumarin-tagged 1,3,4-oxadiazole conjugates against MDA-MB-231 and MCF-7 human breast cancer cells. *Bioorg. Med. Chem.,* **2018**, *26*(21), 5612-5623.
[http://dx.doi.org/10.1016/j.bmc.2018.10.006] [PMID: 30360952]

[98]   Amin, K.M.; Eissa, A.A.M.; Abou-Seri, S.M.; Awadallah, F.M.; Hassan, G.S. Synthesis and biological evaluation of novel coumarin–pyrazoline hybrids endowed with phenylsulfonyl moiety as antitumor agents. *Eur. J. Med. Chem.,* **2013**, *60*, 187-198.
[http://dx.doi.org/10.1016/j.ejmech.2012.12.004] [PMID: 23291120]

[99]   Kurt, B.Z.; Ozten Kandas, N.; Dag, A.; Sonmez, F.; Kucukislamoglu, M. Synthesis and biological evaluation of novel coumarin-chalcone derivatives containing urea moiety as potential anticancer agents. *Arab. J. Chem.,* **2020**, *13*(1), 1120-1129.
[http://dx.doi.org/10.1016/j.arabjc.2017.10.001]

[100] Mokale, S.N.; Begum, A.; Sakle, N.S.; Shelke, V.R.; Bhavale, S.A. Design, synthesis and anticancer screening of 3-(3-(substituted phenyl) acryloyl)-2H-chromen-2ones as selective anti-breast cancer agent. *Biomed. Pharmacother.,* **2017**, *89*, 966-972.
[http://dx.doi.org/10.1016/j.biopha.2017.02.089] [PMID: 28292025]

CHAPTER 3

Progress in Nitrogen and Sulphur-based Heterocyclic Compounds for their Anticancer Activity

Preeti Koli[1] and **Rajesh K. Singh**[1, *]

[1] *Department of Pharmaceutical Chemistry, Shivalik College of Pharmacy, Nangal, Dist. Rupnagar, 140126, Punjab, India*

Abstract: Cancer is a widespread disease worldwide. Researchers and scientists have been giving much attention to the drug design and drug discovery of nitrogen (*N*) and sulfur (*S*)-based heterocyclic compounds in the last decade. These heteroatoms containing heterocyclic compounds have an imperative role in medicinal chemistry in developing new anticancer drugs. These *N* and *S*-based heterocyclic compounds such as pyrrole, quinazoline, thiadiazole, and quinoline are widely used in the rational drug design for anticancer drugs with a favorable therapeutic index. They inhibit the cancerous cells by different mechanisms like inhibiting FGFR, VEGFR, EGFR receptors and inducing apoptosis. They also act as a tyrosine kinase inhibitor, dihydrofolate reductase inhibitor, pancreatic ductal adenocarcinoma inhibitor, and PI3K inhibitor. This chapter highlights the SAR study of recent literature (2016-2020) in which *N* and *S* heterocyclic compounds are present as core structures in molecules. This chapter also emphasizes the benefits of hybrid molecules acting on *multiple* target mechanisms. In the future, *N* and *S*- based heterocyclic compounds will be essential lead compounds for the designing of new anticancer drugs.

Keywords: Cancer, Chalcone, Hybrid molecules, *N*-based heterocyclic compounds, *S*-based heterocyclic compounds, SAR study.

INTRODUCTION

Cancer is a critical disease which become an epidemic nowadays. In 2021 National Cancer Institute (NCI) observes the 50th ceremony of the National Cancer Act 1971. Cancer can damage our immune system because it causes cells to divide uncontrollably.

---
* **Corresponding author Rajesh K. Singh:**Department of Pharmaceutical Chemistry, Shivalik College of Pharmacy, Nangal, Dist. Rupnagar, 140126, Punjab, India; Tel: +919417513730; Email: rksingh244@gmail.com

New retrospective and prospective studies showed that cancer patients are more susceptible to coronavirus disease 2019 as active chemotherapy have higher chances of adverse effect, *i.e.*, respiratory infections [1, 2]. Cancerous patients have a higher risk of Covid 19 than non-cancerous patients. Cancerous patients have a down-regulated immune response known as 'cytokine storm' responsible for various infections [3]. So, there is an urgent need to develop anticancer drugs to treat cancer.

Heterocyclic compounds have always been core parts in the expansion of drug design and development. These compounds exhibit exciting medicinal properties [4], including anticancer. Among all the heterocyclic scaffolds, nitrogen and sulfur-based heterocyclics are the key core structures of anticancer agents [5 - 8]. The *N*-based heterocyclic compound has become an active topic in developing oncology. These are the essential compounds present naturally in the body, including nucleic acid, protein, vitamins. The base pair of RNA and DNA like adenine, guanine, thymine, and cytosine are also made up of *N*-heterocyclic compounds *i.e.,* purine and pyrimidine nucleus. Their vast biological properties are due to the *N* atom's electron-rich nature present in moiety, which can easily form various interactions like H- bonding, Vander wall, dipole-dipole interaction, *etc.* with target molecule [9 - 12].

A quick search of FDA databases demonstrates the structural importance of nitrogen-based heterocycles in pharmaceutical drug design and engineering, with nitrogen heterocycles accounting for over 60% of all small-molecule medications [13].

With the advancement of the *N*-heterocyclic compound, researchers now shifted their interest towards the other heterocyclic rings. Thus, they synthesized *S*-based heterocyclic compounds. These compounds show their significant role in anticancer activity due to the high reactivity of sulfur atoms in the molecule. These heterocyclic compounds can bind suitably to pharmacological targets and receptors *via* intermolecular H-bonds more effectively, giving desired pharmacological effects. They can also alter liposolubility, hence the aqueous solubility of drug molecules to achieve remarkable pharmacokinetic properties. Given the relevance of sulphur in biological systems and its growing popularity as a regulatory agent, the rationale for using sulfur-based heterocycle medicines becomes vibrant. These *N* and *S*-based heterocyclic compounds are used in rational drug design for anticancer drugs with favorable therapeutic index [14, 15]. This chapter focuses on the most recent developments in *N* and *S*-based heterocycle scaffolds, emphasizing their key roles in cancer therapy while also considering their properties as molecule drugs, general mechanisms of action, major biological targets, and structure–activity relationships (SAR).

PYRROLE

Chemistry of Pyrrole

Pyrrole is an aromatic five-membered heterocyclic ring that acts as lead for various anticancer drugs (Fig. **1**). Researchers and chemists have drawn much attention to pyrrole and its derivative for the benefit of mankind. It reacts with other biomolecules through non-covalent bonding like *H*-bonding and anionic bonding through the pyrrole *N* site [16].

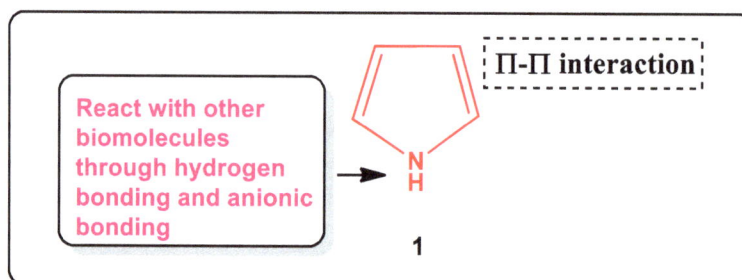

Fig. (1). Chemistry of pyrrole.

Anticancer Activity of Pyrrole Derivatives

Combretastatin A-4 is the natural compound derived from the *Combretum cafferium*. It is used as an antimitotic agent for anticancer drugs by acting on tubulin's colchicine binding site [17]. Several types of research have shown that only *cis* olefin of CA-4 is essential for antimitotic activity. *Trans* isomers, on the other hand, do not bind with the specific site of tubulin and are hence inactive. Therefore, a five-membered pyrrole ring is used as a linker, resulting in a *cis-like* constrained configuration that increases the potency and bioactivity of the drug by inhibiting the conversion of *cis* into *trans* isomer. In 2016, Jung *et al.* synthesized several compounds containing pyrrole as an analog for Combretastatin A-4. The compound **2** (Fig. **2**) was synthesized by aryl Claisen rearrangement, which gives 63% yield and the highest activity. The 3-methoxy-4-hydroxy phenyl group was essential for activity as it binds to the colchicine site of tubulin, which gave potent antitumor activity [18].

Cytochrome P450 is a heme-containing potent tumor biomarker, a diverse family of isoform CYP1A1, CYP1B1, and CYP1A2. These act by phase 1 metabolism of xenobiotics and act as a carcinogen [19]. The pyrrole-chalcones were synthesized by Claisen-Schmidt condensation to give a 24-73% yield. SAR Study of compound **3** (Fig. **3**) revealed that the pyrrole group increases the potency of the drug by interacting with hydrophobic π-π interactions. The 2-methoxy benzene inhibits all the isoforms of CYP1 (IC_{50}=1.2µM) but was not specific to CYP1B1. Therefore, the replacement of the aryl group with 2-chlorobenzene specifically inhibits CYP1B1 (IC_{50}=0.23 µM). The chalcone group in the active scaffold is responsible for selectively inhibiting the CYP1 enzyme [20].

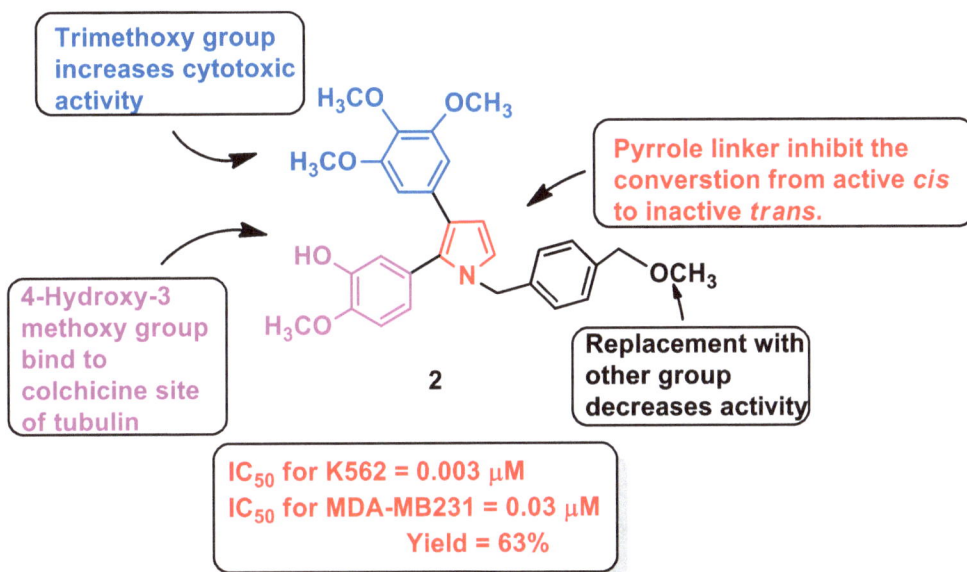

Fig. (2). Structure-activity relationship (SAR) of pyrrole as an analog for Combretastatin A-4.

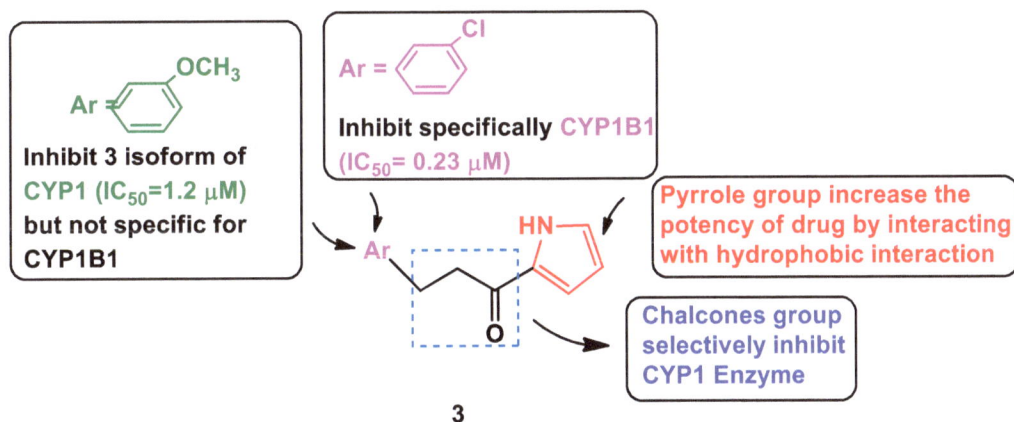

Fig. (3). Structure-activity relationship (SAR) of pyrrole-chalcone hybrid.

Fibroblast growth factors are essential to regulate the various cellular actions, *i.e.*, proliferation and metastasis of cancerous cells. FGFR (fibroblast growth factor receptor) is a subfamily of receptor tyrosine kinase [RTKs] [21]. To develop new anticancer drugs, pyrrole moiety was attached with sulphonamide group based on FGFR binding ligand interaction. This scaffold increases the therapeutic index of the drug and increases the potency. Due to this pyrrole's effective pharmacological effect as active moiety, scientists investigated compound **4** (Fig. **4**) that could bind to FGFR protein and inhibit cell proliferation of MCF-7 and HL60. Its inhibitory activity can be distinguished at different concentrations using cisplatin as a reference drug. This drug causes apoptosis in PC-12 cells by distorting the shape of the cell. Its electronic parameter like chemical hardness, softness, and electronegativity was evaluated by density functional theory (DFT). SAR study shows that replacement of methyl ester group with methyl group decreases the activity. Pyrrole moiety is responsible for antiproliferative activity. The sulphonamide group enhances the antiproliferative activity. Morpholine ring was critical for activity as replacement of morpholine ring by other moieties like barbituric acid and phenyl ring leads to loss of antiproliferative activity [22].

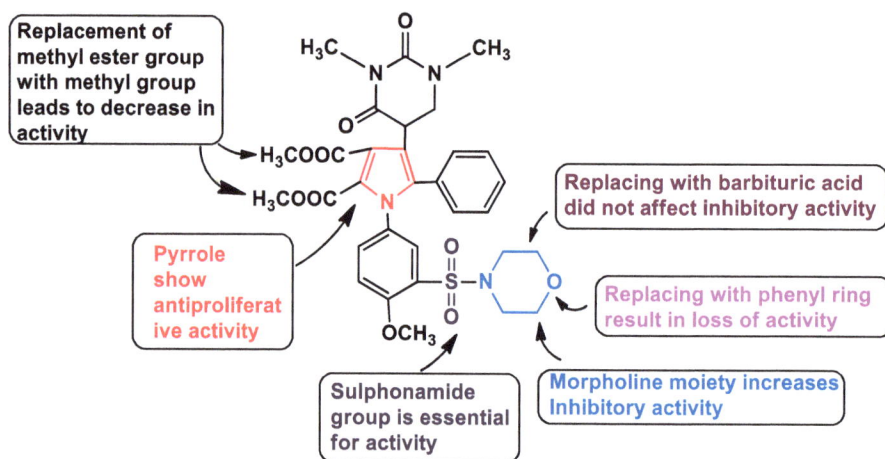

Fig. (4). Structure-activity relationship (SAR) of pyrrole as an analog for FGFR inhibitor.

Various small-molecule kinase inhibitors (SMKI) reduce the toxicity and target specifically for kinase receptors. These are the broad-spectrum inhibitors of the cancerous cells because of their high penetration ability [23]. Due to these versatile pharmacological properties of SMKI, scientists and researchers synthesized several chemical compounds [24]. In 2018 Yang *et al.* reviewed many small molecule kinase inhibitors (SMKI) containing pyrrole as an active molecule. Compound **5** (Fig. **5**) inhibited the vascular endothelial growth factor receptor (VEGFR) and platelet-derived growth factor receptor (PDGFR). The rationale behind attaching the 5-6 membered heterocyclic, *i.e.*, indoline, with pyrrole was to demonstrate the better inhibitory activity against both VEGFR and PDGFR. Substitutions at 5th and 6th positions were found to be more effective in enhancing antiproliferative activity. The active pyrrole-indoline-2-one moiety binds with a hydrophobic pocket of the ATP binding site of the kinase [25].

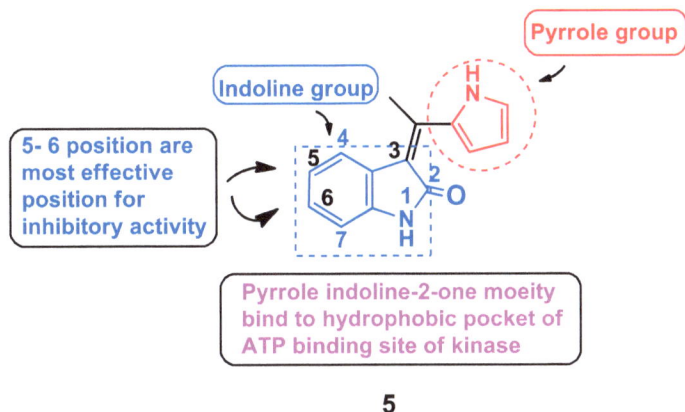

5

Fig. (5). Structure-activity relationship (SAR) of pyrrole-indoline hybrid.

In 2019, Thiriveedhi *et al.* described that pyrrole moiety attached to the pyrimidine group inhibited the excessive proliferation of tumor cells and showed excellent cytotoxic activity. They synthesized compound **6** (Fig. **6**) which was evaluated by MTT assay using murine melanoma cell lines (B16F10) and breast cancer lines (MCF-7). SAR study revealed that the pyrrole group was responsible for the antiproliferative activity. The five-membered ring was attached with pyrrole to act as an MCF-7 inhibitor (IC$_{50}$=18.92 μM). Triazole moiety act as target specific EGFR tyrosine kinase inhibitor [26].

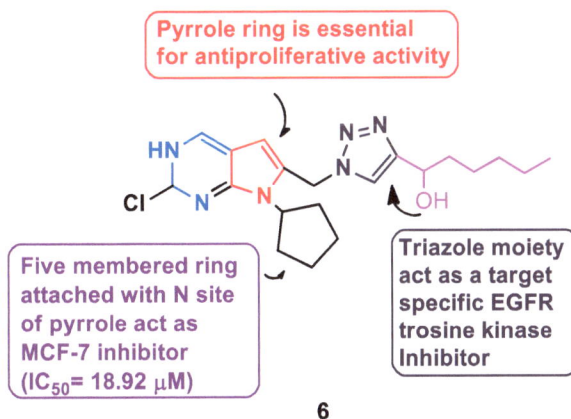

6

Fig. (6). Structure-activity relationship (SAR) of pyrrole and pyrimidine hybrid.

Calixpyrrole **7** (Fig. **7**) is a non-aromatic tetrapyrrolic macrocycle that showed versatile pharmacological activities. These supramolecules displayed better binding affinity and selectivity [27]. Calixpyrrole has a pivotal role in anticancer activity. They act as a pyrrole-containing anion binder. Anions play a key role in the living world. The cytotoxic effect is exerted by the chloride transfer in a biomembrane. Calixpyrrole and anionic binding receptors have shown a comprehensive role in potential drug systems by transferring anion across the membrane. The main target for Calixpyrrole is the G-protein-coupled estrogen receptor, and it acts as an inhibitor of MCF-7 cancerous cell lines [28].

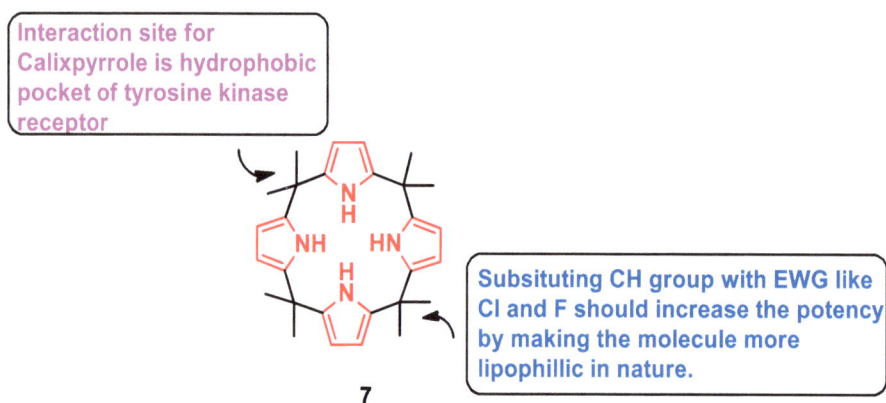

Interaction site for Calixpyrrole is hydrophobic pocket of tyrosine kinase receptor

Subsituting CH group with EWG like Cl and F should increase the potency by making the molecule more lipophillic in nature.

7

Fig. (7). Structure-activity relationship (SAR) of calixpyrrole analog.

In other miscellaneous studies, Koley *et al.* studiedpyrrole-based (II) Schiff-based complex **8** (Fig. **8**). DNA is the primary target for anticancer activity. Pyrrole-based Cu (II) Schiff-based complex are used against the cervical cancer Hela and normal human diploid WI-38 cell lines by binding them with guanine of DNA. It can disrupt the *H* bonding in DNA, which is evaluated by MTT assay and FASC experiment. Pyrrole substituted CuL^4 has higher efficacy for oxidative DNA damage and acts *via* antiproliferative action [29].

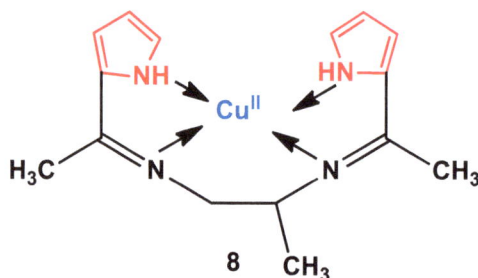

8

Fig. (8). Pyrrole based Cu (II) Schiff based complex.

QUINAZOLINE

Chemistry of Quinazoline

Quinazoline **9** (Fig. **9**) is a medicinally crucial nitrogen-containing heterocyclic. In 1895, Bischlerand Lang first synthesized quinazoline. It is a privileged scaffold for various anticancer drugs. This scaffold can act as a pharmacophore that has a broad spectrum of biological activity [30]. Substitution at the 2nd,3rd,6th positions of quinazoline is essential for anticancer activity. The heterocyclic group attached at the third position shows better inhibitory activity [31].

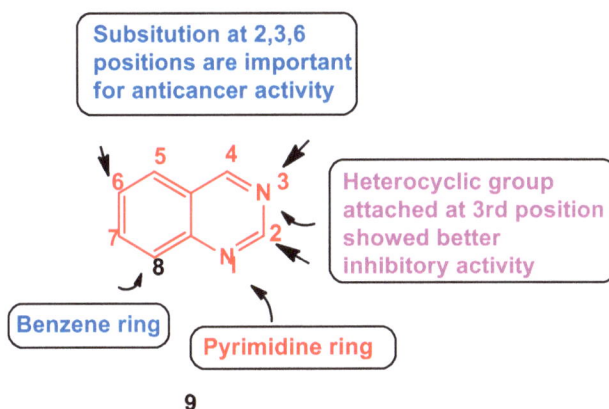

9

Fig. (9). Structure-activity relationship (SAR) quinazoline moiety.

Anticancer Activity of Quinazoline Derivatives

Epidermal growth factor receptor (EGFR) is a type of tyrosine kinase that was overexpressed in many carcinomas. Overactivation of EGFR has been a major cause of cell proliferation, cell growth, and tumor cell survival. The researchers were being adopted various approaches to inhibit the function of EGFR. Therefore, various EGFR inhibitors have been successfully developed and brought to the market [32]. Quinazoline is a potent EGFR inhibitor. FDA approved the various quinazoline moieties as EGFR inhibitors such as erlotinib for metastatic pancreatic cancer and gefitinib for lung cancer. According to the biological investigation of quinazoline, it showed that moiety was substituted with different groups must impart different pharmacological activities.

1st Generation Reversible EGFR Inhibitor

Firstly, reversible first-generation aminoquinazoline derivative **10** (Fig. **10**) was synthesized as EGFR inhibitor. Quinazoline-containing amino group at 4th position increases the binding affinity toward the tyrosine kinase receptor's hydrophobic pocket. SAR study shows that the aniline group attached at the 4th

position of quinazoline bind with a hydrophobic pocket. Replacement of amine at this position of quinazoline with methylene can lead to decrease inactivity. Substitution at phenyl ring with a bulkier and lipophilic group enhances the inhibitory activity. Methoxy group at 6th position increases the activity. Electron donating group at 7th position increases the antitumor activity. Substitution at the 8th position of quinazoline resulted in the loss of activity [33].

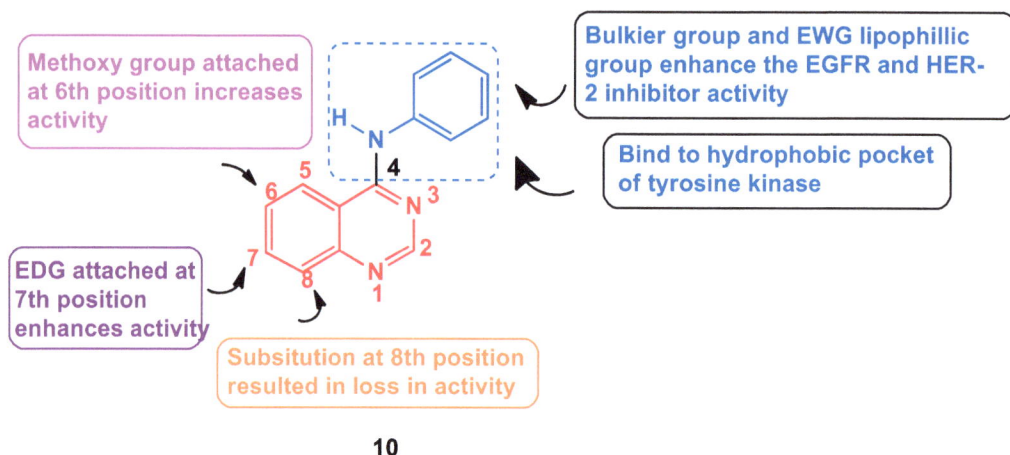

10

Fig. (10). Structure-activity relationship (SAR) quinazoline as 1st generation reversible EGFR inhibitor.

2nd Generation Irreversible EGFR Inhibitor

Further studies showed that first-generation drugs were being limited by some genetic mutation and showed resistance toward EGFR. These inhibitors thus decrease the sensitivity and efficacy of drugs [34]. Consequently, researchers developed irreversible 2nd generation inhibitors to overcome the EGFR mutation and drug resistance which was evaluated for antiproliferative activity. In a clinical trial, these 2nd generation inhibitors have appeared superior to 1st generation inhibitors.

Das *et al.* and his coworkers synthesized various compounds, which showed activity against various cancerous cell lines. It also acted as a dual inhibitor of FGFR and HER-2. This compound was evaluated against afatinib as a reference drug. Afatinib **11** (Fig. **11**) is 2nd generation irreversible inhibitor drug. It was approved by FDA in 2013 for NSCLC treatment. SAR study of compound **12** (Fig. **11**) reveals that **i)** aryl unit at position 4 of quinazoline showed better inhibitory activity for H1975 (IC_{50}=65.6 nM) **ii)** Micheal acceptor at position 6 showed activity against H1975 (IC_{50}=35.23 nM) **iii)** Size of alkoxy alkane at position 7 showed that longer chain above 7 C atom and branched-chain decreases the antitumor activity (IC_{50}=0.31 nM). Compound **13** (Fig. **11**) showed the most potent antiproliferative activity. The inhibitory activity of compound **13** (Fig. **11**) on HER2 was better than the reference drug afatinib. It displayed better bioavailability and pharmacokinetic properties in the human body [35].

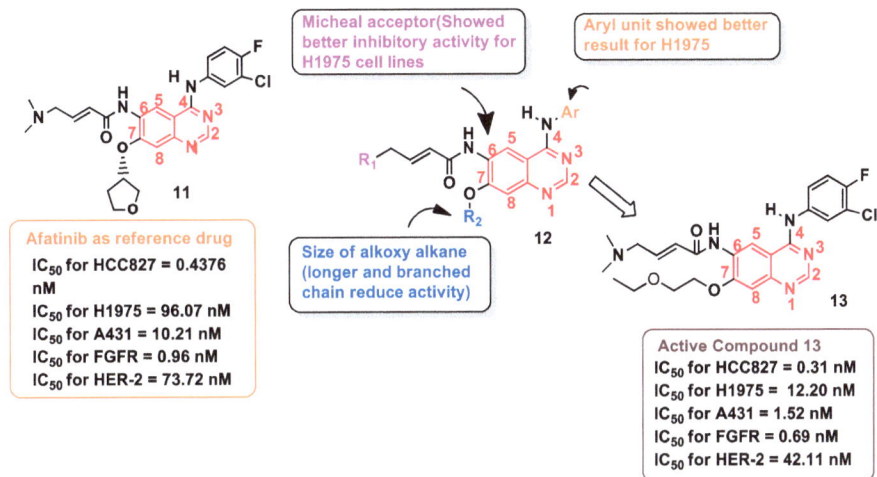

Fig. (11). Structure-activity relationship (SAR) of 2nd generation irreversible EGFR inhibitor.

Alkahtani *et al.* designed new potent EGFR inhibitors, which were evaluated against sorafenib as a reference drug. High potency and selectivity of these drugs were being carried out by MTT assay and various molecular docking examinations. Among all compound **14 (a-b)** (Fig. **12**) were found to be the most potent. SAR study of compound **14b** (Fig. **12**) revealed that acetamide derivative showed significant improvement in cytotoxic activity. The *N* site of the molecule interacts with the receptor *via H*-bonding [36].

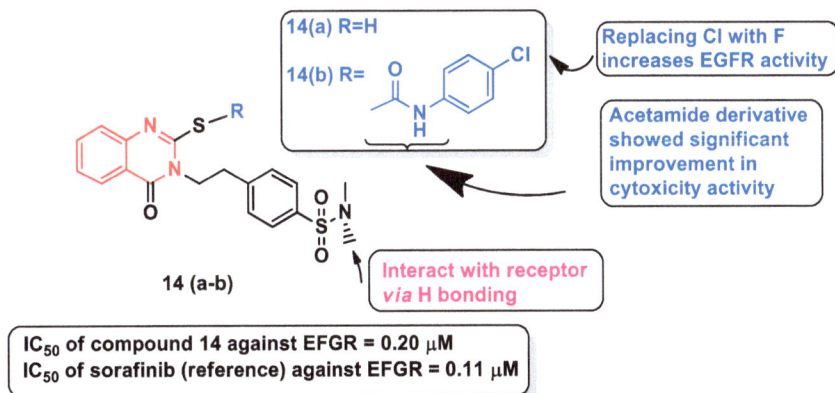

Fig. (12). Structure-activity relationship (SAR) of quinazoline as EGFR inhibitors.

Li *et al.* designed the most potent disubstituted quinazoline derivatives. This moiety has shown good antiproliferative activity against gefitinib as a reference drug. It causes the cell cycle arrest at G2 and thus induces apoptosis in the MCF-7 cancerous cell line (IC$_{50}$ = 5.10 µM). Attachment of EWG was more bioactive than EDG. This moiety constitutes *H*-bonding with Cys797. Molecular hybridization is the linkage criteria between the 4-trifluoromethylbenzyl and sulfhydryl group in moiety (Fig. **13**) [37].

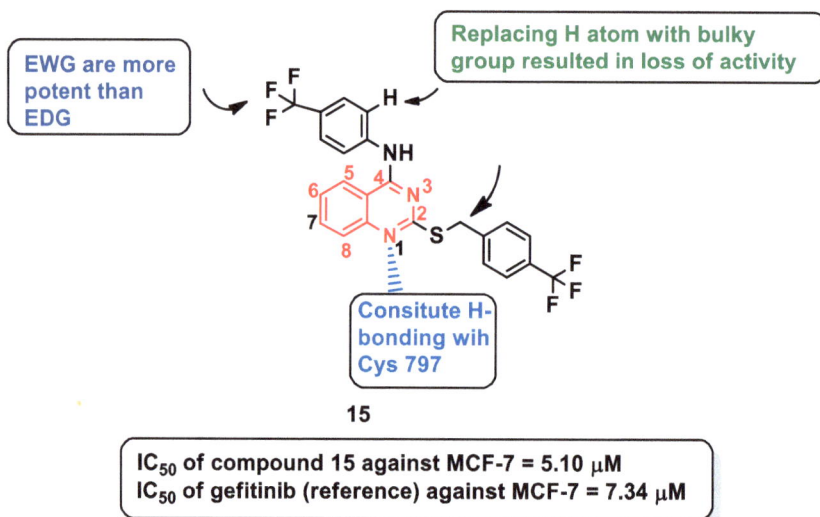

Fig. (13). Structure-activity relationship (SAR) of a disubstituted quinazoline derivative.

The class 1 family of phosphoinositide-3-kinase is the signal transduction pathway essential for various cellular functions like cell survival, cell proliferation, and differentiation. Thus, P13k is the key regulatory role in the production of cancer in the human body. Copanlibsib and duvelisib have been approved as P13k inhibitors for blood cancer [38]. Likewise, HDAC is the critical regulator of gene expression. Histone deacetylases are a class of epigenetic enzymes that are responsible for transcriptional activity. FDA-approved HDAC inhibitors like vorinostat, romidepsin for the treatment of hemoglobin cancer [39]. Co-administration of two or more drugs at the same time causes drug-drug interaction and undesirable pharmacokinetic actions. Due to this limitation, researchers designed new types of drugs that can target multiple mechanisms with a single molecule [40]. However, recent studies revealed a combination of P13k and HDAC to show synergistic anticancer activity. SAR study showed that quinazoline moiety exhibits PI3k inhibitor activity. It acts as a surface recognition domain or capping region. HDAC functionality shown by linker attached with quinazoline ring. It was shown that the 6 C atom chain is responsible for the optimal activity for HCT116 cell lines (IC_{50} = 0.007 μM). Substituting the 6-carbon chain with amino-2-pyrimidinyl moiety increases the antiproliferative activity for HCT116 cell lines (IC_{50} = 0.007 μM) (Fig. **14**) [41].

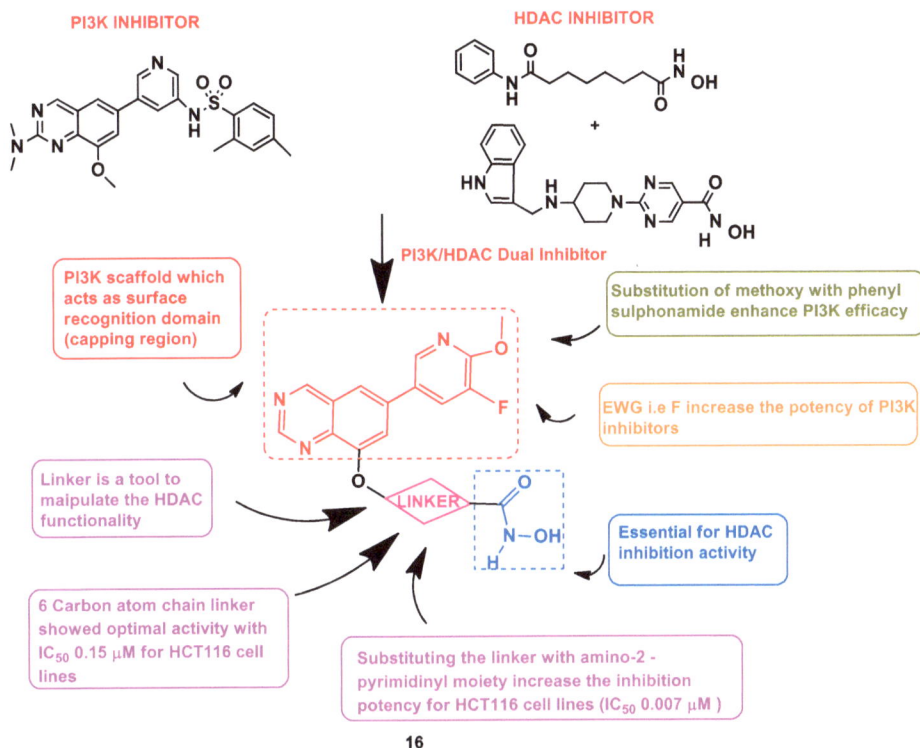

Fig. (14). Structure-activity relationship (SAR) of quinazoline analog as a dual inhibitor of P13k and HDAC.

THIADIAZOLE

Chemistry of Thiadiazole

Thiadiazole 17 (Fig. **15**) is an active scaffold for various pharmacological activities. It is a five-membered heterocyclic ring that contained two nitrogen and one sulfur atom. Thiadiazole has various isomers like 1,3,4 thiadiazole; 1,2,3 thiadiazole; 1,2,4 thiadiazole; 1,2,5 thiadiazole. Among all isomers, the 1,3,4 thiadiazole is the most reactive isomer for a cytotoxic property. The reactivity of the *N* atom depends on the electrophilic reaction and tautomeric equilibrium. Nucleophilic attacks on C atoms at positions 2 and 5 occur readily due to the electron-deficient nature of the ring. *N* is favorable for the anticancer activity due to the electron-donating nature of *N* and forms *H*-bonding with specific receptors [42].

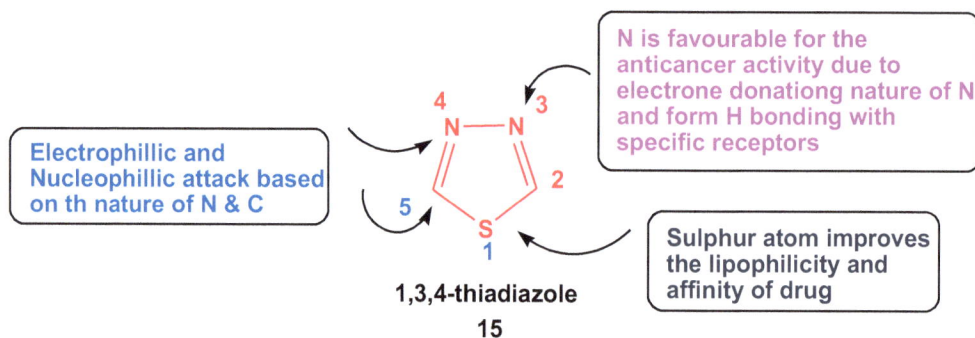

Fig. (15). Structure-activity relationship (SAR) of thiadiazole.

Anticancer Activity of Thiadiazole Derivatives

Bcr-Abl is the activated gene of tyrosine kinase that causes chronic myeloid leukemia (CML). It is a type of blood cancer that begins in bone marrow caused by a chromosomal mutation in the human body [43]. Imatinib is a small molecule kinase inhibitor that acts on a Bcr-Abl tyrosine kinase receptor and is used against CML. Imatinib is the first approved tyrosine kinase inhibitor (Fig. **16**). Further study revealed that imatinib showed resistance as a Bcr-Abl inhibitor. The resistance occurs through point mutation, which interferes with drug binding [44].

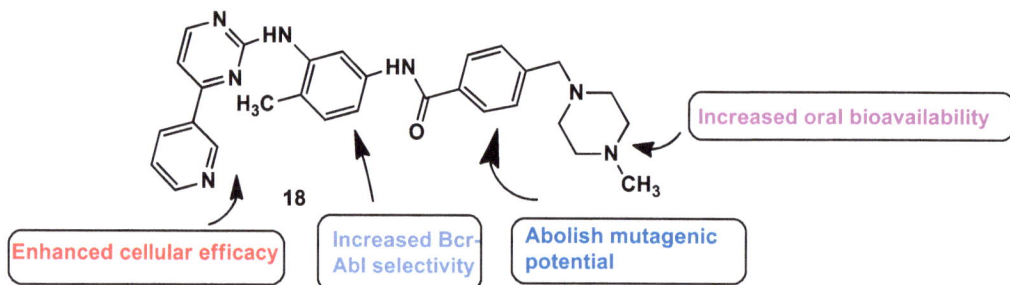

Fig. (16). Structure-activity relationship (SAR) of imatinib (reference drug).

Recently, researchers explored 1, 3, and 4-thiadiazole as a potent scaffold for tyrosine kinase inhibitory activity by taking imatinib as a reference drug. They explored that introduction of hydrophobic and *H*-bonding in the 1, 3, 4-thiadiazole nucleus generates a promising scaffold with Bcr-Abl inhibitory activity. Given that, they introduced a 4-(trifluoromethyl)-phenylamino group as a hydrophobic moiety and *N*-(thiazol-2-yl)-2-mercaptoacetanilide as an *H*-bonding moiety in 1,3,4- thiadiazole ring. Compound **19** (Fig. **17**) was the most active drug molecule that potently inhibited the Bcr-Abl kinase activity (IC_{50}=0.2 μM). It also causes apoptosis in Hela cell lines (IC_{50}=12.4 μM). SAR study showed that the nitro group is crucial for Bcr-Abl kinase inhibitory activity due to its *H*-bonding with a receptor site. The absence of the nitro group abolishes the activity. EWG group attached at hydrophobic substituent site increases the antiproliferative activity. The polar thiazole group has lower potency than the pyrimidine group of imatinib. The sulfur atom in the thiadiazole ring improves the lipophilic character and increases the affinity and bioavailability of drug molecules [45].

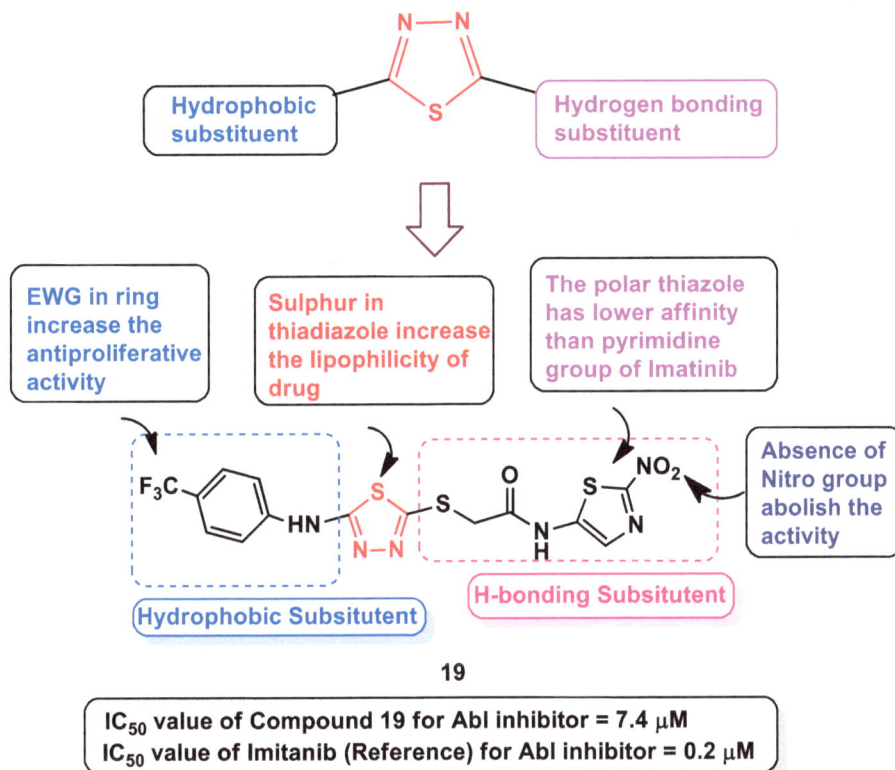

Fig. (17). Structure-activity relationship (SAR) of thiadiazole as Bcr-Abl tyrosine kinase receptor inhibitor.

The 1,3,4-thiadiazole has been fused with many other heterocyclic moieties like thiophene and imidazole to increase the cytotoxic potential of the drug molecules. The hybrid molecules have a synergistic effect on drug molecules because they can act on more than one target. These hybrid molecules are also used to overcome the pharmacokinetic drawbacks conventional drug molecules face [46]. Thiophene has been exhibiting cytotoxic properties for various types of cancers like ovarian cancer, lung cancer, liver cancer, pancreatic cancer, *etc.* Thiadiazole also inhibits the DNA and RNA synthesis, therefore used as a potential anticancer drug target. The wide range of importance of both of these scaffolds could be used for the synthesis of many drug molecules which act as antitumor agents. Encouraged by these facts, researchers and scientists designed *N*-thiophene-

2-carbohydrazonoyl chloride derivative for the synthesis of 1, 3, 4-thiadiazole incorporating thiophene ring as a versatile tool against A-549 and HepG-2 cancerous cell lines. The potential compound **20** (Fig. **18**) was investigated against two cancer cell lines. Human hepatocellular carcinoma HepG-2 (IC$_{50}$ 8.30 µM) and human lung cancer A-549 (IC$_{50}$=1.40 µM) cell lines by using cisplatin as a reference drug. The methoxy group increases the antitumor activity. Substituting the methoxy group with the chloro group decreases the activity [47].

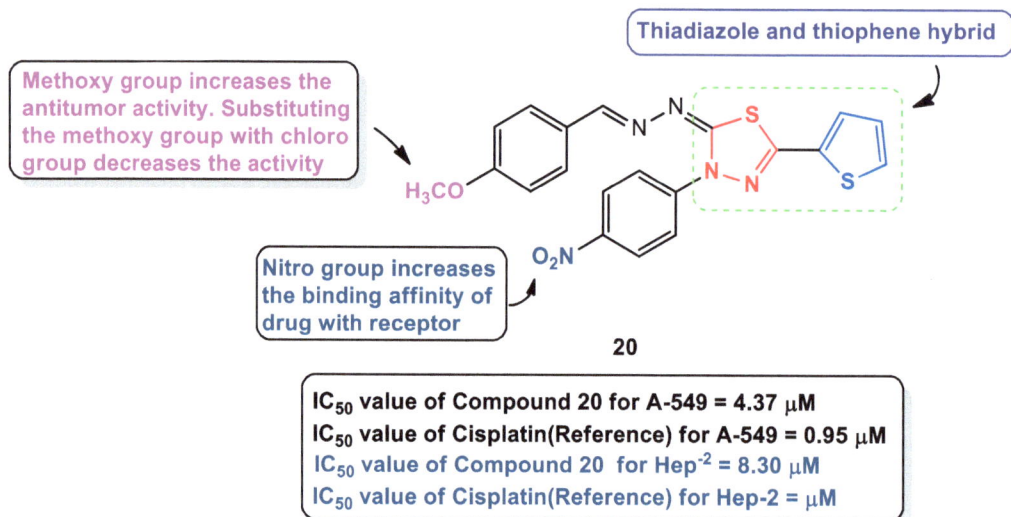

Fig. (18). Structure-activity relationship (SAR) of thiadiazole and thiophene hybrid moiety.

Dihydrofolate reductase is an enzyme known for its key role in DNA and RNA synthesis. DHFR inhibitors are an important class of drugs mainly used as anticancer agents. Its biological mechanism depends on the enzyme selectivity and antiproliferative property [48]. The 1,3,4-thiadiazole has a broad biological activity due to the presence of nitrogen, carbon, and sulfur in the moiety. Compounds **21a-c** (Fig. **19**) were found to be prominent DHFR inhibitors that are used against the prostate cancer (PC-3) cell lines. It was evaluated against doxorubicin as a reference drug. SAR study showed that in **21a** (Fig. **19**) 2-thioxopyrimidine-4,6-dione having benzylidene group have highest cytotoxic activity (IC$_{50}$=4.67 µM). In **21b** (Fig. **19**), the substitution of benzylidene with 2-phenyl hydrazone decreases the activity (IC$_{50}$=6.99 µM). Addition of a new 1,3,4-thiadiazole ring which was substituted with thio-1-phenylethan-1-one group *via* amine linker in **21c** (Fig. **19**) increases the potency of the drug but less than **21a** **(Fig. 19)** (IC$_{50}$=9.66 µM) [49].

21a   R ⟹

2-thioxopyrimidine-4,6-dione having benzylidene group have highest cytotoxic activity.
IC_{50} of doxorubicin (Refernce) against PC-3 = 4.56 μM
IC_{50} of compound 21(a) against PC-3 = 4.67 μM

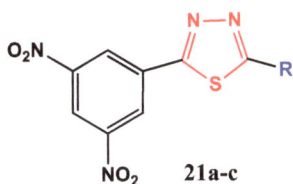

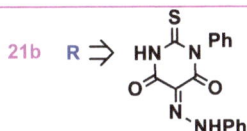

Backbone of DHFR INHIBITOR & has higher anticancer potency

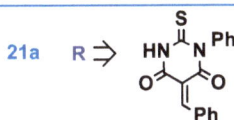

21b   R ⟹

Substitution of benzylidene with 2-phenyl hydrazone must decrease the activity
IC_{50} of doxorubicin (Refernce) against PC-3 = 4.56 μM
IC_{50} of compound 21(b) against PC-3 = 6.99 μM

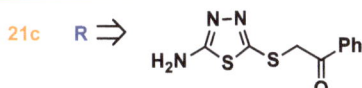

21c   R ⟹

Addition of new 1,3,4- thiadiazole ring which was substituted with thio-1-phenylethan-1-one group via amine linker should increse the potency of drug
IC_{50} of doxorubicin (Refernce) against PC-3 = 4.56 μM
IC_{50} of compound 21(c) against PC-3 = 9.96 μM

Fig. (19). Structure-activity relationship (SAR) of thiadiazole as dihydrofolate reductase inhibitor.

Pancreatic ductal adenocarcinoma (PDAC) is a chronic neoplasm commonly referred to as pancreatic cancer. It causes an increasing mortality rate in both men and women. The increasing death rate is due to a lack of effective treatment against its metastatic behavior [50]. Gemcitabine is a deoxycytidine nucleotide analog that inhibits DNA synthesis and acts as an antiproliferative agent. Gemcitabine monotherapy is the first-line treatment of PDAC, but it can cause resistance to drug therapy [51]. The imidazole and thiadiazole hybrid nucleus has been considered a privileged scaffold for the development of new anticancer drugs. The new imidazothiadiazole derivative **22** (Fig. **20**) was synthesized and used against the PDAC cell lines. SAR study revealed that the thiophene ring is essential for PDAC inhibitors. EWG increases antiproliferative activity. Substituting the F with H atom decreases the activity. The methyl group is essential for antiproliferative activity [52].

QUINOLINE

Chemistry of Quinoline

Quinoline is a heterocyclic aromatic compound having the molecular formula C_9H_7N. In the structure of quinoline, benzene is fused with a pyridine nucleus.

Quinoline is an active pharmacological scaffold for the preparation of many drug molecules like an anticancer agent, antimalarial agent, and antituberculosis agent [53]. Quinoline moiety has been used in various anticancer drugs as an active pharmacophore because of the cytotoxic nature of moiety (Fig. **21**). SAR study showed that substitution of R_1 with heterocyclic moiety often gives better cytotoxic activity. Substitution of R_2 with hydrazone and other groups showed optimum activity. R_3 substituted with a linker, amide and methyl groups give good antitumor activity. Unsubstituted R_4 and R_5 enhance anticancer activity. R_6 substituted with halogen gives potent activity. Unsubstituted R_7 gives good anticancer activity. The presence of the *N* atom increases the basic character facilitating *H*-bonding with target enzymes and thus increasing the water solubility for oral absorption of drug design [54].

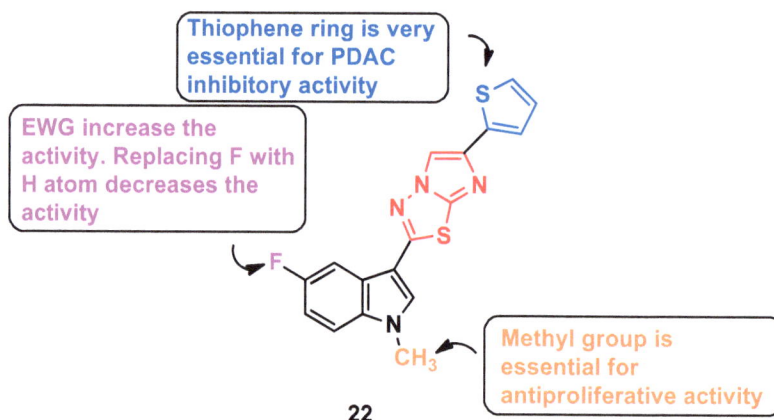

Fig. (20). Structure-activity relationship (SAR) of thiadiazole and imidazole hybrid moiety.

Anticancer Activity of Quinoline Derivatives

Quinoline is the essential moiety among the *N*-based heterocyclic compound for anticancer activity. Quinoline hybridized with chalcone increases the effectiveness by the synergistic effect of the drug. Chalcones are the privileged natural compound acting as cytotoxic agents by inhibiting various cancerous cells by different mechanisms. They act as Micheal acceptors to bind with respective targets and give biological activities [55]. Researchers synthesized a set of quinolone-chalcone compounds, among which hybrid **24** (Fig. **22**) was found to be most potent. It was tested as a potent inhibitor (IC_{50}=1.91 µM) of K549 cancerous cell lines and PI3K gamma isoform (IC_{50} 52.03 nM) by taking cisplatin (IC_{50}=2.71 µM) as a reference drug. SAR study revealed that replacing the hydrogen with a methoxy group at the 4th position of quinoline decreases the activity. Unsubstituted phenyl ring, which was attached with quinoline moiety, decreases the activity. Methoxy group at 4th position of phenyl ring enhances the cytotoxic activity against K562 cancer cell lines. Substitution at the 2nd position of quinoline gives optimal activity [56].

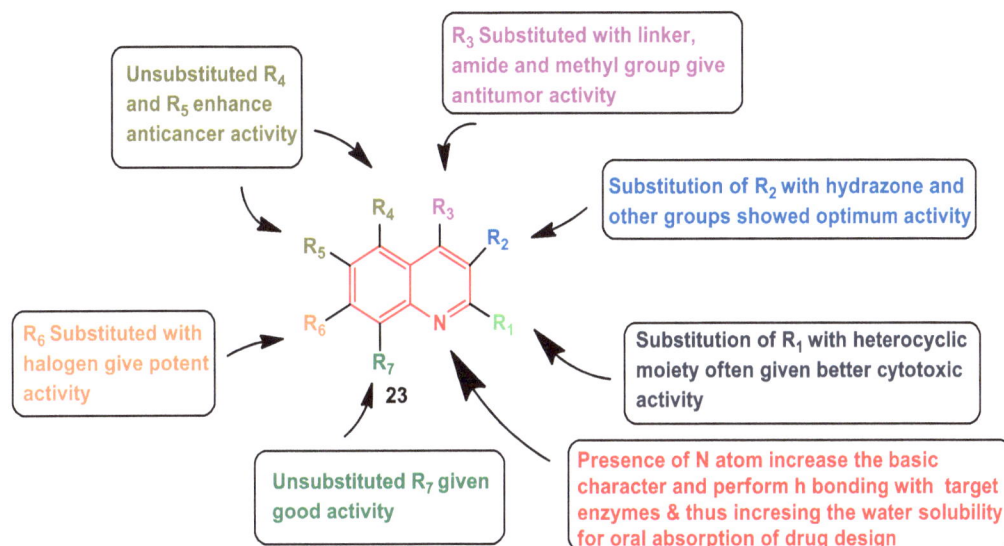

Fig. (21). Structure-activity relationship (SAR) of quinoline ring for anticancer activity.

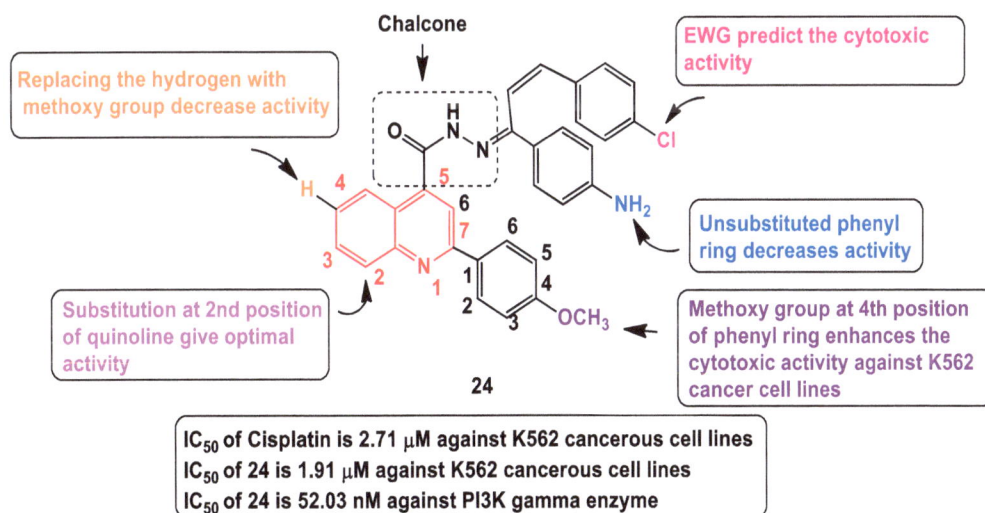

Fig. (22). Structure-activity relationship (SAR) of quinoline-chalcone hybrid structure.

Quinoline-chalcone hybrid derivatives also acted as tubulin polymerization inhibitors. Li *et al*., synthesized several compounds containing quinoline-chalcone hybrid moiety, which showed cytotoxic activities. Compound **25** (Fig. **23**)

(IC$_{50}$=0.009 μM) was found to be more potent than CA-4 as a standard drug (IC$_{50}$=0.012 μM). It binds with the colchicine site of tubulin and showed the potent inhibitor of tubulin polymerization. The Compound **25** (Fig. **23**) improved the safety profile of the drug by i.v injection. According to the SAR study, the *N* atom of the quinoline ring is essential for activity. Steric hindrance showed a critical effect on antiproliferative activity. Substitution with methyl group *i.e.*, the smaller group at position 2nd of quinoline ring was more active than the larger group [57].

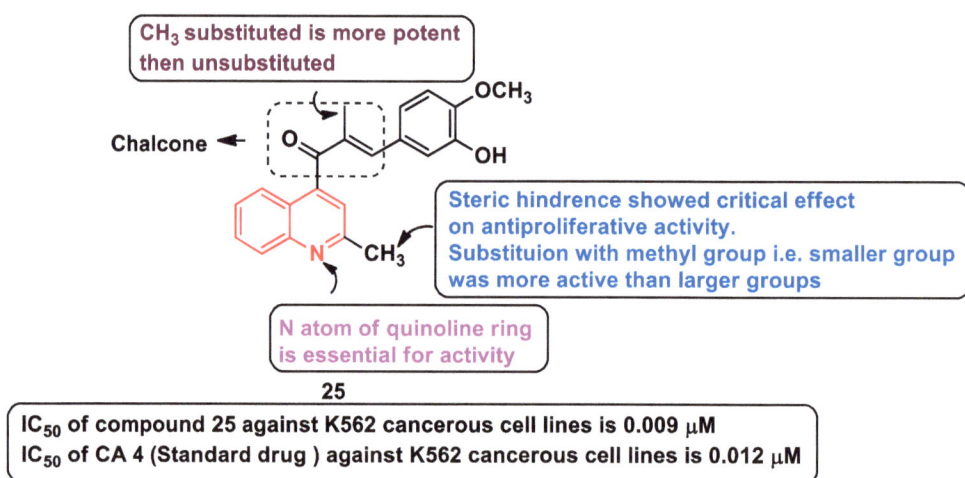

Fig. (23). Structure-activity relationship (SAR) of quinoline-chalcone hybrid structure.

Othman *et al.* synthesized and evaluated a new hybrid compound by combining quinoline with thiophene moiety. Both moieties show cytotoxic properties by inhibiting the various cancerous cell lines like MCF-7, Hep G2, and HCT-116. The compound **26** (Fig. **24**) was the most potent against MCF-7 cell lines (IC$_{50}$=28.36 μM) evaluated by MTT assay. This compound also acted as an inhibitor of EGFR and the Topo II enzyme. SAR study showed that halogen's presence at the 4th position of the phenyl ring enhances the cytotoxic activity. Benzoxy group act as the lipophilic moiety, which had more cytotoxic activity than isoxazolyl and triazolyl ring [58].

Triazole is the most active pharmacophore in oncology drug discovery. It was hybridized with quinoline moiety to show anticancer activities. Mohassab *et al.* synthesized several anticancer drugs containing quinoline and triazole hybrid. They acted on various cancerous cell lines and inhibited growth by blocking different receptors. Mainly these categories of drugs were EGFR inhibitors. Compound **27** (Fig. **25**) (IC$_{50}$=2.1 μM) which was evaluated against erlotinib (IC$_{50}$ 0.08 μM) as a reference drug was the most potent among them. According to the

SAR study, the chloro group imparts better antiproliferative activity than the trimethoxy group. Replacement of allyl group with phenyl group leads to 2.5-fold reduction in activity. Hydrogen group showed potent inhibiting activity H > Cl > OCH₃ [59].

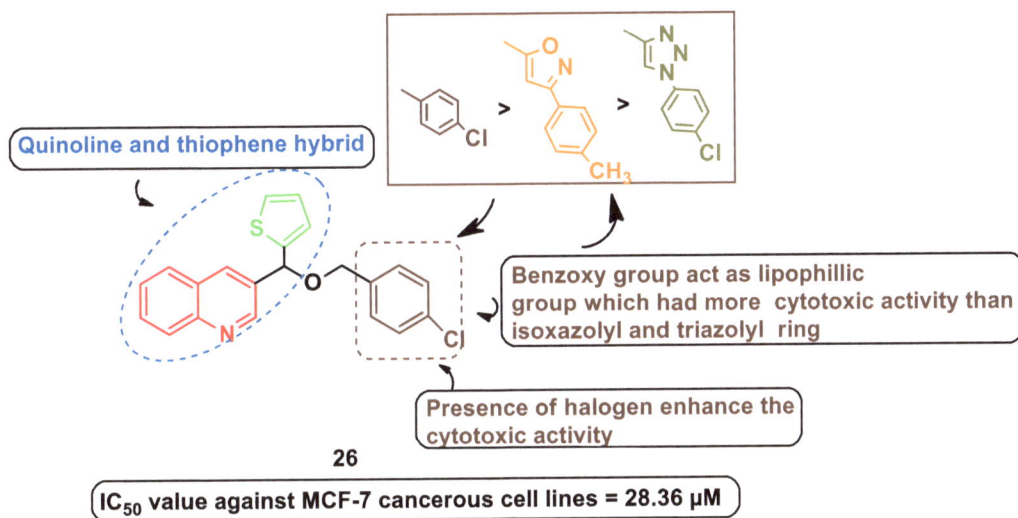

Fig. (24). Structure-activity relationship (SAR) of the quinoline-thiophene hybrid molecule.

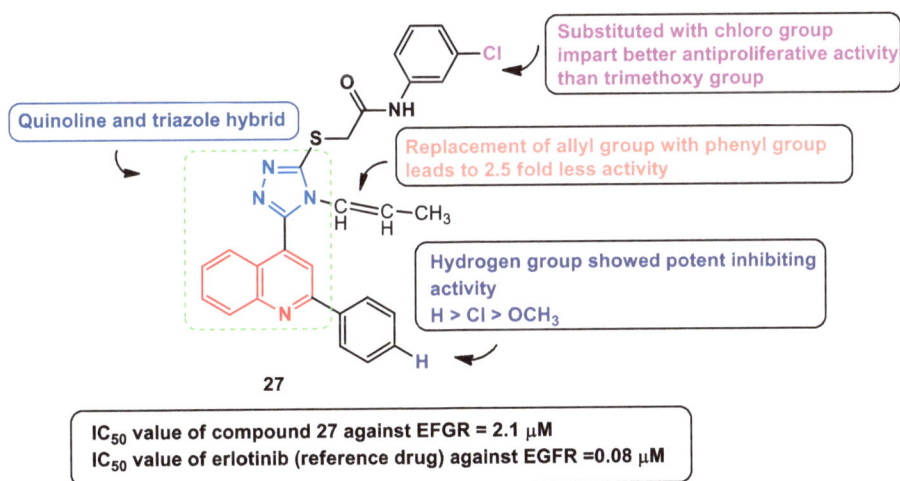

Fig. (25). Structure-activity relationship (SAR) of quinoline and triazole hybrid structure.

CONCLUSION

Cancer is becoming a life-threatening disease nowadays. It is necessary to explore the medication and drug delivery to treat cancer patients. Heterocyclic compounds are the essential key component in the majority of anticancer drugs. Despite heterocycles' pivotal role in rational drug design, new molecular drugs must demonstrate not only their ability to reach the target site of action, but also their therapeutic efficacy. Due to their vast pharmacological properties, researchers are giving continuous momentum for discoveries of heterocyclic drugs in the oncology field. The chapter discusses the last five years' studies on *N* and *S*-heterocyclic compounds and their chemistry, SAR study, and anticancer mechanism. Hybridization of *N* and *S*-heterocyclic rings with other potent pharmacophore has also been reported showing an increase in activity and fewer side effects. On one hand, the high polarity of the *N* atom in heterocyclic rings raises the bioavailability of drug molecules and on the other hand, the sulfur atom is more reactive and easily form interactions with the target receptors. Hence these *N* and *S*-based heterocyclic compounds have a great role in anticancer drug discovery. Chemical study of pyrrole, quinazoline, thiadiazole, and quinoline shows that these are active moieties in chemical compounds. Despite the significant progress made in cancer therapy through the use of heterocyclic chemistry, many of the currently used chemotherapeutic drugs face numerous challenges in terms of pharmacokinetic/pharmacodynamic properties and off-target effects, opening new avenues for improvement through research.

CONSENT FOR PUBLICATION

Not applicable.

CONFLICT OF INTEREST

The author declares no conflict of interest, financial, or otherwise.

ACKNOWLEDGEMENT

The author wishes to acknowledge the Management, Shivalik College of Pharmacy, Nangal for the constant encouragement and support.

REFERENCES

[1]   Singh, R.K.; Kumar, S.; Prasad, D.N.; Bhardwaj, T.R. Therapeutic journey of nitrogen mustard as alkylating anticancer agents: Historic to future perspectives. *Eur. J. Med. Chem.,* **2018**, *151*, 401-433.
       [http://dx.doi.org/10.1016/j.ejmech.2018.04.001] [PMID: 29649739]

[2]   Park, R.; Lee, S.A.; Kim, S.Y.; de Melo, A.C.; Kasi, A. Association of active oncologic treatment and risk of death in cancer patients with COVID-19: A systematic review and meta-analysis of patient data. *Acta Oncol.,* **2021**, *60*(1), 13-19.
       [http://dx.doi.org/10.1080/0284186X.2020.1837946] [PMID: 33131376]

[3]   Giannakoulis, V.G.; Papoutsi, E.; Siempos, I.I. Effect of cancer on clinical outcomes of patients with covid-19: A meta-analysis of patient data. *JCO Glob. Oncol.,* **2020**, *6*(6), 799-808.
       [http://dx.doi.org/10.1200/GO.20.00225] [PMID: 32511066]

[4] Kumar, S.; Singh, R.K.; Patial, B.; Goyal, S.; Bhardwaj, T.R. Recent advances in novel heterocyclic scaffolds for the treatment of drug-resistant malaria. *J. Enzyme Inhib. Med. Chem.*, **2016**, *31*(2), 173-186.
[http://dx.doi.org/10.3109/14756366.2015.1016513] [PMID: 25775094]

[5] Kumari, A.; Singh, R.K. Medicinal chemistry of indole derivatives: Current to future therapeutic prospectives. *Bioorg. Chem.*, **2019**, *89*, 103021.
[http://dx.doi.org/10.1016/j.bioorg.2019.103021] [PMID: 31176854]

[6] Kumari, A.; Singh, R.K. Morpholine as ubiquitous pharmacophore in medicinal chemistry: Deep insight into the structure-activity relationship (SAR). *Bioorg. Chem.*, **2020**, *96*, 103578.
[http://dx.doi.org/10.1016/j.bioorg.2020.103578] [PMID: 31978684]

[7] Sethi, N.S.; Prasad, D.N.; Singh, R.K. An insight into the synthesis and sar of 2,4-thiazolidinediones (2,4-TZD) as multifunctional scaffold: A review. *Mini Rev. Med. Chem.*, **2020**, *20*(4), 308-330.
[http://dx.doi.org/10.2174/1389557519666191029102838] [PMID: 31660809]

[8] Sethi, N.S.; Prasad, D.N.; Singh, R.K. Synthesis, anticancer and antibacterial studies of benzylidene bearing 5-substituted and 3,5-disubstituted-2,4-thiazolidinedione derivatives. *Med. Chem.*, **2020**.
[http://dx.doi.org/10.2174/1573406416666200512073640] [PMID: 32394843]

[9] Kerru, N.; Gummidi, L.; Maddila, S.; Gangu, K.K.; Jonnalagadda, S.B. A review on recent advances in nitrogen-containing molecules and their biological applications. *Molecules*, **2020**, *25*(8), 1909.
[http://dx.doi.org/10.3390/molecules25081909] [PMID: 32326131]

[10] Singh, R.K.; Prasad, D.N.; Bhardwaj, T.R. Hybrid pharmacophore-based drug design, synthesis and antiproliferative activity of 1,4-dihydropyridines linked alkylating anticancer agents. *Med. Chem. Res.*, **2015**, *24*(4), 1534-1541.
[http://dx.doi.org/10.1007/s00044-014-1236-1]

[11] Singh, R.K.; Prasad, D.N.; Bhardwaj, T.R. Design, synthesis and antiproliferative activity of benzodiazepine-mustard conjugates as potential brain antitumour agents. *J. Saudi Chem. Soc.*, **2017**, *14*(S1), S86-S93.
[http://dx.doi.org/10.1016/j.jscs.2013.10.004]

[12] Martins, P; Jesus, J; Santos, S Heterocyclic anticancer compounds: Recent advances and the paradigm shift towards the use of nanomedicine's tool box. *Molecules*, **2015**, *20*, 16852-16891.
[http://dx.doi.org/10.3390/molecules200916852]

[13] Vitaku, E.; Smith, D.T.; Njardarson, J.T. Analysis of the structural diversity, substitution patterns, and frequency of nitrogen heterocycles among U.S. FDA approved pharmaceuticals. *J. Med. Chem.*, **2014**, *57*(24), 10257-10274.
[http://dx.doi.org/10.1021/jm501100b] [PMID: 25255204]

[14] Pathania, S.; Narang, R. K.; Rawal, R. K. Role of sulfur-heterocycles in medicinal chemistry: An update. *Eur. J. Med. Chem.*, **2019**, *180*, 486-508.
[http://dx.doi.org/10.1016/j.ejmech.2019.07.043]

[15] Sharma, P.C.; Bansal, K.K.; Sharma, A.; Sharma, D.; Deep, A. Thiazole-containing compounds as therapeutic targets for cancer therapy. *Eur. J. Med. Chem.*, **2020**, *188*, 112016.
[http://dx.doi.org/10.1016/j.ejmech.2019.112016] [PMID: 31926469]

[16] Maeda, H. Supramolecular chemistry of pyrrole-based π conjugated molecules. *Bull. Chem. Soc. Jpn.*, **2013**, *86*(12), 1359-1399.
[http://dx.doi.org/10.1246/bcsj.20130219]

[17] Tron, G.C.; Pirali, T.; Sorba, G.; Pagliai, F.; Busacca, S.; Genazzani, A.A. Medicinal chemistry of combretastatin A4: Present and future directions. *J. Med. Chem.*, **2006**, *49*(11), 3033-3044.
[http://dx.doi.org/10.1021/jm0512903] [PMID: 16722619]

[18] Jung, E.K.; Leung, E.; Barker, D. Synthesis and biological activity of pyrrole analogues of combretastatin A-4. *Bioorg. Med. Chem. Lett.*, **2016**, *26*(13), 3001-3005.

[http://dx.doi.org/10.1016/j.bmcl.2016.05.026] [PMID: 27212068]

[19]　Guengerich, F.P. Cytochrome p450 and chemical toxicology. *Chem. Res. Toxicol.,* **2008**, *21*(1), 70-83.
[http://dx.doi.org/10.1021/tx700079z] [PMID: 18052394]

[20]　Williams, I.S.; Joshi, P.; Gatchie, L.; Sharma, M.; Satti, N.K.; Vishwakarma, R.A.; Chaudhuri, B.;
Bharate, S.B. Synthesis and biological evaluation of pyrrole-based chalcones as CYP1 enzyme
inhibitors, for possible prevention of cancer and overcoming cisplatin resistance. *Bioorg. Med. Chem.
Lett.,* **2017**, *27*(16), 3683-3687.
[http://dx.doi.org/10.1016/j.bmcl.2017.07.010] [PMID: 28711350]

[21]　Tiong, K.H.; Mah, L.Y.; Leong, C.O. Functional roles of fibroblast growth factor receptors (FGFRs)
signaling in human cancers. *Apoptosis,* **2013**, *18*(12), 1447-1468.
[http://dx.doi.org/10.1007/s10495-013-0886-7] [PMID: 23900974]

[22]　Bavadi, M.; Niknam, K.; Shahraki, O. Novel pyrrole derivatives bearing sulfonamide groups:
Synthesis *in vitro* cytotoxicity evaluation, molecular docking and DFT study. *J. Mol. Struct.,* **2017**,
1146, 242-253.
[http://dx.doi.org/10.1016/j.molstruc.2017.06.003]

[23]　Bhatia, R.; Singh, R.K. Introductory Chapter: Protein kinases as promising targets for drug design
against cancer. In: *Protein Kinases - Promising Targets for Anticancer Drug Research*; Singh, R.K.,
Ed.; IntechOpen: London, **2021**.
[http://dx.doi.org/10.5772/intechopen.100315]

[24]　Zhang, J.; Yang, P.L.; Gray, N.S. Targeting cancer with small molecule kinase inhibitors. *Nat. Rev.
Cancer,* **2009**, *9*(1), 28-39.
[http://dx.doi.org/10.1038/nrc2559] [PMID: 19104514]

[25]　Lee, A-R.; Hsu, R-J.; Huang, W-H.; Lee, A-R. Pyrrole indolin-2-One Based Kinase Inhibitor as Anti-
Cancer Agents. *J. Cancer Treatment Diagn.,* **2018**, *2*(5), 24-29.
[http://dx.doi.org/10.29245/2578-2967/2018/5.1153]

[26]　Thiriveedhi, A.; Nadh, R.V.; Srinivasu, N.; Bobde, Y.; Ghosh, B.; Sekhar, K.V.G.C. Design, synthesis
and anti-tumour activity of new pyrimidine-pyrrole appended triazoles. *Toxicol. In Vitro,* **2019**, *60*,
87-96.
[http://dx.doi.org/10.1016/j.tiv.2019.05.009] [PMID: 31100376]

[27]　Peng, S.; He, Q.; Vargas-Zúñiga, G.I.; Qin, L.; Hwang, I.; Kim, S.K.; Heo, N.J.; Lee, C.H.; Dutta, R.;
Sessler, J.L. Strapped calix[4]pyrroles: From syntheses to applications. *Chem. Soc. Rev.,* **2020**, *49*(3),
865-907.
[http://dx.doi.org/10.1039/C9CS00528E] [PMID: 31957756]

[28]　Kohnke, F.H. Calixpyrroles: From Anion Ligands to Potential Anticancer Drugs. *Eur. J. Org. Chem.,*
2020, *2020*(28), 4261-4272.
[http://dx.doi.org/10.1002/ejoc.202000208]

[29]　Koley Seth, B; Saha, A; Haldar, S; Chakraborty, PP; Saha, P; Basu, S Structure dependent selective
efficacy of pyridine and pyrrole-based Cu(II) Schiff base complexes towards *in vitro* cytotoxicity,
apoptosis and DNA-bases binding in the ground and excited state. *J. Photochem. Photobiol. B.,* **2016**,
162, 463-472.
[http://dx.doi.org/10.1016/j.jphotobiol.2016.07.012]

[30]　Hameed, A.; Al-Rashida, M.; Uroos, M.; Ali, S.A.; Arshia, M.I.; Ishtiaq, M.; Khan, K.M. Quinazoline
and quinazolinone as important medicinal scaffolds: A comparative patent review (2011–2016).
Expert Opin. Ther. Pat., **2018**, *28*(4), 281-297.
[http://dx.doi.org/10.1080/13543776.2018.1432596] [PMID: 29368977]

[31]　Shagufta, S.; Ahmad, I. An insight into the therapeutic potential of quinazoline derivatives as
anticancer agents. *MedChemComm,* **2017**, *8*(5), 871-885.
[http://dx.doi.org/10.1039/C7MD00097A] [PMID: 30108803]

[32] Woodburn, J.R. *The Epidermal Growth Factor Receptor and Its Inhibition in Cancer Therapy*; ZENECA PHARMACEUTICALS, **1999**, pp. 241-250.
[http://dx.doi.org/10.1016/S0163-7258(98)00045-X]

[33] Ismail Rania, S.M.; Ismail Nasser, S.M. Recent advances in 4-aminoquinazoline based scaffold derivatives targeting EGFR kinases as anticancer agents. *Future J. Pharm. Sci.,* **2016**, *2*(1)
[http://dx.doi.org/10.1016/j.fjps.2016.02.001]

[34] Juchum, M.; Günther, M.; Laufer, S.A. Fighting cancer drug resistance: Opportunities and challenges for mutation-specific EGFR inhibitors. *Drug Resist. Updat.,* **2015**, *20*, 12-28.
[http://dx.doi.org/10.1016/j.drup.2015.05.002] [PMID: 26021435]

[35] Das, D.; Xie, L.; Wang, J.; Xu, X.; Zhang, Z.; Shi, J.; Le, X.; Hong, J. Discovery of new quinazoline derivatives as irreversible dual EGFR/HER2 inhibitors and their anticancer activities – Part 1. *Bioorg. Med. Chem. Lett.,* **2019**, *29*(4), 591-596.
[http://dx.doi.org/10.1016/j.bmcl.2018.12.056] [PMID: 30600209]

[36] Alkahtani, HM; Abdalla, AN; Obaidullah, AJ; Alanazi, MM; Almehizia, AA; Alanazi, MG; Ahmed, AY; Alwassil, OI; Darwish, HW; Abdel-Aziz, AA; El-Azab, AS Synthesis, cytotoxic evaluation, and molecular docking studies of novel quinazoline derivatives with benzenesulfonamide and anilide tails: Dual inhibitors of EGFR/HER2. *Bioorg Chem*, **2020**, 103461.
[http://dx.doi.org/10.1016/j.bioorg.2019.103461]

[37] Li, E.; Lin, Q.; Meng, Y.; Zhang, L.; Song, P.; Li, N.; Xin, J.; Yang, P.; Bao, C.; Zhang, D.; Zhang, Y.; Wang, J.; Zhang, Q.; Liu, H. 2,4-Disubstituted quinazolines targeting breast cancer cells *via* EGFR-PI3K. *Eur. J. Med. Chem.,* **2019**, *172*, 36-47.
[http://dx.doi.org/10.1016/j.ejmech.2019.03.030] [PMID: 30939352]

[38] Liu, P.; Cheng, H.; Roberts, T.M.; Zhao, J.J. Targeting the phosphoinositide 3-kinase pathway in cancer. *Nat. Rev. Drug Discov.,* **2009**, *8*(8), 627-644.
[http://dx.doi.org/10.1038/nrd2926] [PMID: 19644473]

[39] West, A.C.; Johnstone, R.W. New and emerging HDAC inhibitors for cancer treatment. *J. Clin. Invest.,* **2014**, *124*(1), 30-39.
[http://dx.doi.org/10.1172/JCI69738] [PMID: 24382387]

[40] Proschak, E.; Stark, H.; Merk, D. Polypharmacology by design: A medicinal chemist's perspective on multitargeting compounds. *J. Med. Chem.,* **2019**, *62*(2), 420-444.
[http://dx.doi.org/10.1021/acs.jmedchem.8b00760] [PMID: 30035545]

[41] Zhang, K.; Lai, F.; Lin, S.; Ji, M.; Zhang, J.; Zhang, Y.; Jin, J.; Fu, R.; Wu, D.; Tian, H.; Xue, N.; Sheng, L.; Zou, X.; Li, Y.; Chen, X.; Xu, H. Design, Synthesis, and Biological Evaluation of 4-Methyl Quinazoline Derivatives as Anticancer Agents Simultaneously Targeting Phosphoinositide 3-Kinases and Histone Deacetylases. *J. Med. Chem.,* **2019**, *62*(15), 6992-7014.
[http://dx.doi.org/10.1021/acs.jmedchem.9b00390] [PMID: 31117517]

[42] Hu, Y.; Li, C.Y.; Wang, X.M.; Yang, Y.H.; Zhu, H.L. 1,3,4-Thiadiazole: Synthesis, reactions, and applications in medicinal, agricultural, and materials chemistry. *Chem. Rev.,* **2014**, *114*(10), 5572-5610.
[http://dx.doi.org/10.1021/cr400131u] [PMID: 24716666]

[43] Druker, B.J.; Guilhot, F.; O'Brien, S.G.; Gathmann, I.; Kantarjian, H.; Gattermann, N.; Deininger, M.W.N.; Silver, R.T.; Goldman, J.M.; Stone, R.M.; Cervantes, F.; Hochhaus, A.; Powell, B.L.; Gabrilove, J.L.; Rousselot, P.; Reiffers, J.; Cornelissen, J.J.; Hughes, T.; Agis, H.; Fischer, T.; Verhoef, G.; Shepherd, J.; Saglio, G.; Gratwohl, A.; Nielsen, J.L.; Radich, J.P.; Simonsson, B.; Taylor, K.; Baccarani, M.; So, C.; Letvak, L.; Larson, R.A. Five-year follow-up of patients receiving imatinib for chronic myeloid leukemia. *N. Engl. J. Med.,* **2006**, *355*(23), 2408-2417.
[http://dx.doi.org/10.1056/NEJMoa062867] [PMID: 17151364]

[44] Shah, N.P.; Tran, C.; Lee, F.Y.; Chen, P.; Norris, D.; Sawyers, C.L. Overriding imatinib resistance with a novel ABL kinase inhibitor. *Science,* **2004**, *305*(5682), 399-401.

[http://dx.doi.org/10.1126/science.1099480] [PMID: 15256671]

[45]   Altıntop, MD; Ciftci, HI; Radwan, MO Design, synthesis, and biological evaluation of novel 1,3,4-thiadiazole derivatives as potential antitumor agents against chronic myelogenous leukemia: Striking effect of nitrothiazole moiety. *Molecules,* **2017**, *23*(1), 59.
[http://dx.doi.org/10.3390/molecules23010059]

[46]   Fortin, S.; Bérubé, G. Advances in the development of hybrid anticancer drugs. *Expert Opin. Drug Discov.,* **2013**, *8*(8), 1029-1047.
[http://dx.doi.org/10.1517/17460441.2013.798296] [PMID: 23646979]

[47]   Gomha, S.; Edrees, M.; Muhammad, Z.; El-Reedy, A. 5-(Thiophen-2-yl)-1,3,4-thiadiazole derivatives: Synthesis, molecular docking and *in vitro* cytotoxicity evaluation as potential anticancer agents. *Drug Des. Devel. Ther.,* **2018**, *12*, 1511-1523.
[http://dx.doi.org/10.2147/DDDT.S165276] [PMID: 29881258]

[48]   Raimondi, M.; Randazzo, O.; La Franca, M.; Barone, G.; Vignoni, E.; Rossi, D.; Collina, S. DHFR Inhibitors: Reading the Past for Discovering Novel Anticancer Agents. *Molecules,* **2019**, *24*(6), 1140.
[http://dx.doi.org/10.3390/molecules24061140] [PMID: 30909399]

[49]   El-Naggar, M; Sallam, HA; Shaban, SS Design, synthesis, and molecular docking study of novel heterocycles incorporating 1,3,4-thiadiazole moiety as potential antimicrobial and anticancer agents. *Molecules,* **2019**, *24*(6), 1066.
[http://dx.doi.org/10.3390/molecules24061066]

[50]   Giovannetti, E.; van der Borden, C.L.; Frampton, A.E.; Ali, A.; Firuzi, O.; Peters, G.J. Never let it go: Stopping key mechanisms underlying metastasis to fight pancreatic cancer. *Semin. Cancer Biol.,* **2017**, *44*, 43-59.
[http://dx.doi.org/10.1016/j.semcancer.2017.04.006] [PMID: 28438662]

[51]   Amrutkar, M.; Gladhaug, I. Pancreatic cancer chemoresistance to gemcitabine. *Cancers (Basel),* **2017**, *9*(12), 157.
[http://dx.doi.org/10.3390/cancers9110157] [PMID: 29144412]

[52]   Cascioferro, S.; Petri, G.L.; Parrino, B.; Carbone, D.; Funel, N.; Bergonzini, C.; Mantini, G.; Dekker, H.; Geerke, D.; Peters, G.J.; Cirrincione, G.; Giovannetti, E.; Diana, P. Imidazo[2,1-b][1,3,4]thiadiazoles with antiproliferative activity against primary and gemcitabine-resistant pancreatic cancer cells. *Eur. J. Med. Chem.,* **2020**, *189*, 112088.
[http://dx.doi.org/10.1016/j.ejmech.2020.112088] [PMID: 32007666]

[53]   Shang, X.F.; Morris-Natschke, S.L.; Liu, Y.Q.; Guo, X.; Xu, X.S.; Goto, M.; Li, J.C.; Yang, G.Z.; Lee, K.H. Biologically active quinoline and quinazoline alkaloids part I. *Med. Res. Rev.,* **2018**, *38*(3), 775-828.
[http://dx.doi.org/10.1002/med.21466] [PMID: 28902434]

[54]   Mandewale, M.C.; Patil, U.C.; Shedge, S.V.; Dappadwad, U.R.; Yamgar, R.S. A review on quinoline hydrazone derivatives as a new class of potent antitubercular and anticancer agents. *Beni. Suef Univ. J. Basic Appl. Sci.,* **2017**, *6*(4), 354-361.
[http://dx.doi.org/10.1016/j.bjbas.2017.07.005]

[55]   Ducki, S. The development of chalcones as promising anticancer agents. *IDrugs,* **2007**, *10*(1), 42-46.
[PMID: 17187314]

[56]   Abbas, SH; Abd El-Hafeez, AA; Shoman, ME; Montano, MM; Hassan, HA New quinoline/chalcone hybrids as anticancer agents: Design, synthesis, and evaluations of cytotoxicity and PI3K inhibitory activity. *Bioorg Chem.,* **2019**, *82*, 360-377.
[http://dx.doi.org/10.1016/j.bioorg.2018.10.064]

[57]   Li, W; Xu, F; Shuai, W; Sun, H; Yao, H; Ma, C; Xu, S; Yao, H; Zhu, Z; Yang, DH; Chen, ZS; Xu, J Discovery of novel quinoline-chalcone derivatives as potent antitumor agents with microtubule polymerization inhibitory activity. *J. Med Chem.,* **2019**, *62*(2), 993-1013.
[http://dx.doi.org/10.1021/acs.jmedchem.8b01755]

[58] Othman, D.I.A.; Selim, K.B.; El-Sayed, M.A.A.; Tantawy, A.S.; Amen, Y.; Shimizu, K.; Okauchi, T.; Kitamura, M. Design, synthesis and anticancer evaluation of new substituted thiophene-quinoline derivatives. *Bioorg. Med. Chem.,* **2019**, *27*(19), 115026.
[http://dx.doi.org/10.1016/j.bmc.2019.07.042] [PMID: 31416740]

[59] Mohassab, AM; Hassan, HA; Abdelhamid, D; Gouda, AM; Youssif, BGM; Tateishi, H; Fujita, M; Otsuka, M; Abdel-Aziz, M Design and synthesis of novel quinoline/chalcone/1,2,4-triazole hybrids as potent antiproliferative agent targeting EGFR and BRAF^{V600E} kinases. *Bioorg Chem.,* **2021**, *106*, 104510.

CHAPTER 4

Imidazole Showing its Therapeutic Voyage as Anticancer Heterocyclic Ring

Ashwani K. Dhingra[1,*], Bhawna Chopra[1], Akram Sidhu[2], Kumar Guarve[1] and **Ashish Gupta[3]**

[1] *Guru Gobind Singh College of Pharmacy, Yamuna Nagar-135001, Haryana, India*

[2] *UNT Health Science Center, Fort Worth, Texas, USA*

[3] *CSIR-National Physical Laboratory, New Delhi-110012, India*

Abstract: In the current era, numerous anticancer drugs are available with potential pharmacological activity. Still, issues like multi-drug resistance, toxicity, solubility *etc.*, were in existence, which finally decreases the overall therapeutic value of indices of the drug molecule. Therefore, in search of new anticancer agents to fight against cancer is not an ending process. Keeping this in view, aromatic diazole heterocyclic nucleus named imidazole was proved with quite promising health benefits. The imidazole nucleus possesses numerous pharmacological activities. Thus, its derivatives/analogs have occupied a distinctive position in medicinal chemistry due to the incorporation of the heterocyclic nucleus, imidazole, to develop the new synthetic strategy in the significant drug discovery process. In addition to this, the significant therapeutic potential of the imidazole containing agents have triggered the medicinal chemist to develop a large number of novel anticancer compounds with a low toxicity profile. This chapter aims ornately pronounced the therapeutic voyage of imidazole and its analogs as anticancer.

Keywords: Anticancer, Benzimidazole, Cancer, Drug discovery, Imidazole.

INTRODUCTION

Cancer is a complex biological disorder mainly progressed by developing multistep carcinogenesis involving an array of physiological systems like cell signalling and apoptosis [1]. At present, diverse heterocyclic moieties were recognized to possess anticancer activity, but they exhibit less therapeutic efficacy, multi-drug resistance, adverse drug effects, and/or poor solubility and bioavailability issues, thus developing a necessity to explore other more effective, potent, less toxic molecules [2]. Literature reveals a variety of N-heterocyclic

---

* **Corresponding author Ashwani K. Dhingra:** Guru Gobind Singh College of Pharmacy, Yamuna Nagar-135001, Haryana, India; Tel: +919996230055; E-mail: ashwani1683@gmail.com

compounds have been explored for their diverse therapeutic activities [3] and especially for anticancer potential [4, 5]. Imidazole, a five-membered heterocyclic nucleus with two nitrogen atoms, that are commonly found in various natural [6, 7] and synthetic [8 - 11] compounds. A number of imidazole molecules like dacarbazine **(1)**, zoledronic acid **(2)**, temozolomide **(3)**, nilotinib **(4)**, mercaptopurine **(5)**, tipifarnib **(6)**, *etc.* Fig. **(1)** have been used clinically to treat several types of cancers. Thus it can be concluded that it appears to be an essential pharmacophore for drug discovery and development as some of the imidazole derivatives shows dual action *i.e.*, on inflammation and cancer affecting the COX and various types of kinases (P13K).

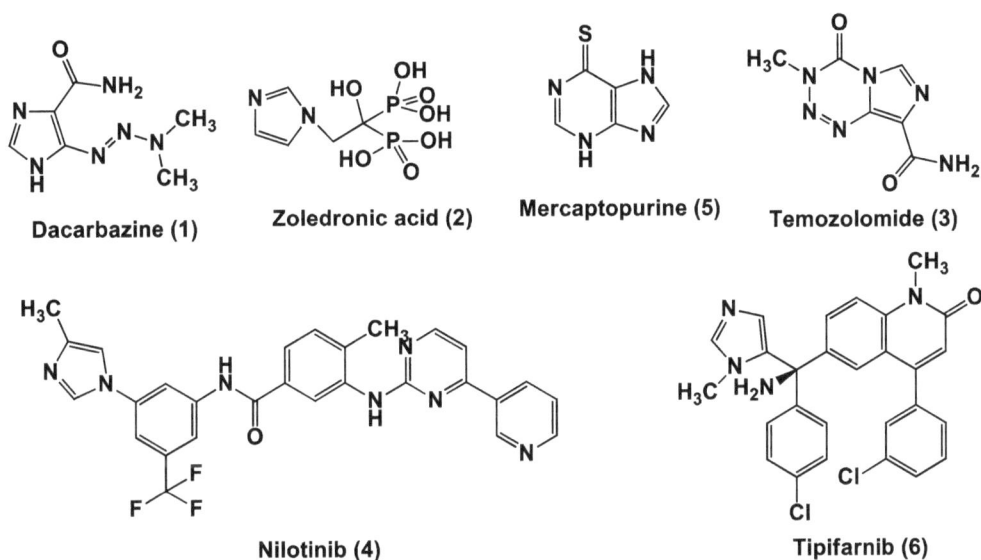

Fig. (1). Structure of some clinically used anticancer imidazoles.

Studies conclude that the cancer development may be due to the variation in the structure and function of the DNA, VEGF, mitotic spindle microtubules, topoisomerases I &II, receptor tyrosinase kinase, histone deacetylases, release of NO and its vasoldilation effect in tumor blood vessels. It can also be achieved by controlling the gene expression [12 - 14]. It was expected that imidazoles might interact with DNA [15] and molecules of protein [16]. Therefore, it inspired the chemist to accelerate the studies to prepare newer analogs with increased efficacy and affinity with a lower toxicity profile. It was also predicted that imidazole analogs might inhibit the cell membrane components like membrane or mitrochondrial potential [17] and thus helps in treating cancer. In the current era, imidazole gains immense importance due to its pharmacological potential.

CHEMISTRY OF IMIDAZOLE

Chemically, imidazole is 1, 3-diaza-2,4-cyclopentadiene having two nitrogen atoms at position 1 and 3, planar five-membered heterocyclic nucleus. It exists in two equivalent tautomeric forms (**7 & 8**) shown in Fig. (**2**) [18 - 21].

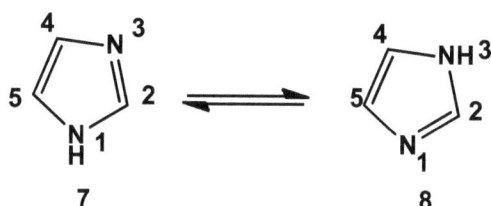

Fig. (2). Tautomeric structures of imidazoles.

It has a delocalized sextet of π-electrons. It may be referred to as an aromatic compound, and its resonance structure (**9-13**) is shown in Fig. (**3**) [22].

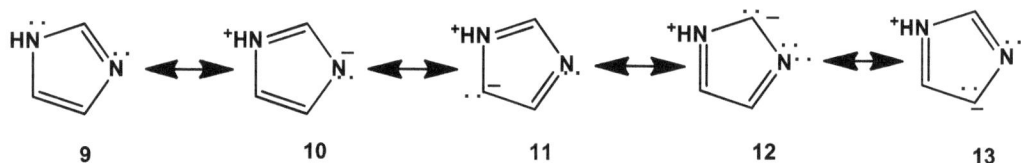

Fig. (3). Resonating structures of imidazoles.

Heinrich Debus first synthesized imidazole in 1858; however, numerous imidazole analogs or derivatives were also discovered in the early 1840s [23]. It was first known as gluoxaline as it was carried out using glyoxal and formaldehyde in the presence of ammonia (Fig. **4a**) [24]. Later, in 1977 Van Leusen reported imidazole synthesis using a three component reaction using aldimines and tosylmethyl isocyanide (Fig. **4b**) [25]. It was also synthesized by Zhang *et al.*, in 1996 *via* Ugi four-component reaction using primary amines, arylglyoxals, isocyanide, and carboxylic acids on a Wang resin (Fig. **4c**) in the presence of $CHCl_3$:MeOH:pyridine (1:1:1) at 65°C for three days [26]. Primarily, ketoamides were formed, which on treatment with ammonium acetate in acetic acid at 100°C for twenty hours, followed by reaction with 10% TFA-DCM at 23°C for 20 minutes undergo cyclization to yield the corresponding imidazoles.

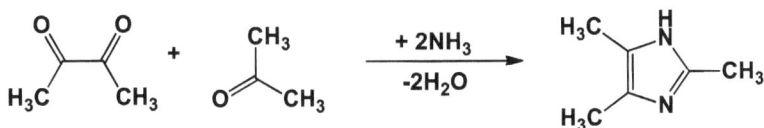

Figure 4a: Heinrich debus synthesis

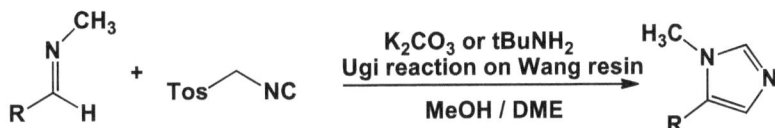

Figure 4b: Van Leusen three-component reaction (vl-3CR)

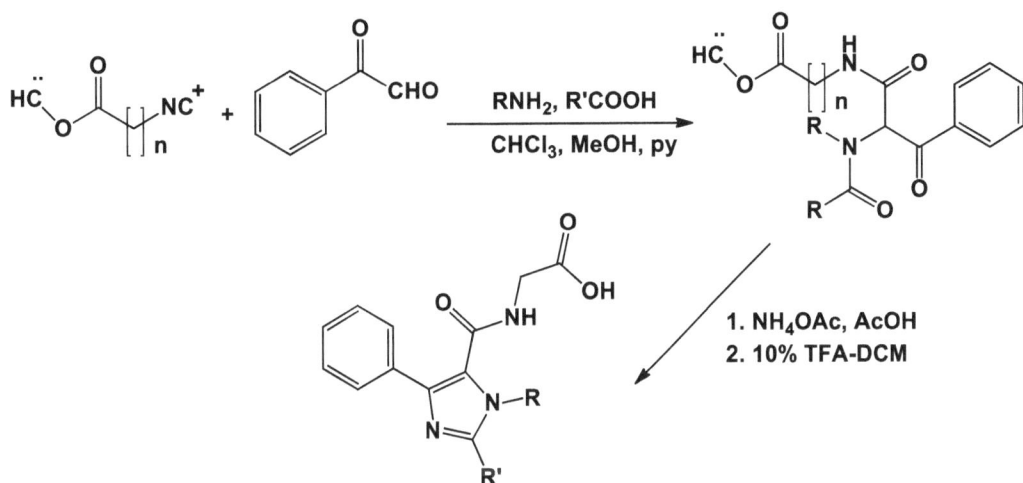

Figure 4c: Ugi reaction on wang resin

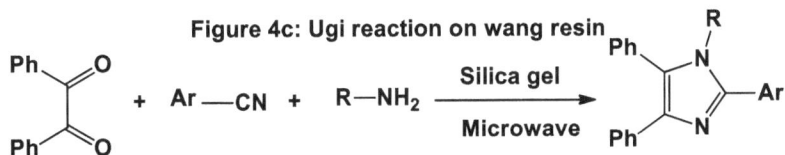

Figure 4d: One pot synthesis under microwave condition with 80-92% yield

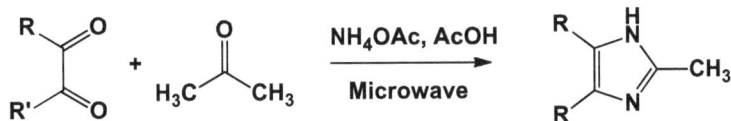

R, R' = alkyl, aryl, heteroaryl

Figure 4e: One pot synthesis under microwave condition with 80-99% yield

Fig. (4). Synthetic methodology for the preparation of imidazole (**4a-4e**).

Furthermore, one-pot synthesis of tetrasubstituted imidazoles by microwave irradiation was reported by Balalaie *et al.* in the year 2003 (Fig. **4d**) with a quite high yield (80–92%) [27]. Wolkenberg *et al.*, in 2003, reported a simple and efficient method for the preparation of imidazoles using 1, 2-diketones and aldehydes in the presence of ammonium acetate with high yield (Fig. **4e**). Apart from this, there are many more methods reported for the synthesis of imidazole analogs with excellent yields [28, 38 - 45], including Radiszewski synthesis [29, 30], dehydrogenation of imidazoline [31], Wallach synthesis [32, 33], Markwald synthesis [34], Oxozolones condensation [35], Benzilic acid rearrangement [36], Tandem oxidation [37] *etc.*

Thus, this exciting heterocyclic moiety can be constructed and derivatized to prepare newer imidazole analogs, imidazolones and others which are recognized to have the diverse era of pharmacological activities like antimicrobial [46 - 48], CNS depressant [49], antidepressant [50], anticonvulsant [50, 51], immunomodulatory [52], anthelmintic [53], cardiovascular activity [54], xanthine oxidase inhibitors [55], anti-inflammatory [56, 57], antifungal [58], neuroprotective [59], antimalarial [60] and antiulcerative [61]. However, it also exhibits anticancer property, and this journey was started with the synthesis of dacarbazine. This triggers medicinal chemist to develop and design imidazole analogs as potential anticancer agents [62]. In addition to this, imidazole analogs also possess the potential to reduce the toxicity/side effect of currently existing clinical molecules. Therefore, an attempt has been made to emphasize some imidazole analogs, which may further develop anticancer drugs. The following section describes the imidazole analogs with variant mechanisms of action.

IMIDAZOLE ANALOGS POSSESSING ANTICANCER POTENTIAL

Imidazoles as Antiangiogenic Agents

The angiogenesis process involves the development of new blood vessels from the pre-existing blood vessels produced by vasculogenesis. Angiogenesis also involves vascular endothelial growth factor (VEGF); it plays a key role and proves to be a vital pathway responsible for the growth of cells and tissues [63 - 66]. Human cancer cells lead to the excess secretion of VEGF along with its receptors on their surface, which leads to the development of vascularized tumors. For the last two decades, a variety of imidazole analogs have been explored as anticancer agents through anti-angiogenesis. Several imidazole analogs like N-methyllevamisoles **(14 and 15)** Fig. **(5)** showed significant inhibition of angiogenesis [67]. In another study, chrome-3-carboxylic acids derived twenty-six imidazole derivatives were synthesized and assessed for *in-vitro* anti-angiogenesis properties. Out of all designed analogs, compound **(16)** Fig. **(5)** reported as potent anti-angiogenic agents. In addition, the molecular docking study also represents the higher binding affinity of compound **(16)** Fig. **(5)** with KRAS/Wnt and VEGF, which concludes that this analog possesses potent anticancer property [68].

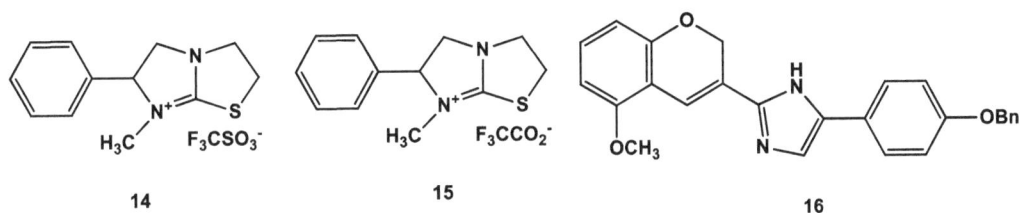

Fig. (5). Structure of some imidazole as antiangiogenic agents.

Imidazoles as Focal Adhesion Kinase Enzyme Inhibitors

The focal adhesion kinase (FAK) enzyme stimulates metastasis and tumor progression through regulation, of the cell migration, extracellular matrix, invasion, and angiogenesis process. The transcriptional and translational levels of various cancers lead to overexpression of this enzyme, which made it a promising therapeutic target [69 - 71]. Literature survey reveals that several imidazoles based heterocyclic compounds showed significant focal adhesion kinase (FAK) inhibition against several cancer cell lines with reference to TAE-226 (standard FAK inhibitor). Out of all prepared analogs, several imidazole analogs **(17-20,** Fig. **(6)** showed significant anticancer activities against U87-MG, HCT-116, and PC-3 cell lines [72].

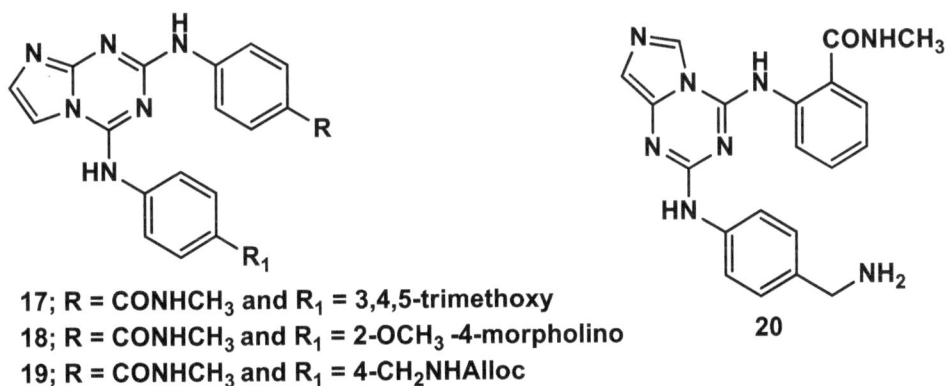

17; R = CONHCH$_3$ and R$_1$ = 3,4,5-trimethoxy
18; R = CONHCH$_3$ and R$_1$ = 2-OCH$_3$ -4-morpholino
19; R = CONHCH$_3$ and R$_1$ = 4-CH$_2$NHAlloc

Fig. (6). Structure of some imidazoles as focal adhesion kinase (FAK) enzyme Inhibitors.

Imidazoles as Anti-proliferative Agents

The anti-proliferative approach is one of the important pathways to cure various types of cancer illness. In this regard, a number of imidazole analogs were prepared, which showed significant anti-proliferative potential. Several imidazole analogs **21-27** Fig. (7) showed significant anti-proliferative activities against human A375 cells and mouse B16 cells melanoma cell lines [73]. The anticancer potential of these analogs were determined by using sulforhodamine B assay. The SAR studies reveal that incorporating an imidazole ring system substituted with electron-withdrawing groups significantly enhances the anti-proliferative effect of 1, 8-acridinones [74]. In another study, several heterocyclic analogs (**28-30**) Fig. (7) bearing imidazole nucleus were investigated by MTT assay for anti-proliferative effect against HeLa (cervical), MCF-7 (breast), LS180 (colon), and Jurk at human cancer cell lines taking cis-platin as a standard drug [75].

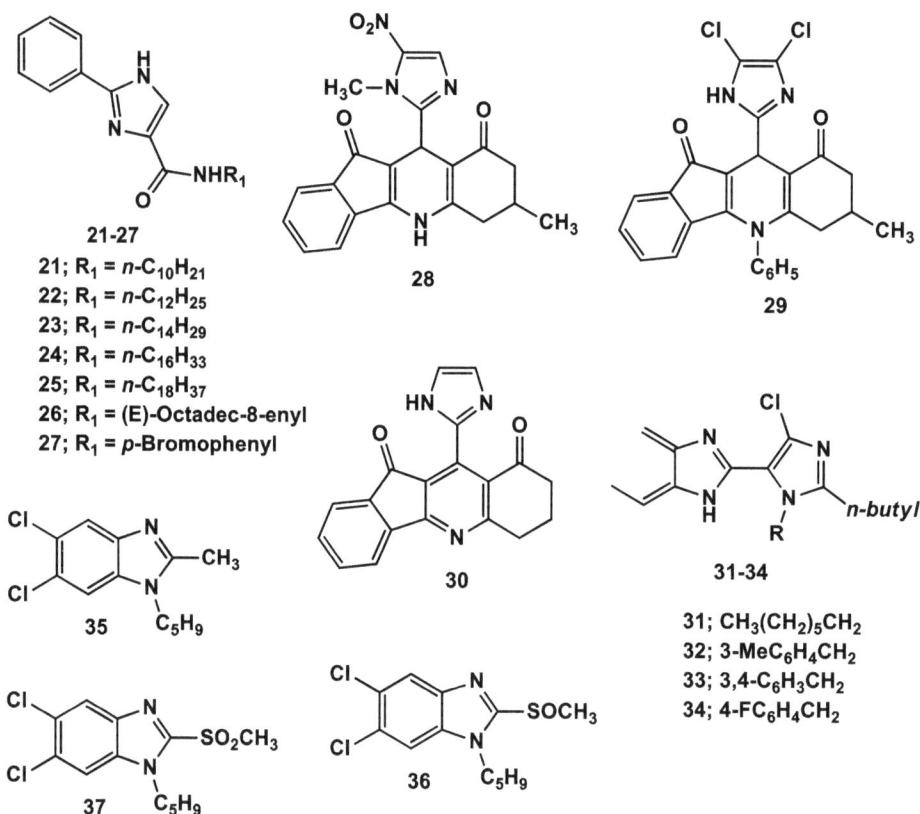

21-27
21; R₁ = *n*-C₁₀H₂₁
22; R₁ = *n*-C₁₂H₂₅
23; R₁ = *n*-C₁₄H₂₉
24; R₁ = *n*-C₁₆H₃₃
25; R₁ = *n*-C₁₈H₃₇
26; R₁ = (E)-Octadec-8-enyl
27; R₁ = *p*-Bromophenyl

31; CH₃(CH₂)₅CH₂
32; 3-MeC₆H₄CH₂
33; 3,4-C₆H₃CH₂
34; 4-FC₆H₄CH₂

Fig. (7). Structure of some imidazoles as antiproliferative agents.

Furthermore, other imidazole derivatives like benzimidazoles were also found to possess potent antitumor activity [76, 77]. Several benzimidazole analogs **31-34** Fig. (7) showed remarkable anti-proliferative activity on Hela cells [78]. In another study, some benzo[d]imidazoles **35–37** Fig. (7) bearing −CH₃, -Cl, −SOCH₃, −SO₂CH₃, and cyclopentyl group showed significant anti-proliferative activity on various cancer cell lines [79].

Imidazoles as CYP26A1 Enzyme Inhibitors

The physiological metabolites of vitamin A, All trans-retinoic acids (ATRAs) were reported for the effective treatment of various types of cancer [80 - 82], particularly acute promyelocytic leukemia (APL) [83 - 86]. However, the easy breakdown of ATRAs into 4-hydroxyl-RA characterized by CYP26A1 enzyme will hamper its clinical applications badly. As a result, the inhibition of the CYP26A1 enzyme leads to a promising strategy for the design and discovery of novel molecules with anticancer activity. The literature survey highlights the possible role of the imidazole nucleus by targeting the CYP26A1 enzyme to develop retinoic acid metabolism blocking agents.

The imidazole based naphthyl compound (38); Fig. (8) and other azoles like ketoconazole (39); Fig. (8) led to the development of second generation CYP26A1 inhibitors (40); Fig. (8) [87 - 90] as RAMBAs. Based on the preclinical and clinical results, some of these second-generation RAMBAs have been preceded for clinical studies [91, 92]. Recently, fifteen imidazole analogs were prepared as RAMBAs and evaluated against CYP26A1 enzyme inhibition [93]. Out of all designed analogs, two analogs, **41 and 42** Fig. (8), showed selective and promising effect towards the CYP26A1 enzyme.

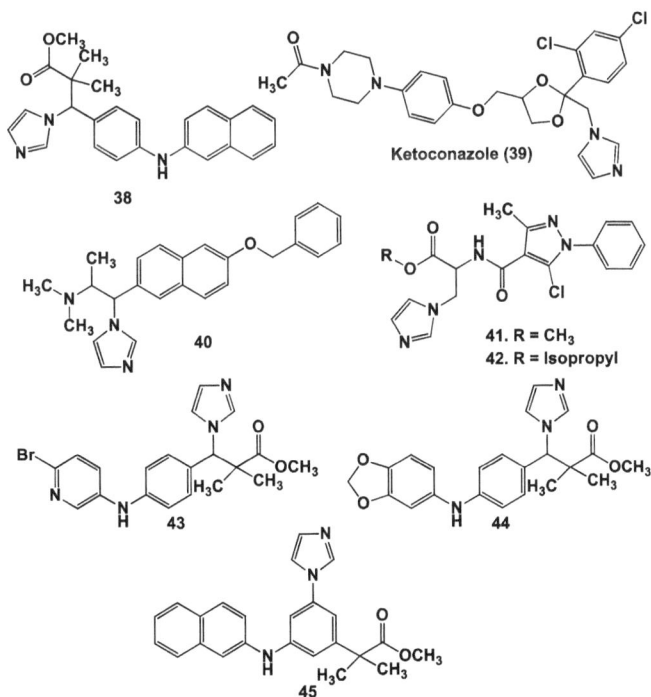

Fig. (8). Structure of some imidazoles as CYP26A1 enzyme inhibitors.

In another study, the two imidazole analogs, **43 and 44** Fig. (**8**) exhibits strong activity through cell-free microsomal assay against the CYP26A1 enzyme [94]. Furthermore, another eleven imidazole analogs were prepared and screened for CYP26A1 inhibition activity through MCF-7 CYP26A1 microsomal assay [95]. Out of all prepared compounds, **45** Fig. (**8**) showed the most promising activity than the standard drug (liarozole and R116010).

Imidazoles as Topoisomerase Inhibitors

Topoisomerases (TOP) enzymes have been reported as one of the important targets in the development of novel anticancer drug [96 - 100]. In addition, about 50% of anticancer compounds used clinically to treat cancer act by inhibiting topoisomerase enzymes [101, 102]. In search of novel effective and safe TOP inhibitors, the imidazole nucleus has been widely considered as a structural fragment in various other bioactive skeletons. In this regard, a novel series of N-fused imidazoles **46–50** Fig. (**9**) have been prepared, which showed a potent DNA non-intercalating topoisomerase IIα inhibitory activity [103]. Recently, three imidazole analogs **51–53** Fig. (**9**) prepared by conjugation with imine/amides under microwave condition showed promising *in-vitro* anticancer activities against (H-460, Hep-G2, and A-459) [104] cancer cell lines.

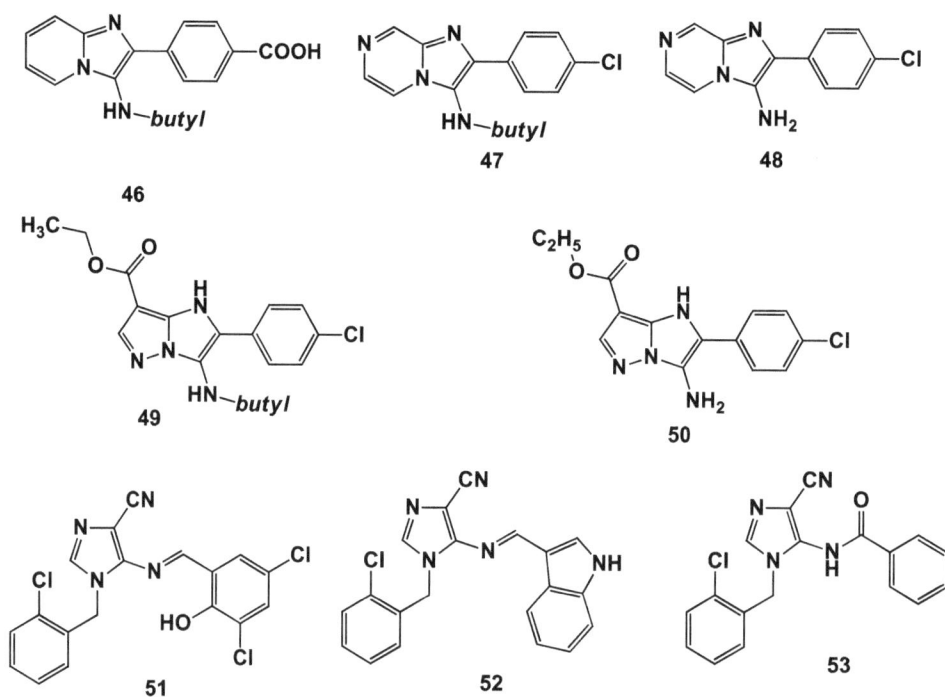

Fig. (9). Structure of some imidazoles as topoisomerase inhibitors.

The other imidazole-based, clinically used anticancer drugs as Top-I inhibitors, include Indimitecan (**54**); Fig. (**10**) [105]. In addition, several camptothecins (CPT) derived imidazoline analogs **55** and **56** Fig. (**10**) showed significant TOP I inhibitory activity against colon (HCT-8) and breast (MCF-7) cancer cell lines [106, 107].

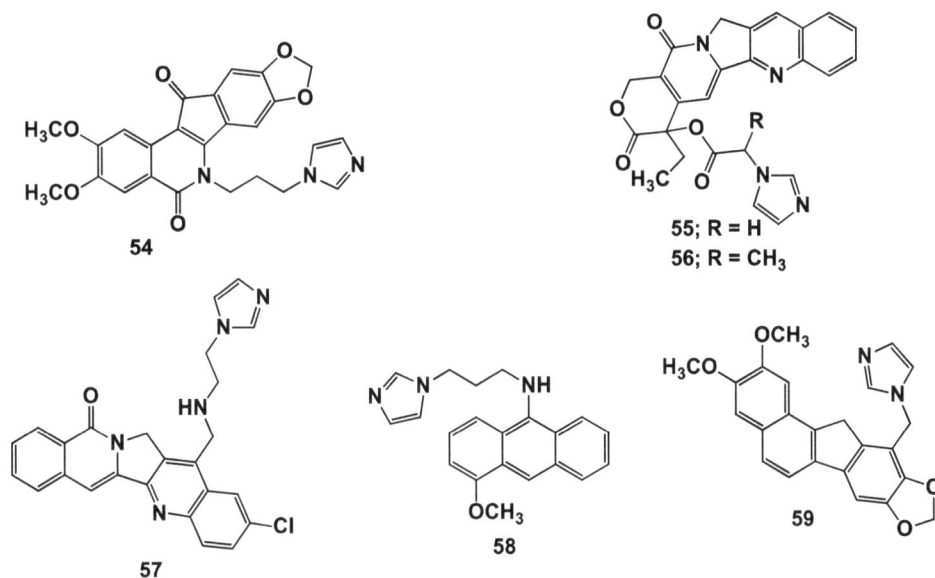

Fig. (10). Structure of some imidazoles as topoisomerase inhibitors.

Furthermore, the imidazole based aromathecin **57** Fig. (**10**) also showed better TOP I inhibitory activity than the parent molecule aromathecin [108]. Moreover, the imidazole derivatives derived from podophyllotoxin showed remarkable anticancer activities *via* inhibiting DNA-TOP II against three human cell lines [109]. In addition, the acridine-based imidazole analog **58** Fig. (**10**) displayed significant anticancer activity *via* inhibiting DNA-TOP II against MCF-7, COLO-205, HEP-2, A-549, HCT-15 and IMR-32 cancer cell lines [110]. Apart from this, the imidazole derivative Norindenoisoquinolines **59** Fig. (**10**) also represented good TOP I inhibitory activity and showed improved anticancer potential against IGROVI, MCF-7, SN12C, and HCT-116 cell lines [111].

Imidazoles as Rapid Accelerated Fibrosarcoma (RAF) Kinase Inhibitors

Currently, sorafenib is used clinically as an RAF kinases inhibitor against renal cancer [112]. However, the two imidazole analogs of sorafenib **60 and 61** Fig. (**11**) displayed remarkable CRAF inhibitory activity as compared to sorafenib against the melanoma cancer cell line WM3629 [113]. These studies revealed the great potential of imidazole analogs for the treatment of cancer *via* RAF inhibitory activity. In addition, another imidazole analog of sorafenib **62** Fig. **(11)** showed excellent RAF inhibitory activity against two human cell lines (A549 and DLD-1) [114]. Furthermore, the molecular docking studies showed that this compound occupies the ATP binding pocket's ribose position. In addition, the imidazole incorporated pyrazole analog **63** Fig. **(11)** exhibit significant CRAF inhibitory activity as compared to sorafenib against two human melanoma (A375P and WM3629) cell lines [115]. Apart from this, imidazole containing pyrazole tricyclic analog **64** Fig. **(11)** showed good cellular activity *via* BRAF inhibitory activity against melanoma [116].

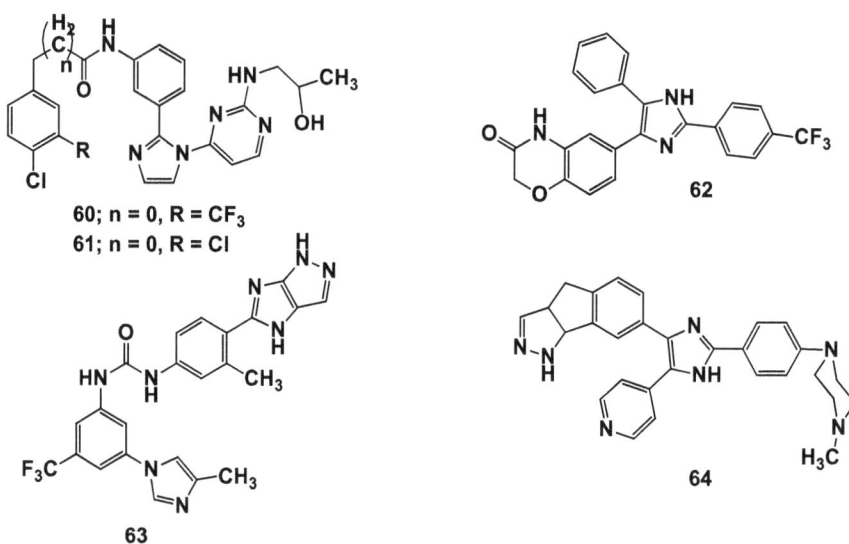

Fig. **(11).** Structure of some imidazoles as rapid accelerated fibrosarcoma (RAF) kinase inhibitors.

Imidazoles as Microtubule Destabilizing Anticancer Agents

Microtubules present in cells that act as important molecular targets for the development of anticancer drugs [117 - 121]. There are a number of clinically useful anticancer drugs like vinca alkaloids (vincristine, vinblastine), combretastatin A-4 phosphate, docetaxel, paclitaxel, *etc.* act by inhibiting the microtubule targeted tubulin binding site [112 - 117]. Literature survey reveals the anticancer potential of imidazole analogs which acts as microtubule destabilizing agents [122 - 127]. In 2010, a series of fourteen 2-amino-1- arylidenaminoimida-zole analogs were prepared and evaluated for cytotoxicity against human gastric NUGC-3 cancer cells using a high throughput screening platform [128]. All the prepared imidazole analogs showed significant anticancer activity *via* a microtubule target mechanism. In addition, the two imidazole analogs **65 and 66** Fig. **(12)** showed remarkable anticancer activity *via* microtubule assembly inhibition against tubulin polymerization assays. Furthermore, some imidazoles *ex-vivo* anticancer assessment showed a significant reduction in the tumor cells on histocultured colorectal (SW-480) and human gastric (MKN-45) tumors by inhibiting tubulin polymerization and thereby interfering with the microtubule assembly.

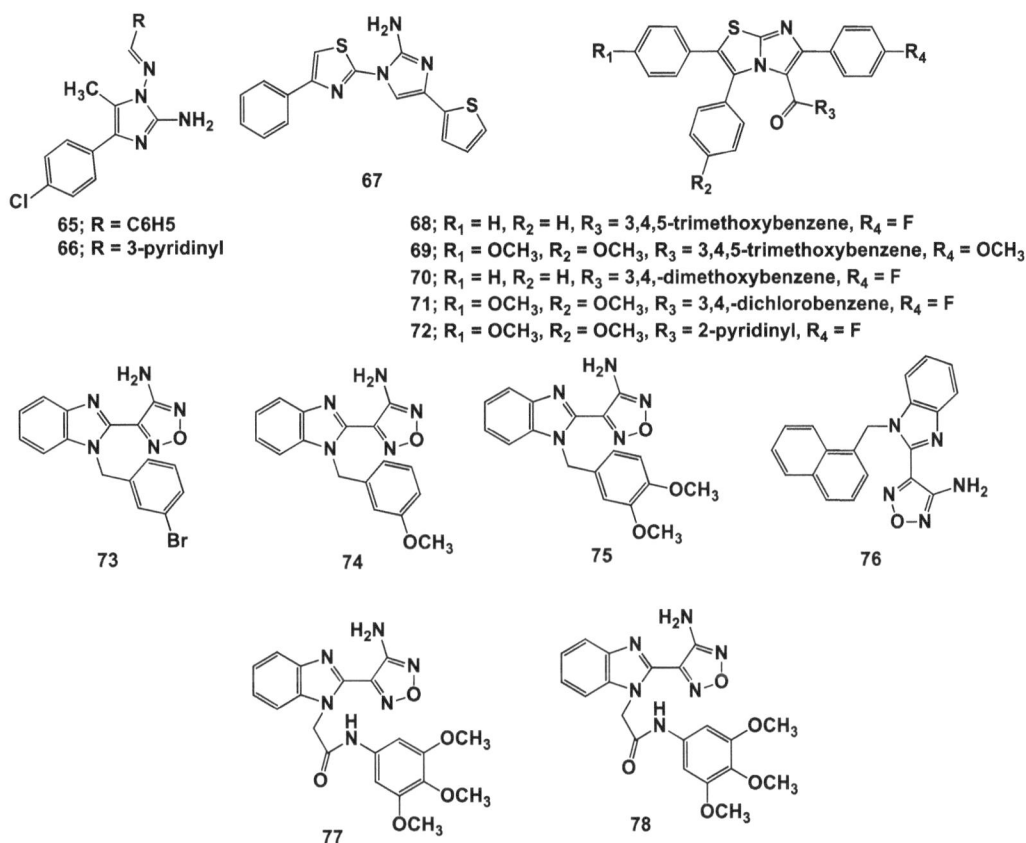

65; R = C6H5
66; R = 3-pyridinyl

67

68; R$_1$ = H, R$_2$ = H, R$_3$ = 3,4,5-trimethoxybenzene, R$_4$ = F
69; R$_1$ = OCH$_3$, R$_2$ = OCH$_3$, R$_3$ = 3,4,5-trimethoxybenzene, R$_4$ = OCH$_3$
70; R$_1$ = H, R$_2$ = H, R$_3$ = 3,4,-dimethoxybenzene, R$_4$ = F
71; R$_1$ = OCH$_3$, R$_2$ = OCH$_3$, R$_3$ = 3,4,-dichlorobenzene, R$_4$ = F
72; R$_1$ = OCH$_3$, R$_2$ = OCH$_3$, R$_3$ = 2-pyridinyl, R$_4$ = F

73   **74**   **75**   **76**

77   **78**

Fig. (12). Structure of some imidazoles as microtubule destabilizing anticancer agents.

In another study, several imidazole analogs (**67**); Fig. (**12**) associated with the thiazole moiety reported as potent microtubule destabilizing antineoplastic candidates due to their remarkable cytotoxic potential against gastric cancer cells [129]. The anticancer activity of this compound was explained on the basis of interfering with the kinetics of microtubule assembly along with colchicine binding sites of tubulins which results in the reticence of tumor resulting tumor cell apoptosis. In addition, several imidazole analogs **68-71** Fig. (**12**) derived from chalcone showed promising anticancer activity against five (MCF-7, DU-145, HeLa, A549, and HT-29) cancer cell lines by inhibiting tubulin polymerization microtubules [130]. Moreover, the flow cytometric analysis of **(72)**; Fig. **(12)** showed G2/M phase cell arrest, which escort to apoptotic cell death. Recently, a series of benzimidazole furazanamines **73-78** Fig. **(12)** showed interesting microtubule destabilizing activity against the sea urchin embryo model along with cultured human cancer cell lines [131]. Furthermore, the prepared analogs cytotoxicities were carried using an *in-vitro* tubulin polymerization assay along with cell cycle distribution analysis. The compounds showed anticancer activity and regarded as active microtubule destabilizing agents [132 - 134].

Imidazoles as CHK-1 and CHK-2 Inhibitors

Over the past decade, checkpoint kinases which are the serine/threonine protein kinases, emerges with prominent targets for the development of novel anticancer agents because they regulates the cellular DNA damage. Recently, three novel checkpoint kinase inhibitors enter the clinic trials [135, 136]. The rationale of using inhibitors of CHK-1 for cancer management includes its selectivity in association with its cytotoxicity. The CHK-1 inhibitor, UCN-01 (7-hydroxystaurosporine), has been reported for significant inhibitory and selectivity as compared to the other kinases CHK-1 inhibitors. As a result, this compound is currently under clinical trials [137 - 146]. On the other hand, the other checkpoint kinase CHK-2 regulates the downstream p53-dependent apoptosis machinery, which triggers the DNA damage characterized by the cytotoxic agent [147]. A series of benzimidazole analogs **79-82** Fig. **(13)** as CHK-1 inhibitors were prepared, which showed remarkable anticancer activity [148]. In another study, two imidazole analogs **83-84** Fig. **(13)** showed potent CHK-2 inhibitory activity [149, 150].

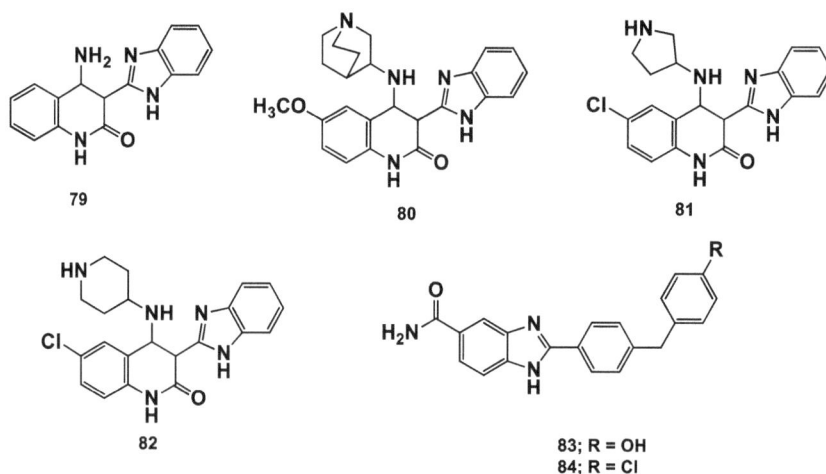

Fig. (13). Structure of some imidazoles as CHK-1 and CHK-2 inhibitors.

Miscellaneous Biological Targets of Imidazoles

Benzimidazole is widely exploded in the search of novel anticancer agents. They act *via* DNA alkylation **85-87** Fig. (**14**) and lead to the breakdown of the G and A bases [151 - 153]. Apart from this, numerous benzimidazole analogs were reported to act as cytotoxic in the management of lung and breast cancers [154, 155]. It was also documented that several conjugated benzimidazoles with pyrimidine showed significant antitumor activity against twelve human cancer cell lines [156]. From a series of derivatives, compound **88-89** Fig. (**14**) were found to be potent anticancer against lung cancer (NCI H460), ovarian carcinoma (SK OV-3), cervical carcinoma (KB), and leukemia (HL60). In addition, the compound **90** Fig. (**14**) having phenylhydrazino group was reported to be the most potent molecule against neuroblastoma (NB-1) and melanoma (G 361) [157]. In another study, two benzimidazole analogs **91-92** Fig. (**14**) were also found to possess significant cytotoxic potential against breast cancer (MCF7) [157].

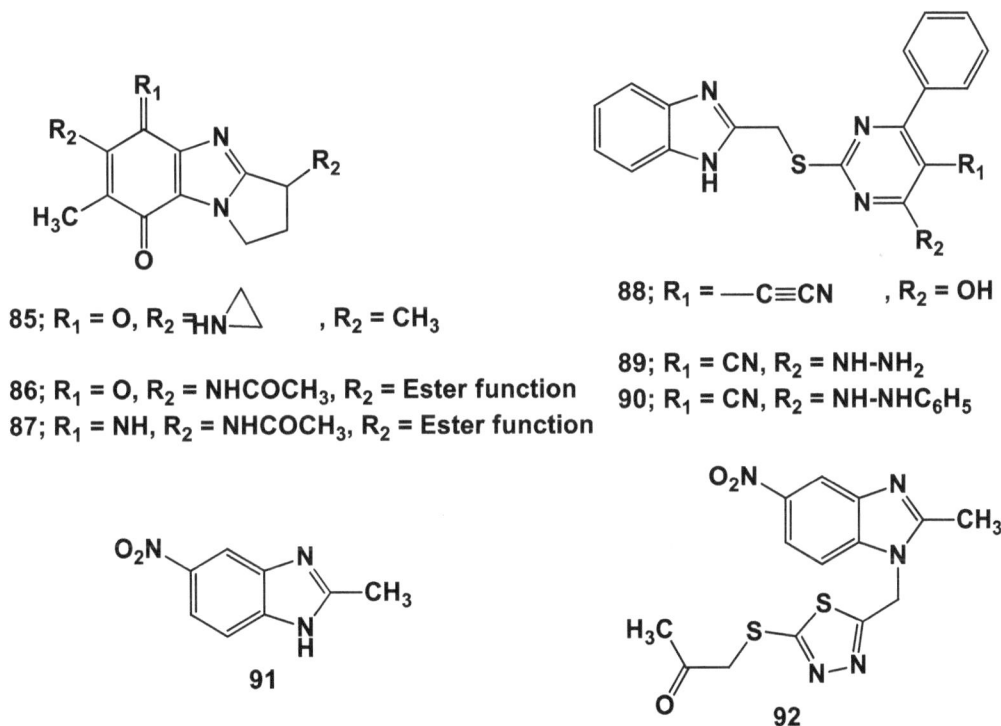

85; R_1 = O, R_2 =HN—△ , R_2 = CH$_3$

86; R_1 = O, R_2 = NHCOCH$_3$, R_2 = Ester function
87; R_1 = NH, R_2 = NHCOCH$_3$, R_2 = Ester function

88; R_1 = —C≡CN , R_2 = OH

89; R_1 = CN, R_2 = NH-NH$_2$
90; R_1 = CN, R_2 = NH-NHC$_6$H$_5$

91

92

Fig. (14). Structure of some anticancer imidazoles.

In addition, the other analogs also showed remarkable inhibition against Burkitt's lymphoma promotion [155], breast cancer and non-small lung cancer [154, 156]. Various other benzimidazole derivatives with pyrazoline [158] and thiazole [159] showed potent anticancer activity against various cancer cell lines. Keeping in view, researchers develop more and more imidazole analogs like 4-amin--thioxothiazole **93** Fig. (**15**), 4-oxothiazolidine **94** Fig. (**15**), 4-fluorobenzylidene **95** Fig. (**15**) [160] and another benzimidazole analog **96** Fig. (**15**) as potent anticancer agents [157]. In another work, some 2, 5, 6-trihalogenobenzimidazole analogs were prepared as androgen receptor antagonists. Out of al prepared analogs, benzimidazole having 1-(4-bromobenzyl) substituent **97** Fig. (**15**) showed the most potent antagonizing activity in prostate cancer [161]. Further extensive research continues, which results in the development of 5-carboxylic acid-containing benzimidazole as potent anti-leukemic agents by inducing apoptosis [162]. Another benzimidazoles containing quinolone ring moiety also proved themselves as potent anticancer compounds [163].

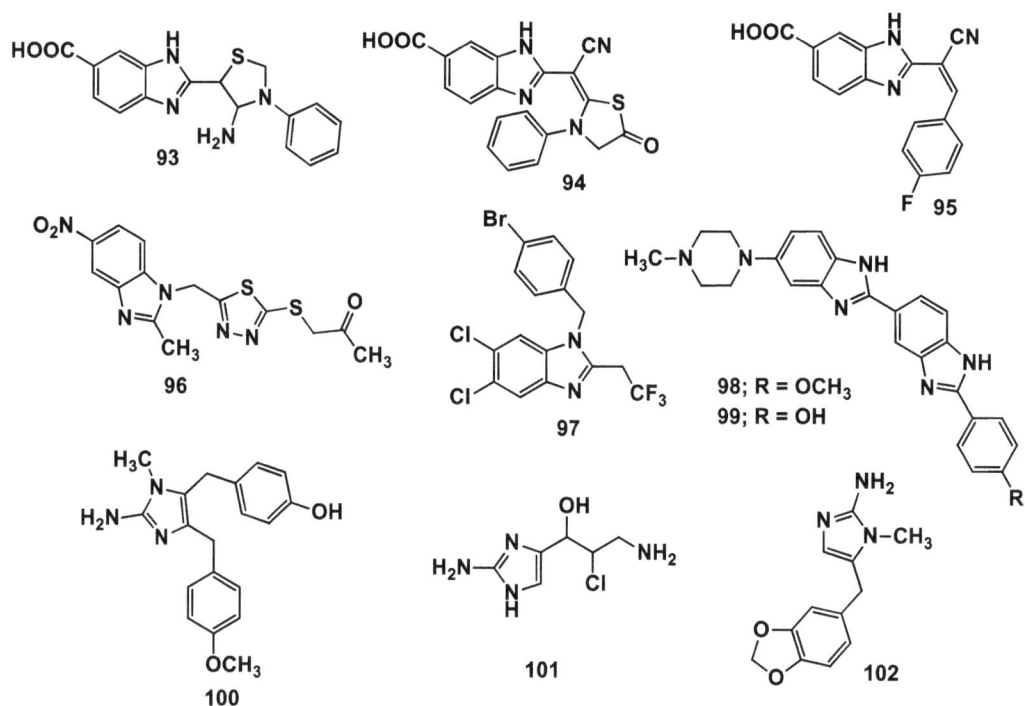

Fig. (15). Structure of some anticancer imidazoles.

Bis-benzimidazoles, another class of compounds, were also explored, which result in the development of Hoechst-33342 **98** Fig. (**15**) and Hoechst-33258 **99** Fig. (**15**) exhibiting anticancer activity *via* DNA top I inhibitory activities [164 - 168]. Apart from this, novel hybrid compounds derived from 2-phenylbenzofuran and 2-bromobenzyl were prepared, which showed remarkable anticancer activity as compare to cisplatin.

Furthermore, the acetamide derivatives [169], 2-benzylbenzofurane analogs [170], regioselective imidazole conjugate [171] were also reported as anticancer agents. Apart from this, the natural bioactive alkaloid naamidine A **100** Fig. (**15**) having 2-aminoimidazole moiety were also reported as epidermal growth factor (EGF) receptor inhibitor [172] and thus affecting mitochondrial mutations. In addition, it also reveals a mild cytotoxic effect against human cervix carcinoma (HeLa), and lymphoma (L5178Y) cell lines [173]. Moreover, nature also provides abundantly imidazole containing anticancer compounds like girolline **101** Fig. (**15**) (**63**) and preclathridine A **102** Fig. (**15**), and many more [174 - 176]. Recently in 2020s, Liu *et al.* synthesized a series of complexes in which the existence of benzene ring connected imidazole ring at different locations can effectively enhances the anticancer activity towards A549 cells in comparison to cisplatin. The anti cancer potential is due to the catalytic conversion of NADH to NAD+, changing mitochondrial membrane potential, disrupting the process of cell cycle, production of ROS and thus induction of apoptosis [177]. In addition to this, literature also reports that imidazole-based metal complexes improves the stability, redox potentiality, membrane permeability and thus increases the biological activity. Furthermore, the redox potential of metal compounds can interact with the balanced cellular redox state, thus causing significant modification in cell viability [178].

MARKET STATUS OF IMIDAZOLE-BASED ANTICANCER DRUGS

The literature describes the remarkable potential of imidazole based anticancer agents because of their capability to hamper the DNA synthesis and, therefore help in the inhibition of cell division and growth. As a result, a number of imidazole-derived anticancer drugs have been developed, which played a key role in the clinical therapeutics of cancer [179]. Some of these marketed imidazole nucleus containing anticancer drugs was depicted in Table **1**.

Table 1. Some of the marketed imidazole nucleus containing anticancer drugs.

S. No.	Name	Type	Application	References
1	Dacarbazine	alkylating agent	Hodgkin lymphoma, Metastatic malignant melanoma, and sarcoma	[180]
2	Azathioprine	Mercaptopurine Prodrug	Childhood acute lymphoblastic leukemia	[181]
3	Misonidazole, Etanidazole	2-nitroimidazoles	Hypoxic tumor cells radiosensitizers	[182]
4	Pimonidazole	2-nitroimidazoles	Hypoxia marker	[183]

S. No.	Name	Type	Application	References
5	Bendamustine	alkylating agent	Chronic lymphocytic leukemia and lymphomas	[184, 185]
6	Etanidazole	-	Inhibits glutathione transferase	[186]
7	Zoledronic acid	-	Inhibitor of osteoclast-mediated bone resorption	[187]
8	Nilotinib	selective small-molecule Bcr-Abl	Potent farnesyl transferase inhibitor	[188]
9	Tipifarnib	non-peptidomimetic quinolone analog	Potent farnesyl transferase inhibitor	[188]
10	Fadrozole	-	Breast cancer (first-line drug)	[189]
11	Indimitecan	-	Inhibit topoisomerase-I enzyme	[190]

CONCLUSION

This book chapter critically assesses the five-member heterocyclic nucleus, imidazole, demonstrating its number of anticancer analogs synthesized by various synthetic procedures. In addition to that, the chapter also describes the available marketed drugs having an imidazole nucleus bearing distinct substituents. These prepared analogs possess a higher potential against cancer but have toxicity and other issues with them. Therefore, there is a need to develop anticancer imidazole analogs exhibiting good therapeutic value with low toxicity and a better safety index. This possible improvement can be achieved by modification in the substituents present on the imidazole nucleus. Furthermore, still, studies are required to determine the specific mechanism of action and SAR studies. These parameters pave work to analyze different new cancer targets opted by drugs having a potent therapeutic profile, and this also helps the medicinal chemist and pharmaceutical industries.

CONSENT FOR PUBLICATION

Not applicable.

CONFLICT OF INTEREST

The author declares no conflict of interest, financial, or otherwise.

ACKNOWLEDGEMENT

The authors extend their heartful thanks to the Principal and Management of Guru Gobind Singh College of Pharmacy, Yamuna Nagar, for moral support.

REFERENCES

[1]   a) Reichert, J.; Wenger, J.B. Development trends for new cancer therapeutics and vaccines. *Drug Discov. Today,* **2008**, *13*(1-2), 30-37.
[http://dx.doi.org/10.1016/j.drudis.2007.09.003] [PMID: 18190861]
b) Singh, R.K.; Kumar, S.; Prasad, D.N.; Bhardwaj, T.R. Therapeutic journery of nitrogen mustard as alkylating anticancer agents: Historic to future perspectives. *Eur. J. Med. Chem.,* **2018**, *151*, 401-433.
[http://dx.doi.org/10.1016/j.ejmech.2018.04.001] [PMID: 29649739]

[2]   Rana, A.; Alex, J.M.; Chauhan, M.; Joshi, G.; Kumar, R. A review on pharmacophoric designs of antiproliferative agents. *Med. Chem. Res.,* **2015**, *24*(3), 903-920.
[http://dx.doi.org/10.1007/s00044-014-1196-5]

[3]   a) Kumari, A.; Singh, R.K. Medicinal chemistry of indole derivatives: Current to future therapeutic prospectives. *Bioorg. Chem.,* **2019**, *89*, 103021.
[http://dx.doi.org/10.1016/j.bioorg.2019.103021] [PMID: 31176854]
b) Kumari, A.; Singh, R.K. Morpholine as ubiquitous pharmacophore in medicinal chemistry: Deep insight into the structure-activity relationship (SAR). *Bioorg. Chem.,* **2020**, *96*, 103578.
[http://dx.doi.org/10.1016/j.bioorg.2020.103578] [PMID: 31978684]
c) Sethi, N.S.; Prasad, D.N.; Singh, R.K. An insight into the synthesis and sar of 2,4-thiazolidinediones (2,4-TZD) as multifunctional scaffold: A review. *Mini Rev. Med. Chem.,* **2020**, *20*(4), 308-330.
[http://dx.doi.org/10.2174/1389557519666191029102838] [PMID: 31660809]
d) Kumar, S.; Singh, R.K.; Patial, B.; Goyal, S.; Bhardwaj, T.R. Recent advances in novel heterocyclic scaffolds for the treatment of drug-resistant malaria. *J. Enzyme Inhib. Med. Chem.,* **2016**, *31*(2), 173-186.
[http://dx.doi.org/10.3109/14756366.2015.1016513] [PMID: 25775094]

[4]   Lang, D.K.; Kaur, R.; Arora, R.; Saini, B.; Arora, S. Nitrogen-containing heterocycles as anticancer agents: An overview. *Anticancer. Agents Med. Chem.,* **2020**, *20*(18), 2150-2168.
[http://dx.doi.org/10.2174/1871520620666200705214917] [PMID: 32628593]

[5]   Mohareb, R.M.; Milad, Y.R.; Mostafa, B.M.; El-Ansary, R.A. New Approaches for the Synthesis of Heterocyclic Compounds Corporating benzo[d]imidazole as Anticancer Agents, Tyrosine, Pim-1 Kinases Inhibitions and their PAINS Evaluations. *Anticancer. Agents Med. Chem.,* **2020**.
[http://dx.doi.org/10.2174/1871520620666200721111230] [PMID: 32698742]

[6]   Jochims, J.; Katritzky, A.; Rees, C.; Scriven, E. *Comprehensive Heterocyclic Chemistry II*; Pergamon Press: Oxford, **1996**, 4, p. 179.
[http://dx.doi.org/10.1016/B978-008096518-5.00082-4]

[7]   Ho, J.Z.; Mohareb, R.M.; Ahn, J.H.; Sim, T.B.; Rapoport, H. Enantiospecific synthesis of carbapentostatins. *J. Org. Chem.,* **2003**, *68*(1), 109-114.
[http://dx.doi.org/10.1021/jo020612x] [PMID: 12515468]

[8]   Zhang, S.Q.; Gao, L.H.; Zhao, H.; Wang, K.Z. Recent progress in polynuclear ruthenium complex-based DNA binders/structural probes and anticancer agents. *Curr. Med. Chem.,* **2020**, *27*(22), 3735-3752.
[http://dx.doi.org/10.2174/0929867326666181203143422] [PMID: 30501596]

[9]   Chopra, P.N.; Sahu, J.K. Biological Significance of Imidazole-based Analogues in New Drug Development. *Curr. Drug Discov. Technol.,* **2020**, *17*(5), 574-584.
[http://dx.doi.org/10.2174/1570163816666190320123340] [PMID: 30894111]

[10]   Fan, C.; Zhong, T.; Yang, H.; Yang, Y.; Wang, D.; Yang, X.; Xu, Y.; Fan, Y. Design, synthesis, biological evaluation of 6-(2-amino-1H-benzo[d]imidazole-6-yl)quinazolin-4(3H)-one derivatives as novel anticancer agents with Aurora kinase inhibition. *Eur. J. Med. Chem.,* **2020**, *190*, 112108.
[http://dx.doi.org/10.1016/j.ejmech.2020.112108] [PMID: 32058239]

[11]   Lo, Y.S.; Nolan, J.C.; Maren, T.H.; Welstead, W.J., Jr; Gripshover, D.F.; Shamblee, D.A. Synthesis and physiochemical properties of sulfamate derivatives as topical antiglaucoma agents. *J. Med. Chem.,* **1992**, *35*(26), 4790-4794.

[http://dx.doi.org/10.1021/jm00104a003] [PMID: 1479580]

[12]   Li, X.L.; Hu, Y.J.; Wang, H.; Yu, B.Q.; Yue, H.L. Molecular spectroscopy evidence of berberine binding to DNA: Comparative binding and thermodynamic profile of intercalation. *Biomacromolecules,* **2012**, *13*(3), 873-880.
[http://dx.doi.org/10.1021/bm2017959] [PMID: 22316074]

[13]   Kang, Y.; Kim, J.; Park, J.; Lee, Y.M.; Saravanakumar, G.; Park, K.M.; Choi, W.; Kim, K.; Lee, E.; Kim, C.; Kim, W.J. Tumor vasodilation by N-Heterocyclic carbene-based nitric oxide delivery triggered by high-intensity focused ultrasound and enhanced drug homing to tumor sites for anticancer therapy. *Biomaterials,* **2019**, *217*, 119297.
[http://dx.doi.org/10.1016/j.biomaterials.2019.119297] [PMID: 31255980]

[14]   Ketron, A.C.; Denny, W.A.; Graves, D.E.; Osheroff, N. Amsacrine as a topoisomerase II poison: Importance of drug-DNA interactions. *Biochemistry,* **2012**, *51*(8), 1730-1739.
[http://dx.doi.org/10.1021/bi201159b] [PMID: 22304499]

[15]   Wang, X.; Li, Y.; Gong, S.; Fu, D. A spectroscopic study on the DNA binding behavior of the anticancer drug dacarbazine. *Spectrosc. Lett.,* **2002**, *35*(6), 751-756.
[http://dx.doi.org/10.1081/SL-120016277]

[16]   Groessl, M.; Reisner, E.; Hartinger, C.G.; Eichinger, R.; Semenova, O.; Timerbaev, A.R.; Jakupec, M.A.; Arion, V.B.; Keppler, B.K. Structure-activity relationships for NAMI-A-type complexes (HL)[trans-RuCl4L(S-dmso)ruthenate(III)] (L = imidazole, indazole, 1,2,4-triazole, 4-amino-1,2-4-triazole, and 1-methyl-1,2,4-triazole): Aquation, redox properties, protein binding, and antiproliferative activity. *J. Med. Chem.,* **2007**, *50*(9), 2185-2193.
[http://dx.doi.org/10.1021/jm061081y] [PMID: 17402720]

[17]   Shalini, K.; Sharma, P.K.; Kumar, N. Imidazole and its biological activities: A review. *Chem. Sin.,* **2010**, *1*, 36-47.

[18]   Eicher, T.; Hauptmann, S. *The Chemistry of Heterocycles: Structures, Reactions, Synthesis and Applications,* 2nd ed; Wiley-VCH Verlag Gmbh& Co., **2003**, pp. 165-166.
[http://dx.doi.org/10.1002/352760183X]

[19]   Finar, I.L. *Organic Chemistry: Stereochemistry and the Chemistry of Natural Products,* 3rd ed; Longmans, Green and Co. Ltd., **1964**, pp. 428-429.

[20]   Obot, I.B.; Obi-Egbedi, N.O.; Umoren, S.A. Adsorption characteristics and corrosion inhibitive properties of clotrimazole for aluminium corrosion in hydrochloric acid. *Int. J. Electrochem. Sci.,* **2009**, *4*, 863-877.

[21]   Siwach, A.; Verma, P.K. Synthesis and therapeutic potential of imidazole containing compounds. *BMC Chem,* **2021**, *15*(1), 12.
[http://dx.doi.org/10.1186/s13065-020-00730-1] [PMID: 33602331]

[22]   Nidhi, R.; Ajay, S.; Randhir, S. Trisubstituted Imidazole Synthesis: A Review Mini-Rev. *Org.Chem.,* *12*(1).
[http://dx.doi.org/10.2174/1570193X11666141028235010]

[23]   Chawla, A.; Sharma, A.; Sharma, A.K. Review: A convenient approach for the synthesis of imidazole derivatives using microwaves. *Pharma Chem.,* **2012**, *4*(1), 116-140.

[24]   Debus, H. Ueber die Einwirkung des Ammoniaks auf GlyoxalAnnalen. *Der. Chemieund. Pharmacie.,* **1858**, *107*(2), 199-208.

[25]   Vanleusen, A.M.; Wildeman, J.; Oldenziel, O. Base induced cycloaddition of sulfonylmethyl isocyanides to c, n double-bonds-synthesis of 1, 5-disubstituted and 1, 4, 5-trisubstituted imidazoles from aldimines and imidoylchlorides. *J. Org. Chem.,* **1977**, *42*(7), 1153-1159.
[http://dx.doi.org/10.1021/jo00427a012]

[26]   Zhang, C.; Moran, E.J.; Woiwode, T.F.; Short, K.M.; Mjalli, A.M.M. Synthesis of tetrasubstituted imidazoles *via* α-(N-acyl-N-alkylamino)-β-ketoamides on Wang resin. *Tetrahedron Lett.,* **1996**, *37*(6),

751-754.
[http://dx.doi.org/10.1016/0040-4039(95)02310-0]

[27]   Balalaie, S.; Hashemi, M.M.; Akhbari, M. A novel one-pot synthesis of tetrasubstituted imidazoles under solvent-free conditions and microwave irradiation. *Tetrahedron Lett.,* **2003**, *44*(8), 1709-1711.
[http://dx.doi.org/10.1016/S0040-4039(03)00018-2]

[28]   Chopra, B.; Dhingra, A.K.; Prasad, D.N. Imidazole: An emerging scaffold showing its therapeutic voyage to develop valuable molecular entities. *Curr. Drug Res. Rev.,* **2021**, *12*(2), 103-117.
[http://dx.doi.org/10.2174/2589977511666191129152038] [PMID: 31782364]

[29]   Lunt, E.; Newton, C.G.; Smith, C.; Stevens, G.P.; Stevens, M.F.G.; Straw, C.G.; Walsh, R.J.A.; Warren, P.J.; Fizames, C.; Lavelle, F. Antitumor imidazotetrazines. 14. Synthesis and antitumor activity of 6- and 8-substituted imidazo[5,1-d]-1,2,3,5-tetrazinones and 8-substituted pyrazolo[5,1-d--1,2,3,5-tetrazinones. *J. Med. Chem.,* **1987**, *30*(2), 357-366.
[http://dx.doi.org/10.1021/jm00385a018] [PMID: 3806616]

[30]   Bredereck, H.; Gompper, R.; Hayer, D. Formamid-Reaktionen, XIII. Imidazole aus α-Diketonen. *Chem. Ber.,* **1959**, *92*(2), 338-343.
[http://dx.doi.org/10.1002/cber.19590920214]

[31]   Robert, C.E. 5- membered heterocycles combining two heteroatoms & their benzo derivatives. Heterocyc. *Compound,* **1957**, *V-5*, 744.

[32]   Wallach, O.; Schulze, E. Ueber Basen der Oxalsäurereihe. *Ber. Dtsch. Chem. Ges.,* **1881**, *14*(1), 420-428.
[http://dx.doi.org/10.1002/cber.18810140195]

[33]   Shabalin, D.A; Camp, J.E Recent advances in the synthesis of imidazoles. *Org. Biomol. Chem,* **2020**, *18*, 3950-3964.
[http://dx.doi.org/10.1039/D0OB00350F]

[34]   Robert, C. E. 5-membered heterocycles combining two heteroatoms & their benzo derivatives. *Heterocyclic Compound,* **1957**, *V-5*, 744.

[35]   Rogoski, J.M.; Nagornyy, P.A. Stereoselective synthesis of piperine *via* a horner wadsworth-emmons reaction. Available from: http://www.geocities.ws/justin_m_r/papers/piperine.pdf

[36]   Sheth, A.H.; Prajapati, P.M.; Shah, Y.R.; Sen, D.J. Synthesis of bispyrimido imidazole fused ring heterocyclic adductwithureas of mannich base for CNS depression. *Int. J. Drug Dev. Res.,* **2009**, *1*(1), 75-80.

[37]   Shaabani, A.; Maleki, A.; Behnam, M. Tandem oxidation process using cerric ammonium nitrate: Three-component synthesis of trisubstitutedimidazoles under aerobic oxidation conditions. *Synth. Commun.,* **2008**, *39*(1), 102-110.
[http://dx.doi.org/10.1080/00397910802369661]

[38]   Lantos, I.; Zhang, W.Y.; Shui, X.; Eggleston, D.S. Synthesis of imidazoles *via* hetero-Cope rearrangements. *J. Org. Chem.,* **1993**, *58*(25), 7092-7095.
[http://dx.doi.org/10.1021/jo00077a033]

[39]   Bleicher, K.H.; Gerber, F.; Wüthrich, Y.; Alanine, A.; Capretta, A. Parallel synthesis of substituted imidazoles from 1,2-aminoalcohols. *Tetrahedron Lett.,* **2002**, *43*(43), 7687-7690.
[http://dx.doi.org/10.1016/S0040-4039(02)01839-7]

[40]   Balalaie, S.; Hashemi, M.M.; Akhbari, M. A novel one-pot synthesis of tetrasubstituted imidazoles under solvent-free conditions and microwave irradiation. *Tetrahedron Lett.,* **2003**, *44*(8), 1709-1711.
[http://dx.doi.org/10.1016/S0040-4039(03)00018-2]

[41]   Balalaie, S.; Arabanian, A. One-pot synthesis of tetrasubstituted imidazoles catalyzed by zeolite HY and silica gel under microwave irradiation. *Green Chem.,* **2000**, *2*(6), 274-276.
[http://dx.doi.org/10.1039/b006201o]

[42]   D'Souza, D.M.; Müller, T.J.J. Multi-component syntheses of heterocycles by transition-metal catalysis. *Chem. Soc. Rev.,* **2007**, *36*(7), 1095-1108.
[http://dx.doi.org/10.1039/B608235C] [PMID: 17576477]

[43]   Zaman, S.; Mitsuru, K.; Abell, A.D. Synthesis of trisubstituted imidazoles by palladium-catalyzed cyclization of O-pentafluorobenzoylamidoximes: Application to amino acid mimetics with a C-terminal imidazole. *Org. Lett.,* **2005**, *7*(4), 609-611.
[http://dx.doi.org/10.1021/ol047628p] [PMID: 15704906]

[44]   Sparks, R.B.; Combs, A.P. Microwave-assisted synthesis of 2,4,5-triaryl-imidazole; a novel thermally induced N-hydroxyimidazole N-O bond cleavage. *Org. Lett.,* **2004**, *6*(14), 2473-2475.
[http://dx.doi.org/10.1021/ol049124x] [PMID: 15228307]

[45]   Chopra, B.; Dhingra, A.K.; Kapoor, R.P.; Parsad, D.N. Microwave assisted novel synthesis and biological evaluation of 1-(Substituted phenyl)-2-phenyl-4-(Substituted benzylidene)-imidazole-5-ones. *Innov. Pharm. Pharmacotherm,* **2015**, *3*(3), 664-672.

[46]   Khan, M.S.; Hayat, M.U.; Khanam, M.; Saeed, H.; Owais, M.; Khalid, M.; Shahid, M.; Ahmad, M. Role of biologically important imidazole moiety on the antimicrobial and anticancer activity of Fe(III) and Mn(II) complexes. *J. Biomol. Struct. Dyn.,* **2020**, 1-14.
[http://dx.doi.org/10.1080/07391102.2020.1776156] [PMID: 32496965]

[47]   Solankee, A.; Kapadia, K.; Patel, J.; Thakor, I. Synthesis and Antimicrobial Activity of 1-Phenyl/Substituted Phenyl/Benzyl/Naphthyl-2-Phenyl-4-(3′-Phenoxy Benzylidene)-Imidazoline-5-ones. *Asian J. Chem.,* **2002**, *14*(2), 699.

[48]   Zhang, H.Z.; Gan, L.L.; Wang, H.; Zhou, C.H. New Progress in Azole Compounds as Antimicrobial Agents. *Mini Rev. Med. Chem.,* **2016**, *17*(2), 122-166.
[http://dx.doi.org/10.2174/1389557516666160630120725] [PMID: 27484625]

[49]   Wright, W.B., Jr; Brabander, H.J.; Hardy, R.A., Jr; Osterberg, A.C. Central nervous system depressants. I. 1-aminoalkyl-3-aryl derivatives of 2-imidazolidinone, 2-imidazolidinethione, and tetrahydro-2(1H)-pyrimidinone. *J. Med. Chem.,* **1966**, *9*(6), 852-857.
[http://dx.doi.org/10.1021/jm00324a017] [PMID: 5972045]

[50]   Soni, J.; Sethiya, A.; Sahiba, N.; Agarwal, D.K.; Agarwal, S. Contemporary Progress in the Synthetic Strategies of Imidazole and its Biological Activities. *Curr. Org. Synth.,* **2020**, *16*(8), 1078-1104.
[http://dx.doi.org/10.2174/1570179416666191007092548] [PMID: 31984918]

[51]   Upadhyay, P.; Pandya, A.; Parekh, H. Possible anticonvulsant imidazoinones. Synthesis and anticonvulsant activity of 1n-(ϒ′-picolinyl)-4-subsituted-benzylidene-2-methyl/-henyl-5-imidazolinone. *J. Indian Chem. Soc.,* **1991**, *68*, 296.

[52]   Visnjic, D.; Dembitz, V.; Lalic, H. The Role of AMPK/mTOR Modulators in the Therapy of Acute Myeloid Leukemia. *Curr. Med. Chem.,* **2019**, *26*(12), 2208-2229.
[http://dx.doi.org/10.2174/0929867325666180117105522] [PMID: 29345570]

[53]   Blanco, M.G.; Vela Gurovic, M.S.; Silbestri, G.F.; Garelli, A.; Giunti, S.; Rayes, D.; De Rosa, M.J. Diisopropylphenyl-imidazole (DII): A new compound that exerts anthelmintic activity through novel molecular mechanisms. *PLoS Negl. Trop. Dis.,* **2018**, *12*(12), e0007021.
[http://dx.doi.org/10.1371/journal.pntd.0007021] [PMID: 30557347]

[54]   Jasim, S.H.; Abu Sheikha, G.M.; Abuzaid, H.M.; Al-Qirim, T.M.; Shattat, G.F.; Sabbah, D.A.; Ala, S.A.; Aboumair, M.S.; Sweidan, K.A.; Bkhaitan, M.M.; Bkhaitan, M.M. synthesis and *in vivo* lipid-lowering activity of novel imidazoles-5-carboxamide derivatives in triton-WR-1339-induced hyperlipidemic wistar rats. *Chem. Pharm. Bull. (Tokyo),* **2018**, *66*(10), 953-958.
[http://dx.doi.org/10.1248/cpb.c18-00346] [PMID: 30270241]

[55]   Chopra, B.; Dhingra, A.K.; Kapoor, R.P.; Parsad, D.N. Microwave assisted synthesis of some 5-substituted imidazolone analogs as a new class of non purine xanthine oxidase inhibitors. *Pharma Chem.,* **2015**, *7*(9), 145-152.

[56] Dhingra, A.K.; Chopra, B.; Dass, R.; Mittal, S.K. Synthesis, antimicrobial and anti-inflammatory activities of some novel 5-substituted imidazolone analogs. *Chin. Chem. Lett.,* **2016**, *27*(5), 707-710. [http://dx.doi.org/10.1016/j.cclet.2016.01.049]

[57] Dhingra, A.K.; Chopra, B.; Dua, J.S.; Prasad, D.N. Therapeutic potential of N-heterocyclic analogs as anti-inflammatory agents. *Antiinflamm. Antiallergy Agents Med. Chem.,* **2018**, *16*(3), 136-152. [http://dx.doi.org/10.2174/1871523017666180126150901] [PMID: 29376495]

[58] Sennequier, N.; Wolan, D.; Stuehr, D.J. Antifungal imidazoles block assembly of inducible NO synthase into an active dimer. *J. Biol. Chem.,* **1999**, *274*(2), 930-938. [http://dx.doi.org/10.1074/jbc.274.2.930] [PMID: 9873034]

[59] Yamada, Y.; Nishii, K.; Kuwata, K.; Nakamichi, M.; Nakanishi, K.; Sugimoto, A.; Ikemoto, K. Effects of pyrroloquinoline quinone and imidazole pyrroloquinoline on biological activities and neural functions. *Heliyon,* **2020**, *6*(1), e03240. [http://dx.doi.org/10.1016/j.heliyon.2020.e03240] [PMID: 32021931]

[60] Jain, R.; Vangapandu, S.; Jain, M.; Kaur, N.; Singh, S.; Pal Singh, P. Antimalarial activities of ring-substituted bioimidazoles. *Bioorg. Med. Chem. Lett.,* **2002**, *12*(13), 1701-1704. [http://dx.doi.org/10.1016/S0960-894X(02)00289-5] [PMID: 12067541]

[61] Yang, W.C.; Li, J.; Li, J.; Chen, Q.; Yang, G.F. Novel synthetic methods for N-cyano-1H-imidazo-e-4-carboxamides and their fungicidal activity. *Bioorg. Med. Chem. Lett.,* **2012**, *22*(3), 1455-1458. [http://dx.doi.org/10.1016/j.bmcl.2011.11.115] [PMID: 22189134]

[62] Ali, I.; Lone, M.; Al-Othman, Z.; Al-Warthan, A.; Sanagi, M. Heterocyclic Scaffolds: Centrality in Anticancer Drug Development. *Curr. Drug Targets,* **2015**, *16*(7), 711-734. [http://dx.doi.org/10.2174/1389450116666150309115922] [PMID: 25751009]

[63] Ameratunga, M.; Pavlakis, N.; Wheeler, H.; Grant, R.; Simes, J.; Khasraw, M. Anti-angiogenic therapy for high-grade glioma. *Cochrane Database Syst. Rev.,* **2018**, *11*(11), CD008218. [PMID: 30480778]

[64] Carmeliet, P. Angiogenesis in life, disease and medicine. *Nature,* **2005**, *438*(7070), 932-936. [http://dx.doi.org/10.1038/nature04478] [PMID: 16355210]

[65] Coultas, L.; Chawengsaksophak, K.; Rossant, J. Endothelial cells and VEGF in vascular development. *Nature,* **2005**, *438*(7070), 937-945. [http://dx.doi.org/10.1038/nature04479] [PMID: 16355211]

[66] Bao, P.; Kodra, A.; Tomic-Canic, M.; Golinko, M.S.; Ehrlich, H.P.; Brem, H. The role of vascular endothelial growth factor in wound healing. *J. Surg. Res.,* **2009**, *153*(2), 347-358. [http://dx.doi.org/10.1016/j.jss.2008.04.023] [PMID: 19027922]

[67] Hansen, A.N.; Bendiksen, C.D.; Sylvest, L.; Friis, T.; Staerk, D.; Jørgensen, F.S.; Olsen, C.A.; Houen, G. Synthesis and antiangiogenic activity of N-alkylated levamisole derivatives. *PLoS One,* **2012**, *7*(9), e45405. [http://dx.doi.org/10.1371/journal.pone.0045405] [PMID: 23024819]

[68] Gudipudi, G.; Sagurthi, S.R.; Perugu, S.; Achaiah, G.; David Krupadanam, G.L. Rational design and synthesis of novel 2-(substituted-2H-chromen-3-yl)-5-aryl-1H-imidazole derivatives as an anti-angiogenesis and anti-cancer agent. *RSC Advances,* **2014**, *4*(99), 56489-56501. [http://dx.doi.org/10.1039/C4RA09945A]

[69] Zhang, J.; Hochwald, S.N. The role of FAK in tumor metabolism and therapy. *Pharmacol. Ther.,* **2014**, *142*(2), 154-163. [http://dx.doi.org/10.1016/j.pharmthera.2013.12.003] [PMID: 24333503]

[70] Li Petri, G.; Pecoraro, C.; Randazzo, O.; Zoppi, S.; Cascioferro, S.M.; Parrino, B.; Carbone, D.; El Hassouni, B.; Cavazzoni, A.; Zaffaroni, N.; Cirrincione, G.; Diana, P.; Peters, G.J.; Giovannetti, E. New Imidazo [2,1- *b*] [1,3,4] Thiadiazole derivatives inhibit FAK phosphorylation and potentiate the antiproliferative effects of gemcitabine through modulation of the human equilibrative nucleoside

transporter-1 in peritoneal mesothelioma. *Anticancer Res.,* **2020**, *40*(9), 4913-4919.
[http://dx.doi.org/10.21873/anticanres.14494] [PMID: 32878779]

[71] Lechertier, T.; Hodivala-Dilke, K. Focal adhesion kinase and tumour angiogenesis. *J. Pathol.,* **2012**, *226*(2), 404-412.
[http://dx.doi.org/10.1002/path.3018] [PMID: 21984450]

[72] Dao, P.; Smith, N.; Tomkiewicz-Raulet, C.; Yen-Pon, E.; Camacho-Artacho, M.; Lietha, D.; Herbeuval, J.P.; Coumoul, X.; Garbay, C.; Chen, H. Design, synthesis, and evaluation of novel imidazo[1,2-a][1,3,5]triazines and their derivatives as focal adhesion kinase inhibitors with antitumor activity. *J. Med. Chem.,* **2015**, *58*(1), 237-251.
[http://dx.doi.org/10.1021/jm500784e] [PMID: 25180654]

[73] Chen, J.; Wang, Z.; Lu, Y.; Dalton, J.T.; Miller, D.D.; Li, W. Synthesis and antiproliferative activity of imidazole and imidazoline analogs for melanoma. *Bioorg. Med. Chem. Lett.,* **2008**, *18*(11), 3183-3187.
[http://dx.doi.org/10.1016/j.bmcl.2008.04.073] [PMID: 18477505]

[74] Jamalian, A.; Shafiee, A.; Hemmateenejad, B.; Khoshneviszadeh, M.; Miri, R.; Madadkar-Sobhani, A.; Bathaie, S.Z.; Moosavi-Movahedi, A.A. Novel imidazolyl derivatives of 1,8-acridinedione as potential DNA-intercalating agents. *J. Indian Chem. Soc.,* **2011**, *8*(4), 1098-1112.
[http://dx.doi.org/10.1007/BF03246568]

[75] Sarkarzadeh, H.; Miri, R.; Firuzi, O.; Amini, M.; Razzaghi-Asl, N.; Edraki, N.; Shafiee, A. Synthesis and antiproliferative activity evaluation of imidazole-based indeno[1,2-b]quinoline-9,11-dione derivatives. *Arch. Pharm. Res.,* **2013**, *36*(4), 436-447.
[http://dx.doi.org/10.1007/s12272-013-0032-7] [PMID: 23440577]

[76] Wang, Z.; Deng, X.; Xiong, S.; Xiong, R.; Liu, J.; Zou, L.; Lei, X.; Cao, X.; Xie, Z.; Chen, Y.; Liu, Y.; Zheng, X.; Tang, G. Design, synthesis and biological evaluation of chrysin benzimidazole derivatives as potential anticancer agents. *Nat. Prod. Res.,* **2018**, *32*(24), 2900-2909.
[http://dx.doi.org/10.1080/14786419.2017.1389940] [PMID: 29063798]

[77] Abonia, R.; Cortés, E.; Insuasty, B.; Quiroga, J.; Nogueras, M.; Cobo, J. Synthesis of novel 1,2,5-trisubstituted benzimidazoles as potential antitumor agents. *Eur. J. Med. Chem.,* **2011**, *46*(9), 4062-4070.
[http://dx.doi.org/10.1016/j.ejmech.2011.06.006] [PMID: 21719162]

[78] Roopashree, R.; Mohan, C.D.; Swaroop, T.R.; Jagadish, S.; Rangappa, K.S. Synthesis, characterization and *in vivo* biological evaluation of novel benzimidazoles as potential anticancer agents. *Asian J. Pharm. Clin. Res.,* **2014**, *7*(5), 309-313.

[79] Alkahtani, H.M.; Abbas, A.Y.; Wang, S. Synthesis and biological evaluation of benzo[d]imidazole derivatives as potential anti-cancer agents. *Bioorg. Med. Chem. Lett.,* **2012**, *22*(3), 1317-1321.
[http://dx.doi.org/10.1016/j.bmcl.2011.12.088] [PMID: 22225635]

[80] Smith, M.A.; Parkinson, D.R.; Cheson, B.D.; Friedman, M.A. Retinoids in cancer therapy. *J. Clin. Oncol.,* **1992**, *10*(5), 839-864.
[http://dx.doi.org/10.1200/JCO.1992.10.5.839] [PMID: 1569455]

[81] Gudas, L.J.; Wagner, J.A. Retinoids regulate stem cell differentiation. *J. Cell. Physiol.,* **2011**, *226*(2), 322-330.
[http://dx.doi.org/10.1002/jcp.22417] [PMID: 20836077]

[82] Lee, J.S.; Newman, R.A.; Lippman, S.M.; Huber, M.H.; Minor, T.; Raber, M.N.; Krakoff, I.H.; Hong, W.K. Phase I evaluation of all-trans-retinoic acid in adults with solid tumors. *J. Clin. Oncol.,* **1993**, *11*(5), 959-966.
[http://dx.doi.org/10.1200/JCO.1993.11.5.959] [PMID: 8487058]

[83] Armstrong, J.L.; Ruiz, M.; Boddy, A.V.; Redfern, C.P.F.; Pearson, A.D.J.; Veal, G.J. Increasing the intracellular availability of all-trans retinoic acid in neuroblastoma cells. *Br. J. Cancer,* **2005**, *92*(4), 696-704.
[http://dx.doi.org/10.1038/sj.bjc.6602398] [PMID: 15714209]

[84]   Ozpolat, B.; Mehta, K.; Lopez-Berestein, G. Regulation of a highly specific retinoic acid--hydroxylase (CYP26A1) enzyme and all- *trans* -retinoic acid metabolism in human intestinal, liver, endothelial, and acute promyelocytic leukemia cells. *Leuk. Lymphoma,* **2005**, *46*(10), 1497-1506.
[http://dx.doi.org/10.1080/10428190500174737] [PMID: 16194896]

[85]   Feng, R.; Fang, L.; Cheng, Y.; He, X.; Jiang, W.; Dong, R.; Shi, H.; Jiang, D.; Sun, L.; Wang, D. Retinoic acid homeostasis through aldh1a2 and cyp26a1 mediates meiotic entry in Nile tilapia (Oreochromis niloticus). *Sci. Rep.,* **2015**, *5*(1), 10131.
[http://dx.doi.org/10.1038/srep10131] [PMID: 25976364]

[86]   Sun, B.; Liu, K.; Han, J.; Zhao, L.; Su, X.; Lin, B.; Zhao, D.M.; Cheng, M.S. Design, synthesis, and biological evaluation of amide imidazole derivatives as novel metabolic enzyme CYP26A1 inhibitors. *Bioorg. Med. Chem.,* **2015**, *23*(20), 6763-6773.
[http://dx.doi.org/10.1016/j.bmc.2015.08.019] [PMID: 26365710]

[87]   Gomaa, M.S.; Bridgens, C.E.; Aboraia, A.S.; Veal, G.J.; Redfern, C.P.F.; Brancale, A.; Armstrong, J.L.; Simons, C. Small molecule inhibitors of retinoic acid 4-hydroxylase (CYP26): Synthesis and biological evaluation of imidazole methyl 3-(4-(aryl-2-ylamino)phenyl)propanoates. *J. Med. Chem.,* **2011**, *54*(8), 2778-2791.
[http://dx.doi.org/10.1021/jm101583w] [PMID: 21428449]

[88]   Stoppie, P.; Borgers, M.; Borghgraef, P.; Dillen, L.; Goossens, J.; Sanz, G.; Szel, H.; Van Hove, C.; Van Nyen, G.; Nobels, G.; Vanden Bossche, H.; Venet, M.; Willemsens, G.; Van Wauwe, J. R115866 inhibits all-trans-retinoic acid metabolism and exerts retinoidal effects in rodents. *J. Pharmacol. Exp. Ther.,* **2000**, *293*(1), 304-312.
[PMID: 10734183]

[89]   Van heusden, J.; Van Ginckel, R.; Bruwiere, H.; Moelans, P.; Janssen, B.; Floren, W.; van der Leede, B.J.; van Dun, J.; Sanz, G.; Venet, M.; Dillen, L.; Van Hove, C.; Willemsens, G.; Janicot, M.; Wouters, W. Inhibition of all-TRANS-retinoic acid metabolism by R116010 induces antitumour activity. *Br. J. Cancer,* **2002**, *86*(4), 605-611.
[http://dx.doi.org/10.1038/sj.bjc.6600056] [PMID: 11870544]

[90]   Mulvihill, M.J.; Kan, J.L.C.; Beck, P.; Bittner, M.; Cesario, C.; Cooke, A.; Keane, D.M.; Nigro, A.I.; Nillson, C.; Smith, V.; Srebernak, M.; Sun, F.L.; Vrkljan, M.; Winski, S.L.; Castelhano, A.L.; Emerson, D.; Gibson, N. Potent and selective [2-imidazol-1-yl-2-(6-alkoxy-naphthal-n-2-yl)-1-methyl-ethyl]-dimethyl-amines as retinoic acid metabolic blocking agents (RAMBAs). *Bioorg. Med. Chem. Lett.,* **2005**, *15*(6), 1669-1673.
[http://dx.doi.org/10.1016/j.bmcl.2005.01.044] [PMID: 15745819]

[91]   Verfaille, C.J.; Thissen, C.A.C.B.; Bovenschen, H.J.; Mertens, J.; Steijlen, P.M.; van de Kerkhof, P.C.M. Oral R115866 in the treatment of moderate to severe plaque-type psoriasis. *J. Eur. Acad. Dermatol. Venereol.,* **2007**, *21*(8), 1038-1046.
[http://dx.doi.org/10.1111/j.1468-3083.2007.02158.x] [PMID: 17714122]

[92]   Geria, A.N.; Scheinfeld, N.S. Talarozole, a selective inhibitor of P450-mediated all-trans retinoic acid for the treatment of psoriasis and acne. *Curr. Opin. Investig. Drugs,* **2008**, *9*(11), 1228-1237.
[PMID: 18951302]

[93]   Sun, B.; Liu, K.; Han, J.; Zhao, L.; Su, X.; Lin, B.; Zhao, D.M.; Cheng, M.S. Design, synthesis, and biological evaluation of amide imidazole derivatives as novel metabolic enzyme CYP26A1 inhibitors. *Bioorg. Med. Chem.,* **2015**, *23*(20), 6763-6773.
[http://dx.doi.org/10.1016/j.bmc.2015.08.019] [PMID: 26365710]

[94]   Gomaa, M.S.; Lim, A.S.T.; Wilson Lau, S.C.; Watts, A.M.; Illingworth, N.A.; Bridgens, C.E.; Veal, G.J.; Redfern, C.P.F.; Brancale, A.; Armstrong, J.L.; Simons, C. Synthesis and CYP26A1 inhibitory activity of novel methyl 3-[4-(arylamino)phenyl]-3-(azole)-2,2-dimethylpropanoates. *Bioorg. Med. Chem.,* **2012**, *20*(20), 6080-6088.
[http://dx.doi.org/10.1016/j.bmc.2012.08.044] [PMID: 22989911]

[95]   Gomaa, M.S.; Bridgens, C.E.; Veal, G.J.; Redfern, C.P.F.; Brancale, A.; Armstrong, J.L.; Simons, C. Synthesis and biological evaluation of 3-(1H-imidazol- and triazol-1-yl)-2,2-dimethy-3-[4-(naphthalen-2-ylamino)phenyl]propyl derivatives as small molecule inhibitors of retinoic acid 4-hydroxylase (CYP26). *J. Med. Chem.,* **2011**, *54*(19), 6803-6811.
[http://dx.doi.org/10.1021/jm200695m] [PMID: 21838328]

[96]   Andoh, T. *DNA Topoisomerases in Cancer Therapy: Present and Future*; Springer Science & Business Media, **2003**.
[http://dx.doi.org/10.1007/978-1-4615-0141-1]

[97]   Jeannot, F.; Taillier, T.; Despeyroux, P.; Renard, S.; Rey, A.; Mourez, M.; Poeverlein, C.; Khichane, I.; Perrin, M.A.; Versluys, S.; Stavenger, R.A.; Huang, J.; Germe, T.; Maxwell, A.; Cao, S.; Huseby, D.L.; Hughes, D.; Bacqué, E. Imidazopyrazinones (IPYs): Non-Quinolone Bacterial Topoisomerase Inhibitors Showing Partial Cross-Resistance with Quinolones. *J. Med. Chem.,* **2018**, *61*(8), 3565-3581.
[http://dx.doi.org/10.1021/acs.jmedchem.7b01892] [PMID: 29596745]

[98]   Wang, H.K.; Morris-Natschke, S.L.; Lee, K.H. Recent advances in the discovery and development of topoisomerase inhibitors as antitumor agents. *Med. Res. Rev.,* **1997**, *17*(4), 367-425.
[http://dx.doi.org/10.1002/(SICI)1098-1128(199707)17:4<367::AID-MED3>3.0.CO;2-U]   [PMID: 9211397]

[99]   Haglof, K.J.; Popa, E.; Hochster, H.S. Recent developments in the clinical activity of topoisomerase-1 inhibitors. *Update Cancer Ther.,* **2006**, *1*(2), 117-145.
[http://dx.doi.org/10.1016/j.uct.2006.05.010]

[100] Hashem, H.E.; Amr, A.E.G.E.; Nossier, E.S.; Elsayed, E.A.; Azmy, E.M. Synthesis, antimicrobial activity and molecular docking of novel thiourea derivatives tagged with thiadiazole, imidazole and triazine moieties as potential DNA gyrase and topoisomerase IV inhibitors. *Molecules,* **2020**, *25*(12), 2766.
[http://dx.doi.org/10.3390/molecules25122766] [PMID: 32549386]

[101] Hande, K.R. Clinical applications of anticancer drugs targeted to topoisomerase II. *Biochim. Biophys. Acta Gene Struct. Expr.,* **1998**, *1400*(1-3), 173-184.
[http://dx.doi.org/10.1016/S0167-4781(98)00134-1] [PMID: 9748560]

[102] Hande, K.R. Etoposide: Four decades of development of a topoisomerase II inhibitor. *Eur. J. Cancer,* **1998**, *34*(10), 1514-1521.
[http://dx.doi.org/10.1016/S0959-8049(98)00228-7] [PMID: 9893622]

[103] Baviskar, A.T.; Madaan, C.; Preet, R.; Mohapatra, P.; Jain, V.; Agarwal, A.; Guchhait, S.K.; Kundu, C.N.; Banerjee, U.C.; Bharatam, P.V. N-fused imidazoles as novel anticancer agents that inhibit catalytic activity of topoisomerase IIα and induce apoptosis in G1/S phase. *J. Med. Chem.,* **2011**, *54*(14), 5013-5030.
[http://dx.doi.org/10.1021/jm200235u] [PMID: 21644529]

[104] Negi, A.; Alex, J.M.; Amrutkar, S.M.; Baviskar, A.T.; Joshi, G.; Singh, S.; Banerjee, U.C.; Kumar, R. Imine/amide–imidazole conjugates derived from 5-amino-4-cyano- N 1-substituted benzyl imidazole: Microwave-assisted synthesis and anticancer activity *via* selective topoisomerase-II-α inhibition. *Bioorg. Med. Chem.,* **2015**, *23*(17), 5654-5661.
[http://dx.doi.org/10.1016/j.bmc.2015.07.020] [PMID: 26216018]

[105] Holleran, J.L.; Parise, R.A.; Yellow-Duke, A.E.; Egorin, M.J.; Eiseman, J.L.; Covey, J.M.; Beumer, J.H. Liquid chromatography–tandem mass spectrometric assay for the quantitation in human plasma of the novel indenoisoquinoline topoisomerase I inhibitors, NSC 743400 and NSC 725776. *J. Pharm. Biomed. Anal.,* **2010**, *52*(5), 714-720.
[http://dx.doi.org/10.1016/j.jpba.2010.02.020] [PMID: 20236781]

[106] Li, Q.; Deng, X.; Zu, Y.; Lv, H.; Su, L.; Yao, L.; Zhang, Y.; Li, L. Cytotoxicity and Topo I targeting activity of substituted 10--nitrogenous heterocyclic aromatic group derivatives of SN-38. *Eur. J. Med. Chem.,* **2010**, *45*(7), 3200-3206.

[http://dx.doi.org/10.1016/j.ejmech.2010.03.013] [PMID: 20392545]

[107] Li, Q.; Lv, H.; Zu, Y.; Qu, Z.; Yao, L.; Su, L.; Liu, C.; Wang, L. Synthesis and antitumor activity of novel 20s-camptothecin analogues. *Bioorg. Med. Chem. Lett.,* **2009**, *19*(2), 513-515.
[http://dx.doi.org/10.1016/j.bmcl.2008.11.031] [PMID: 19056266]

[108] Cinelli, M.A.; Morrell, A.E.; Dexheimer, T.S.; Agama, K.; Agrawal, S.; Pommier, Y.; Cushman, M. The structure–activity relationships of A-ring-substituted aromathecin topoisomerase I inhibitors strongly support a camptothecin-like binding mode. *Bioorg. Med. Chem.,* **2010**, *18*(15), 5535-5552.
[http://dx.doi.org/10.1016/j.bmc.2010.06.040] [PMID: 20630766]

[109] Shang, H.; Chen, H.; Zhao, D.; Tang, X.; Liu, Y.; Pan, L.; Cheng, M. Synthesis and biological evaluation of 4α/4β-imidazolyl podophyllotoxin analogues as antitumor agents. *Arch. Pharm. (Weinheim),* **2012**, *345*(1), 43-48.
[http://dx.doi.org/10.1002/ardp.201100094] [PMID: 21956645]

[110] Sondhi, S.M.; Singh, J.; Rani, R.; Gupta, P.P.; Agrawal, S.K.; Saxena, A.K. Synthesis, anti-inflammatory and anticancer activity evaluation of some novel acridine derivatives. *Eur. J. Med. Chem.,* **2010**, *45*(2), 555-563.
[http://dx.doi.org/10.1016/j.ejmech.2009.10.042] [PMID: 19926172]

[111] Song, Y.; Shao, Z.; Dexheimer, T.S.; Scher, E.S.; Pommier, Y.; Cushman, M. Structure-based design, synthesis, and biological studies of new anticancer norindenoisoquinoline topoisomerase I inhibitors. *J. Med. Chem.,* **2010**, *53*(5), 1979-1989.
[http://dx.doi.org/10.1021/jm901649x] [PMID: 20155916]

[112] Brendel, E.; Ludwig, M.; Lathia, C.; Robert, C.; Ropert, S.; Soria, J.C.; Armand, J.P. Pharmacokinetic results of a phase I trial of sorafenib in combination with dacarbazine in patients with advanced solid tumors. *Cancer Chemother. Pharmacol.,* **2011**, *68*(1), 53-61.
[http://dx.doi.org/10.1007/s00280-010-1423-9] [PMID: 20821331]

[113] Lee, J.; Kim, H.; Yu, H.; Chung, J.Y.; Oh, C.H.; Yoo, K.H.; Sim, T.; Hah, J.M. Discovery and initial SAR of pyrimidin-4-yl-1H-imidazole derivatives with antiproliferative activity against melanoma cell lines. *Bioorg. Med. Chem. Lett.,* **2010**, *20*(5), 1573-1577.
[http://dx.doi.org/10.1016/j.bmcl.2010.01.064] [PMID: 20149658]

[114] Rajitha, C.; Dubey, P.K.; Sunku, V.; Javier Piedrafita, F.; Veeramaneni, V.R.; Pal, M. Synthesis and pharmacological evaluations of novel 2H-benzo[b][1,4]oxazin-3(4H)-one derivatives as a new class of anti-cancer agents. *Eur. J. Med. Chem.,* **2011**, *46*(10), 4887-4896.
[http://dx.doi.org/10.1016/j.ejmech.2011.07.045] [PMID: 21862183]

[115] Yu, H.; Jung, Y.; Kim, H.; Lee, J.; Oh, C.H.; Yoo, K.H.; Sim, T.; Hah, J.M. 1,4-Dihydropyrazolo[4,-d]imidazole phenyl derivatives: A novel type II Raf kinase inhibitors. *Bioorg. Med. Chem. Lett.,* **2010**, *20*(12), 3805-3808.
[http://dx.doi.org/10.1016/j.bmcl.2010.04.039] [PMID: 20466542]

[116] Niculescu-Duvaz, D.; Niculescu-Duvaz, I.; Suijkerbuijk, B.M.J.M.; Ménard, D.; Zambon, A.; Nourry, A.; Davies, L.; Manne, H.A.; Friedlos, F.; Ogilvie, L.; Hedley, D.; Takle, A.K.; Wilson, D.M.; Pons, J.F.; Coulter, T.; Kirk, R.; Cantarino, N.; Whittaker, S.; Marais, R.; Springer, C.J. Novel tricyclic pyrazole BRAF inhibitors with imidazole or furan central scaffolds. *Bioorg. Med. Chem.,* **2010**, *18*(18), 6934-6952.
[http://dx.doi.org/10.1016/j.bmc.2010.06.031] [PMID: 20667740]

[117] Kanthou, C.; Tozer, G.M. Microtubule depolymerizing vascular disrupting agents: Novel therapeutic agents for oncology and other pathologies. *Int. J. Exp. Pathol.,* **2009**, *90*(3), 284-294.
[http://dx.doi.org/10.1111/j.1365-2613.2009.00651.x] [PMID: 19563611]

[118] Olatunde, O.Z.; Yong, J.; Lu, C. The progress of the anticancer agents related to the microtubules target. *Mini Rev. Med. Chem.,* **2021**, *20*(20), 2165-2192.
[http://dx.doi.org/10.2174/1389557520666200729162510] [PMID: 32727327]

[119] Gupta, A.K.; Tulsyan, S.; Bharadwaj, M.; Mehrotra, R. Systematic review on cytotoxic and anticancer

potential of N-substituted isatins as novel class of compounds useful in multidrug-resistant cancer therapy: *In silico* and *in vitro* analysis. *Top. Curr. Chem. (Cham),* **2019**, *377*(3), 15.
[http://dx.doi.org/10.1007/s41061-019-0240-9] [PMID: 31073777]

[120] Ruan, W.; Venkatachalam, G.; Sobota, R.M.; Chen, L.; Wang, L.C.; Jacobson, A.; Paramasivam, K.; Surana, U. Resistance to anti-microtubule drug-induced cell death is determined by regulation of BimEL expression. *Oncogene,* **2019**, *38*(22), 4352-4365.
[http://dx.doi.org/10.1038/s41388-019-0727-4] [PMID: 30770899]

[121] Wang, L.G.; Liu, X.M.; Kreis, W.; Budman, D.R. The effect of antimicrotubule agents on signal transduction pathways of apoptosis: A review. *Cancer Chemother. Pharmacol.,* **1999**, *44*(5), 355-361.
[http://dx.doi.org/10.1007/s002800050989] [PMID: 10501907]

[122] Simoni, D.; Romagnoli, R.; Baruchello, R.; Rondanin, R.; Rizzi, M.; Pavani, M.G.; Alloatti, D.; Giannini, G.; Marcellini, M.; Riccioni, T.; Castorina, M.; Guglielmi, M.B.; Bucci, F.; Carminati, P.; Pisano, C. Novel combretastatin analogues endowed with antitumor activity. *J. Med. Chem.,* **2006**, *49*(11), 3143-3152.
[http://dx.doi.org/10.1021/jm0510732] [PMID: 16722633]

[123] Zhou, J.; Giannakakou, P. Targeting microtubules for cancer chemotherapy. *Curr. Med. Chem. Anticancer Agents,* **2005**, *5*(1), 65-71.
[http://dx.doi.org/10.2174/1568011053352569] [PMID: 15720262]

[124] Carlson, R.O. New tubulin targeting agents currently in clinical development. *Expert Opin. Investig. Drugs,* **2008**, *17*(5), 707-722.
[http://dx.doi.org/10.1517/13543784.17.5.707] [PMID: 18447597]

[125] Budman, D.R. Vinorelbine (Navelbine): A third-generation vinca alkaloid. *Cancer Invest.,* **1997**, *15*(5), 475-490.
[http://dx.doi.org/10.3109/07357909709047587] [PMID: 9316630]

[126] Katsumata, N. Docetaxel: An alternative taxane in ovarian cancer. *Br. J. Cancer,* **2003**, *89*(S3) Suppl. 3, S9-S15.
[http://dx.doi.org/10.1038/sj.bjc.6601495] [PMID: 14661041]

[127] Kamath, K.; Jordan, M.A. Suppression of microtubule dynamics by epothilone B is associated with mitotic arrest. *Cancer Res.,* **2003**, *63*(18), 6026-6031.
[PMID: 14522931]

[128] Li, W.T.; Hwang, D.R.; Song, J.S.; Chen, C.P.; Chuu, J.J.; Hu, C.B.; Lin, H.L.; Huang, C.L.; Huang, C.Y.; Tseng, H.Y.; Lin, C.C.; Chen, T.W.; Lin, C.H.; Wang, H.S.; Shen, C.C.; Chang, C.M.; Chao, Y.S.; Chen, C.T. Synthesis and biological activities of 2-amino-1-arylidenamino imidazoles as orally active anticancer agents. *J. Med. Chem.,* **2010**, *53*(6), 2409-2417.
[http://dx.doi.org/10.1021/jm901501s] [PMID: 20170097]

[129] Li, W.T.; Hwang, D.R.; Song, J.S.; Chen, C.P.; Chen, T.W.; Lin, C.H.; Chuu, J.J.; Lien, T.W.; Hsu, T.A.; Huang, C.L.; Tseng, H.Y.; Lin, C.C.; Lin, H.L.; Chang, C.M.; Chao, Y.S.; Chen, C.T. Synthesis and biological evaluation of 2-amino-1-thiazolyl imidazoles as orally active anticancer agents. *Invest. New Drugs,* **2012**, *30*(1), 164-175.
[http://dx.doi.org/10.1007/s10637-010-9547-7] [PMID: 20890633]

[130] Kamal, A.; Balakrishna, M.; Nayak, V.L.; Shaik, T.B.; Faazil, S.; Nimbarte, V.D. Design and synthesis of imidazo[2,1-b]thiazole-chalcone conjugates: Microtubule-destabilizing agents. *ChemMedChem,* **2014**, *9*(12), 2766-2780.
[http://dx.doi.org/10.1002/cmdc.201402310] [PMID: 25313981]

[131] Stepanov, A.I.; Astrat'ev, A.A.; Sheremetev, A.B.; Lagutina, N.K.; Palysaeva, N.V.; Tyurin, A.Y.; Aleksandrova, N.S.; Sadchikova, N.P.; Suponitsky, K.Y.; Atamanenko, O.P.; Konyushkin, L.D.; Semenov, R.V.; Firgang, S.I.; Kiselyov, A.S.; Semenova, M.N.; Semenov, V.V. A facile synthesis and microtubule-destabilizing properties of 4-(1H-benzo[d]imidazol-2-yl)-furazan-3-amines. *Eur. J. Med. Chem.,* **2015**, *94*, 237-251.

[http://dx.doi.org/10.1016/j.ejmech.2015.02.051] [PMID: 25768706]

[132] Semenova, M.N.; Kiselyov, A.; Semenov, V.V. Sea urchin embryo as a model organism for the rapid functional screening of tubulin modulators. *Biotechniques,* **2006**, *40*(6), 765-774. [http://dx.doi.org/10.2144/000112193] [PMID: 16774120]

[133] Semenova, M.N.; Kiselyov, A.S.; Titov, I.Y.; Raihstat, M.M.; Molodtsov, M.; Grishchuk, E.; Spiridonov, I.; Semenov, V.V. *In vivo* evaluation of indolyl glyoxamides in the phenotypic sea urchin embryo assay. *Chem. Biol. Drug Des.,* **2007**, *70*(6), 485-490. [http://dx.doi.org/10.1111/j.1747-0285.2007.00591.x] [PMID: 17991295]

[134] Kiselyov, A.S.; Semenova, M.N.; Chernyshova, N.B.; Leitao, A.; Samet, A.V.; Kislyi, K.A.; Raihstat, M.M.; Oprea, T.; Lemcke, H.; Lantow, M.; Weiss, D.G.; Ikizalp, N.N.; Kuznetsov, S.A.; Semenov, V.V. Novel derivatives of 1,3,4-oxadiazoles are potent mitostatic agents featuring strong microtubule depolymerizing activity in the sea urchin embryo and cell culture assays. *Eur. J. Med. Chem.,* **2010**, *45*(5), 1683-1697. [http://dx.doi.org/10.1016/j.ejmech.2009.12.072] [PMID: 20110137]

[135] Gesner, T.G.; Harrison, S.D. Intracellular signaling targets for cancer chemosensitization. *Annu. Rep. Med. Chem.,* **2002**, *37*, 115-124. [http://dx.doi.org/10.1016/S0065-7743(02)37013-1]

[136] Sharma, V.; Hupp, C.; Tepe, J. Enhancement of chemotherapeutic efficacy by small molecule inhibition of NF-kappaB and checkpoint kinases. *Curr. Med. Chem.,* **2007**, *14*(10), 1061-1074. [http://dx.doi.org/10.2174/092986707780362844] [PMID: 17456020]

[137] Li, Q.; Zhu, G.D. Targeting serine/threonine protein kinase B/Akt and cell-cycle checkpoint kinases for treating cancer. *Curr. Top. Med. Chem.,* **2002**, *2*(9), 939-971. [http://dx.doi.org/10.2174/1568026023393318] [PMID: 12171565]

[138] Zhao, H.; Watkins, J.L.; Piwnica-Worms, H. Disruption of the checkpoint kinase 1/cell division cycle 25A pathway abrogates ionizing radiation-induced S and G$_2$ checkpoints. *Proc. Natl. Acad. Sci. USA,* **2002**, *99*(23), 14795-14800. [http://dx.doi.org/10.1073/pnas.182557299] [PMID: 12399544]

[139] Xiao, Z.; Chen, Z.; Gunasekera, A.H.; Sowin, T.J.; Rosenberg, S.H.; Fesik, S.; Zhang, H. Chk1 mediates S and G2 arrests through Cdc25A degradation in response to DNA-damaging agents. *J. Biol. Chem.,* **2003**, *278*(24), 21767-21773. [http://dx.doi.org/10.1074/jbc.M300229200] [PMID: 12676925]

[140] Zhao, B.; Bower, M.J.; McDevitt, P.J.; Zhao, H.; Davis, S.T.; Johanson, K.O.; Green, S.M.; Concha, N.O.; Zhou, B.B.S. Structural basis for Chk1 inhibition by UCN-01. *J. Biol. Chem.,* **2002**, *277*(48), 46609-46615. [http://dx.doi.org/10.1074/jbc.M201233200] [PMID: 12244092]

[141] Takahashi, I.; Kobayashi, E.; Asano, K.; Yoshida, M.; Nakano, H. UCN-01, a selective inhibitor of protein kinase C from Streptomyces. *J. Antibiot. (Tokyo),* **1987**, *40*(12), 1782-1784. [http://dx.doi.org/10.7164/antibiotics.40.1782] [PMID: 3429345]

[142] Graves, P.R.; Yu, L.; Schwarz, J.K.; Gales, J.; Sausville, E.A.; O'Connor, P.M.; Piwnica-Worms, H. The Chk1 protein kinase and the Cdc25C regulatory pathways are targets of the anticancer agent UCN-01. *J. Biol. Chem.,* **2000**, *275*(8), 5600-5605. [http://dx.doi.org/10.1074/jbc.275.8.5600] [PMID: 10681541]

[143] Bunch, R.T.; Eastman, A. Enhancement of cisplatin-induced cytotoxicity by 7-hydroxystaurosporine (UCN-01), a new G2-checkpoint inhibitor. *Clin. Cancer Res.,* **1996**, *2*(5), 791-797. [PMID: 9816232]

[144] Busby, E.C.; Leistritz, D.F.; Abraham, R.T.; Karnitz, L.M.; Sarkaria, J.N. The radiosensitizing agent 7-hydroxystaurosporine (UCN-01) inhibits the DNA damage checkpoint kinase hChk1. *Cancer Res.,* **2000**, *60*(8), 2108-2112. [PMID: 10786669]

[145]   Wang, Q.; Fan, S.; Eastman, A.; Worland, P.J.; Sausville, E.A.; O'Connor, P.M. UCN-01: A potent abrogator of G2 checkpoint function in cancer cells with disrupted p53. *J. Natl. Cancer Inst.,* **1996**, *88*(14), 956-965.
[http://dx.doi.org/10.1093/jnci/88.14.956] [PMID: 8667426]

[146]   Sausville, E.A.; Arbuck, S.G.; Messmann, R.; Headlee, D.; Bauer, K.S.; Lush, R.M.; Murgo, A.; Figg, W.D.; Lahusen, T.; Jaken, S.; Jing, X.; Roberge, M.; Fuse, E.; Kuwabara, T.; Senderowicz, A.M. Phase I trial of 72-hour continuous infusion UCN-01 in patients with refractory neoplasms. *J. Clin. Oncol.,* **2001**, *19*(8), 2319-2333.
[http://dx.doi.org/10.1200/JCO.2001.19.8.2319] [PMID: 11304786]

[147]   Falck, J.; Mailand, N.; Syljuåsen, R.G.; Bartek, J.; Lukas, J. The ATM–Chk2–Cdc25A checkpoint pathway guards against radioresistant DNA synthesis. *Nature,* **2001**, *410*(6830), 842-847.
[http://dx.doi.org/10.1038/35071124] [PMID: 11298456]

[148]   Ni, Z.J.; Barsanti, P.; Brammeier, N.; Diebes, A.; Poon, D.J.; Ng, S.; Pecchi, S.; Pfister, K.; Renhowe, P.A.; Ramurthy, S.; Wagman, A.S.; Bussiere, D.E.; Le, V.; Zhou, Y.; Jansen, J.M.; Ma, S.; Gesner, T.G. 4-(Aminoalkylamino)-3-benzimidazole-quinolinones as potent CHK-1 inhibitors. *Bioorg. Med. Chem. Lett.,* **2006**, *16*(12), 3121-3124.
[http://dx.doi.org/10.1016/j.bmcl.2006.03.059] [PMID: 16603354]

[149]   Martínez, R.; Di Geronimo, B.; Pastor, M.; Zapico, J.M.; Coderch, C.; Panchuk, R.; Skorokhyd, N.; Maslyk, M.; Ramos, A.; de Pascual-Teresa, B. Multitarget Anticancer Agents Based on Histone Deacetylase and Protein Kinase CK2 Inhibitors. *Molecules,* **2020**, *25*(7), 1497.
[http://dx.doi.org/10.3390/molecules25071497] [PMID: 32218358]

[150]   McClure, K.J.; Huang, L.; Arienti, K.L.; Axe, F.U.; Brunmark, A.; Blevitt, J.; Guy Breitenbucher, J. Novel non-benzimidazole chk2 kinase inhibitors. *Bioorg. Med. Chem. Lett.,* **2006**, *16*(7), 1924-1928.
[http://dx.doi.org/10.1016/j.bmcl.2005.12.096] [PMID: 16442290]

[151]   Skibo, E.B.; Schulz, W.G. Pyrrolo[1,2-a]benzimidazole-based aziridinyl quinones. A new class of DNA cleaving agent exhibiting G and A base specificity. *J. Med. Chem.,* **1993**, *36*(21), 3050-3055.
[http://dx.doi.org/10.1021/jm00073a002] [PMID: 8230090]

[152]   Skibo, E.B.; Islam, I.; Heileman, M.J.; Schulz, W.G. Structure-activity studies of benzimidazole-based DNA-cleaving agents. Comparison of benzimidazole, pyrrolobenzimidazole, and tetrahydropyridobenzimidazole analogs. *J. Med. Chem.,* **1994**, *37*(1), 78-92.
[http://dx.doi.org/10.1021/jm00027a010] [PMID: 8289204]

[153]   Boruah, R.C.; Skibo, E.B. A comparison of the cytotoxic and physical properties of aziridinyl quinone derivatives based on the pyrrolo[1,2-a]benzimidazole and pyrrolo[1,2-a]indole ring systems. *J. Med. Chem.,* **1994**, *37*(11), 1625-1631.
[http://dx.doi.org/10.1021/jm00037a013] [PMID: 8201596]

[154]   Tahlan, S.; Narasimhan, B.; Lim, S.M.; Ramasamy, K.; Mani, V.; Shah, S.A.A. Design, Synthesis, SAR Study, Antimicrobial and Anticancer Evaluation of Novel 2-Mercaptobenzimidazole Azomethine Derivatives. *Mini Rev. Med. Chem.,* **2020**, *20*(15), 1559-1571.
[http://dx.doi.org/10.2174/1389557518666180903151849] [PMID: 30179132]

[155]   Ramla, M.M.; Omar, M.A.; Tokuda, H.; El-Diwani, H.I. Synthesis and inhibitory activity of new benzimidazole derivatives against Burkitt's lymphoma promotion. *Bioorg. Med. Chem.,* **2007**, *15*(19), 6489-6496.
[http://dx.doi.org/10.1016/j.bmc.2007.04.010] [PMID: 17643992]

[156]   Abdel-Mohsen, H.T.; Ragab, F.A.F.; Ramla, M.M.; El Diwani, H.I. Novel benzimidazole–pyrimidine conjugates as potent antitumor agents. *Eur. J. Med. Chem.,* **2010**, *45*(6), 2336-2344.
[http://dx.doi.org/10.1016/j.ejmech.2010.02.011] [PMID: 20356655]

[157]   Ramla, M.M.; Omar, M.A.; El-Khamry, A.M.M.; El-Diwani, H.I. Synthesis and antitumor activity of 1-substituted-2-methyl-5-nitrobenzimidazoles. *Bioorg. Med. Chem.,* **2006**, *14*(21), 7324-7332.
[http://dx.doi.org/10.1016/j.bmc.2006.06.033] [PMID: 16860558]

[158] Shaharyar, M.; Abdullah, M.M.; Bakht, M.A.; Majeed, J. Pyrazoline bearing benzimidazoles: Search for anticancer agent. *Eur. J. Med. Chem.,* **2010**, *45*(1), 114-119.
[http://dx.doi.org/10.1016/j.ejmech.2009.09.032] [PMID: 19883957]

[159] Luo, Y.; Xiao, F.; Qian, S.; Lu, W.; Yang, B. Synthesis and *in vitro* cytotoxic evaluation of some thiazolylbenzimidazole derivatives. *Eur. J. Med. Chem.,* **2011**, *46*(1), 417-422.
[http://dx.doi.org/10.1016/j.ejmech.2010.11.014] [PMID: 21115212]

[160] Refaat, H.M. Synthesis and anticancer activity of some novel 2-substituted benzimidazole derivatives. *Eur. J. Med. Chem.,* **2010**, *45*(7), 2949-2956.
[http://dx.doi.org/10.1016/j.ejmech.2010.03.022] [PMID: 20399544]

[161] Ng, R.A.; Guan, J.; Alford, V.C., Jr; Lanter, J.C.; Allan, G.F.; Sbriscia, T.; Lundeen, S.G.; Sui, Z. 2-(2,2,2-Trifluoroethyl)-5,6-dichlorobenzimidazole derivatives as potent androgen receptor antagonists. *Bioorg. Med. Chem. Lett.,* **2007**, *17*(4), 955-958.
[http://dx.doi.org/10.1016/j.bmcl.2006.11.047] [PMID: 17134895]

[162] Gowda, N.R.T.; Kavitha, C.V.; Chiruvella, K.K.; Joy, O.; Rangappa, K.S.; Raghavan, S.C. Synthesis and biological evaluation of novel 1-(4-methoxyphenethyl)-1H-benzimidazole-5-carboxylic acid derivatives and their precursors as antileukemic agents. *Bioorg. Med. Chem. Lett.,* **2009**, *19*(16), 4594-4600.
[http://dx.doi.org/10.1016/j.bmcl.2009.06.103] [PMID: 19616939]

[163] Hranjec, M.; Pavlović, G.; Marjanović, M.; Kralj, M.; Karminski-Zamola, G. Benzimidazole derivatives related to 2,3-acrylonitriles, benzimidazo[1,2-a]quinolines and fluorenes: Synthesis, antitumor evaluation *in vitro* and crystal structure determination. *Eur. J. Med. Chem.,* **2010**, *45*(6), 2405-2417.
[http://dx.doi.org/10.1016/j.ejmech.2010.02.022] [PMID: 20207049]

[164] Chen, A.Y.; Yu, C.; Gatto, B.; Liu, L.F. DNA minor groove-binding ligands: A different class of mammalian DNA topoisomerase I inhibitors. *Proc. Natl. Acad. Sci. USA,* **1993**, *90*(17), 8131-8135.
[http://dx.doi.org/10.1073/pnas.90.17.8131] [PMID: 7690143]

[165] Chen, A.Y.; Yu, C.; Bodley, A.; Peng, L.F.; Liu, L.F. A new mammalian DNA topoisomerase I poison Hoechst 33342: Cytotoxicity and drug resistance in human cell cultures. *Cancer Res.,* **1993**, *53*(6), 1332-1337.
[PMID: 8383008]

[166] Kraut, E.; Fleming, T.; Segal, M.; Neidhart, J.; Behrens, B.; MacDonald, J. Phase II study of pibenzimol in pancreatic cancer. *Invest. New Drugs,* **1991**, *9*(1), 95-96.
[http://dx.doi.org/10.1007/BF00194556] [PMID: 1709154]

[167] Tolner, B.; Hartley, J.A.; Hochhauser, D. Transcriptional regulation of topoisomerase II α at confluence and pharmacological modulation of expression by bis-benzimidazole drugs. *Mol. Pharmacol.,* **2001**, *59*(4), 699-706.
[http://dx.doi.org/10.1124/mol.59.4.699] [PMID: 11259613]

[168] Beerman, T.A.; McHugh, M.M.; Sigmund, R.; Lown, J.W.; Rao, K.E.; Bathini, Y. Effects of analogs of the DNA minor groove binder Hoechst 33258 on topoisomerase II and I mediated activities. *Biochim. Biophys. Acta Gene Struct. Expr.,* **1992**, *1131*(1), 53-61.
[http://dx.doi.org/10.1016/0167-4781(92)90098-K] [PMID: 1374646]

[169] Lungu, C.N.; Bratanovici, B.I.; Grigore, M.M.; Antoci, V.; Mangalagiu, I.I. Hybrid imidazole-pyridine derivatives: An approach to novel anticancer DNA intercalators. *Curr. Med. Chem.,* **2020**, *27*(1), 154-169.
[http://dx.doi.org/10.2174/0929867326666181220094229] [PMID: 30569842]

[170] Wang, X.Q.; Liu, L.X.; Li, Y.; Sun, C.J.; Chen, W.; Li, L.; Zhang, H.B.; Yang, X.D. Design, synthesis and biological evaluation of novel hybrid compounds of imidazole scaffold-based 2-benzylbenzofuran as potent anticancer agents. *Eur. J. Med. Chem.,* **2013**, *62*, 111-121.
[http://dx.doi.org/10.1016/j.ejmech.2012.12.040] [PMID: 23353748]

[171] Singh, K.; Verma, V.; Yadav, K.; Sreekanth, V.; Kumar, D.; Bajaj, A.; Kumar, V. Design, regioselective synthesis and cytotoxic evaluation of 2-aminoimidazole–quinoline hybrids against cancer and primary endothelial cells. *Eur. J. Med. Chem.,* **2014**, *87*, 150-158.
       [http://dx.doi.org/10.1016/j.ejmech.2014.09.055] [PMID: 25247771]

[172] Copp, B.R.; Fairchild, C.R.; Cornell, L.; Casazza, A.M.; Robinson, S.; Ireland, C.M. Naamidine A is an antagonist of the epidermal growth factor receptor and an *in vivo* active antitumor agent. *J. Med. Chem.,* **1998**, *41*(20), 3909-3911.
       [http://dx.doi.org/10.1021/jm980294n] [PMID: 9748366]

[173] Hassan, W.; Edrada, R.; Ebel, R.; Wray, V.; Berg, A.; van Soest, R.; Wiryowidagdo, S.; Proksch, P. New imidazole alkaloids from the Indonesian sponge Leucetta chagosensis. *J. Nat. Prod.,* **2004**, *67*(5), 817-822.
       [http://dx.doi.org/10.1021/np0305223] [PMID: 15165143]

[174] Newman, D.J.; Cragg, G.M. Advanced preclinical and clinical trials of natural products and related compounds from marine sources. *Curr. Med. Chem.,* **2004**, *11*(13), 1693-1713.
       [http://dx.doi.org/10.2174/0929867043364982] [PMID: 15279577]

[175] Alvi, K.A.; Crews, P.; Loughhead, D.G. Structures and total synthesis of 2-aminoimidazoles from a Notodoris nudibranch. *J. Nat. Prod.,* **1991**, *54*(6), 1509-1515.
       [http://dx.doi.org/10.1021/np50078a004]

[176] Alvi, K.A.; Peters, B.M.; Lisa, H.M.; Phillip, C. 2-Aminoimidazoles and their zinc complexes from indo-pacific leucetta sponges and notodoris nudibranchs. *Tetrahedron,* **1993**, *49*(2), 329-336.
       [http://dx.doi.org/10.1016/S0040-4020(01)80302-1]

[177] Liu, X.; Han, Y.; Ge, X.; Liu, Z. Imidazole and Benzimidazole Modified Half-Sandwich IridiumIIIN-Heterocyclic Carbene Complexes: Synthesis, Anticancer Application, and Organelle Targeting. *Front Chem.,* **2020**, *8*, 182.
       [http://dx.doi.org/10.3389/fchem.2020.00182]

[178] Zhang, L.; Peng, X.M.; Damu, G.L.V.; Geng, R.X.; Zhou, C.H. Comprehensive review in current developments of imidazole-based medicinal chemistry. *Med. Res. Rev.,* **2014**, *34*(2), 340-437.
       [http://dx.doi.org/10.1002/med.21290] [PMID: 23740514]

[179] Ali, I.; Lone, M.N.; Aboul-Enein, H.Y. Imidazoles as potential anticancer agents. *MedChemComm,* **2017**, *8*(9), 1742-1773.
       [http://dx.doi.org/10.1039/C7MD00067G] [PMID: 30108886]

[180] Pectasides, D.; Yianniotis, H.; Alevizakos, N.; Bafaloukos, D.; Barbounis, V.; Varthalitis, J.; Dimitriadis, M.; Athanassiou, A. Treatment of metastatic malignant melanoma with dacarbazine, vindesine and cisplatin. *Br. J. Cancer,* **1989**, *60*(4), 627-629.
       [http://dx.doi.org/10.1038/bjc.1989.327] [PMID: 2803936]

[181] Hawwa, A.F.; Millership, J.S.; Collier, P.S.; Vandenbroeck, K.; McCarthy, A.; Dempsey, S.; Cairns, C.; Collins, J.; Rodgers, C.; McElnay, J.C. Pharmacogenomic studies of the anticancer and immunosuppressive thiopurines mercaptopurine and azathioprine. *Br. J. Clin. Pharmacol.,* **2008**, *66*(4), 517-528.
       [http://dx.doi.org/10.1111/j.1365-2125.2008.03248.x] [PMID: 18662289]

[182] Josephy, P.D.; Palcic, B.; Skarsgard, L.D. *In vitro* metabolism of misonidazole. *Br. J. Cancer,* **1981**, *43*(4), 443-450.
       [http://dx.doi.org/10.1038/bjc.1981.65] [PMID: 7236487]

[183] Varia, M.A.; Calkins-Adams, D.P.; Rinker, L.H.; Kennedy, A.S.; Novotny, D.B.; Fowler, W.C., Jr; Raleigh, J.A. Pimonidazole: A novel hypoxia marker for complementary study of tumor hypoxia and cell proliferation in cervical carcinoma. *Gynecol. Oncol.,* **1998**, *71*(2), 270-277.
       [http://dx.doi.org/10.1006/gyno.1998.5163] [PMID: 9826471]

[184] Hartmann, M.; Zimmer, C. Investigation of cross-link formation in DNA by the alkylating cytostatica

IMET 3106, 3393 and 3943. *Biochim. Biophys. Acta Nucleic Acids Protein Synth.,* **1972**, *287*(3), 386-389.
[http://dx.doi.org/10.1016/0005-2787(72)90282-1] [PMID: 4629776]

[185] Kath, R.; Blumenstengel, K.; Fricke, H.J.; Höffken, K. Bendamustine monotherapy in advanced and refractory chronic lymphocytic leukemia. *J. Cancer Res. Clin. Oncol.,* **2001**, *127*(1), 48-54.
[http://dx.doi.org/10.1007/s004320000180] [PMID: 11206271]

[186] Yang, Y.; Jin, C.; Li, H.; He, Y.; Liu, Z.; Bai, L.; Dou, K. Improved radiosensitizing effect of the combination of etanidazole and paclitaxel for hepatocellular carcinoma *in vivo. Exp. Ther. Med.,* **2012**, *3*(2), 299-303.
[http://dx.doi.org/10.3892/etm.2011.389] [PMID: 22969885]

[187] Li, E.C.; Davis, L.E. Zoledronic acid: A new parenteral bisphosphonate. *Clin. Ther.,* **2003**, *25*(11), 2669-2708.
[http://dx.doi.org/10.1016/S0149-2918(03)80327-2] [PMID: 14693298]

[188] Thomas, X.; Elhamri, M. Tipifarnib in the treatment of acute myeloid leukemia. *Biologics,* **2007**, *1*(4), 415-424.
[PMID: 19707311]

[189] Raats, J.I.; Falkson, G.; Falkson, H.C. A study of fadrozole, a new aromatase inhibitor, in postmenopausal women with advanced metastatic breast cancer. *J. Clin. Oncol.,* **1992**, *10*(1), 111-116.
[http://dx.doi.org/10.1200/JCO.1992.10.1.111] [PMID: 1530798]

[190] Beck, D.E.; Agama, K.; Marchand, C.; Chergui, A.; Pommier, Y.; Cushman, M. Synthesis and biological evaluation of new carbohydrate-substituted indenoisoquinoline topoisomerase I inhibitors and improved syntheses of the experimental anticancer agents indotecan (LMP400) and indimitecan (LMP776). *J. Med. Chem.,* **2014**, *57*(4), 1495-1512.
[http://dx.doi.org/10.1021/jm401814y] [PMID: 24517248]

CHAPTER 5

Morpholine: Pharmacophore Modulating Pharmacokinetic Properties of Anticancer Leads

Archana Kumari[1] and **Rajesh K. Singh**[2,*]

[1] *School of Pharmaceutical Sciences, Lovely Professional University, Phagwara, 144001, Punjab, India*

[2] *Department of Pharmaceutical Chemistry, Shivalik College of Pharmacy, Nangal, Dist. Rupnagar, 140126, Punjab, India*

Abstract: The morpholine ring is considered the most preferred and versatile heterocylic ring in medicinal chemistry due to its distinctive mechanistic activities that give it various biological activities. The eminence of the morpholine ring to modulate the pharmacokinetic properties of the compound, further makes it a fundamental pharmacophore in developing lead molecules. Multi-drug resistance in cancer leads to discovering selective and potent chemotherapeutic agents. Researchers are designing and synthesizing morpholine derivatives as potential anticancer drugs those act by targeting various signaling pathways driven by various protein kinases in the cell, *i.e.* Ras-Raf-MEK-ERK (ERK) and PI3K/Akt/mTOR, thereby inhibiting cell proliferation and growth. The potency of natural and synthetic derivatives of morpholine makes it a drug of choice for cancer treatment. Many of the morpholine containing anticancer drugs are under clinical trials. Hence, morpholine ring synthesis also becomes a central target for various scientists using green synthesis by straightforward one-step methods. A substantial literature is available on synthetic techniques of morpholine and substituted morpholine. The present chapter updates diverse new synthetic strategies of the morpholine ring and morpholine derivatives with potent anticancer activity. The chapter will also highlight the clinical data of morpholine derivatives with anticancer activity and mechanism of action. The latest information on novel anticancer morpholine derivatives with structural activity relationship (SAR) is also included. This chapter provides information about the necessary structural modifications required in drugs' chemical structure and contribute to the anticancer drug discovery program.

Keywords: Anticancer, Morpholine, Pharmacokinetic, PI3K/Akt/mTOR, Protein kinase, Ras-Raf-MEK-ERK (ERK), Structure-activity relationship (SAR).

---

[*] **Corresponding author Rajesh K. Singh:** Department of Pharmaceutical Chemistry, Shivalik College of Pharmacy, Nangal, Dist. Rupnagar, 140126, Punjab, India; Tel: +919417513730; E-mail: rksingh244@gmail.com

Rajesh Kumar Singh (Ed.)

INTRODUCTION

The versatility of heterocyclic compounds makes them an attractive target for researchers all over the world [1, 2]. Both natural and synthetic compounds are found to be pharmacologically active [3, 4]. Therefore, people's get motivated to prepare synthetic analogues of natural compounds with implausible activity. Morpholine is an organic chemical, structurally six-membered ring containing two hetero atoms, nitrogen and oxygen, hence, considered as an important nucleus in the field of medicinal chemistry, catalyst, rubber chemical, corrosion inhibitor [5]. It was commercially available in the USA in 1935, and wide pharmacological and industrial applications made it very popular molecule. Pharmacologically, it is used as an analgesic, anticancer, antimicrobial, anti-inflammatory, anti-viral agents, antidepressant, HIV-protease inhibitors, *etc*. [6]. Industrially, it acts as rubber chemical, corrosion inhibitor, wax emulsifier, optical brighteners, separating agent, surface-active agents, and also act as catalyst such as chiral organocatalysis, chiral auxiliaries, chiral models α-hydroxy acid and oxacycle synthesis in the laboratory [7, 8]. Various miscellaneous applications can also be seen of morpholine derivatives in medicinal chemistry [9 - 14].

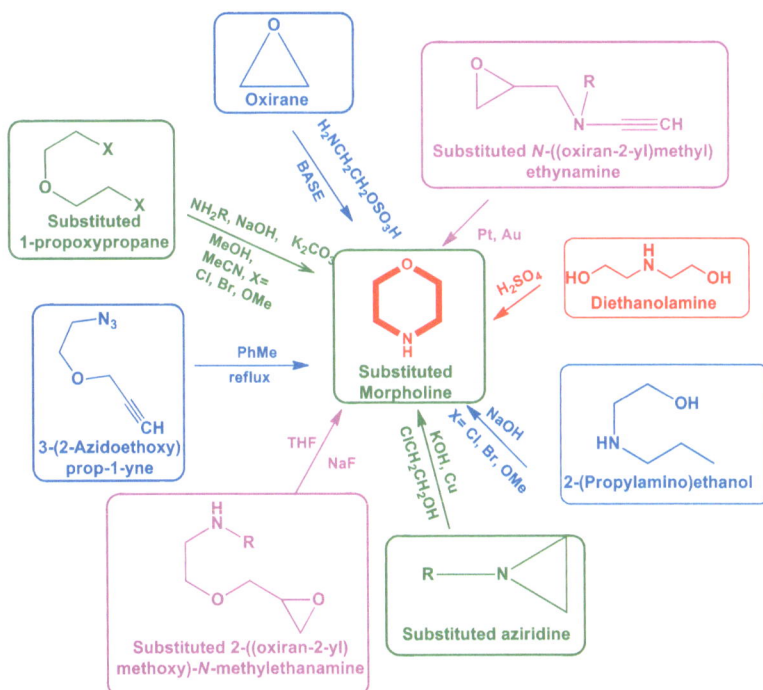

Scheme 1. Morpholine ring synthesis by different chemical reactions.

Different Strategies for Morpholine Ring Synthesis

The morpholine ring synthesis performed by intramolecular cyclization, requiring a variety of conditions [15]. Various strategies followed of the synthesis of the morpholine nucleus have been presented in Scheme (**1**) [16]. However, some limitations on the reaction conditions, time and yield, led to the design of new techniques for synthesizing morpholine nucleus as presented in Scheme (**2**) [17 - 24].

Natural and Synthetic Sources of Morpholine

Various natural products contain an essential pharmacologically active moiety-morpholine. Marine sponge Chelonaplysilla, have important morpholine containing alkaloids *i.e.*, Chelonin A 1 & Chelonin C 2 (Fig. **1**), having potent anti-inflammatory and antimicrobial effect [25, 26]. Similarly essential alkaloid, syn-3-isopropyl-6-(4-methoxybenzyl)-4-methylmorpholine-2,5-dione 3 (Fig. **1**) obtained from Thai sea hare, *Bursatella leachii*, found to be a potent anticancer compound [26]. Marine sponge *Monanchora pulchra* secrete the chemical Monanchocidin A 4 (Fig. **1**), has good antitumor activity [27]. In view of the pharmacological activity of various natural derivatives of morpholine, the researchers are motivated and oriented towards the synthesis of a variety of non-steroidal anti-inflammatory drugs of compounds of morpholine. At the nuclear level, morpholine conjugated drugs are found to suppress the activity of antiapoptotic kinases *i.e.*, Bcr-Abl, leads to increased differentiation and apoptosis [28]. In 1978, Timolol 5 (Fig. **1**) comes on the market. By means of the β-adrenoceptor blocking mechanism, it is used to treat angina and hypertension [29]. Merlion pharmaceuticals and Alcon Company developed Finafloxacin 6 (Fig. **1**), and approved by FDA as a potential drug for the treatment of *P. aerugenosa* and *S. aureus* bacterial infections [30]. Pfizer developed Reboxetine 7 (Fig. **1**) as an antidepressant drug [31]. In 1996, Levofloxacin 8 (Fig. **1**), was approved by the US against various infections [32]. In 1950, the German pharmaceutical company Ravensberg made improvements to Morazone 9 (Fig. **1**) and having nonsteroidal anti-inflammatory activity [33, 34]. Moclobemide 10 (Fig. **1**) used in the treatment of depression and anxiety, was first marketed in 1992 [35].

For decades, morpholine has been incorporated by medicinal chemists as a lead molecule and various marketed clinical medicines with different therapeutic effects [36]. The present chapter provides an overview of different synthetic strategies of morpholine derivatives along with structure-activity relationship studies depicting anticancer activity. The chapter also highlights the role of morpholine in altering the potency and pharmacokinetics of various morpholine drugs in clinical trials (Table **1**).

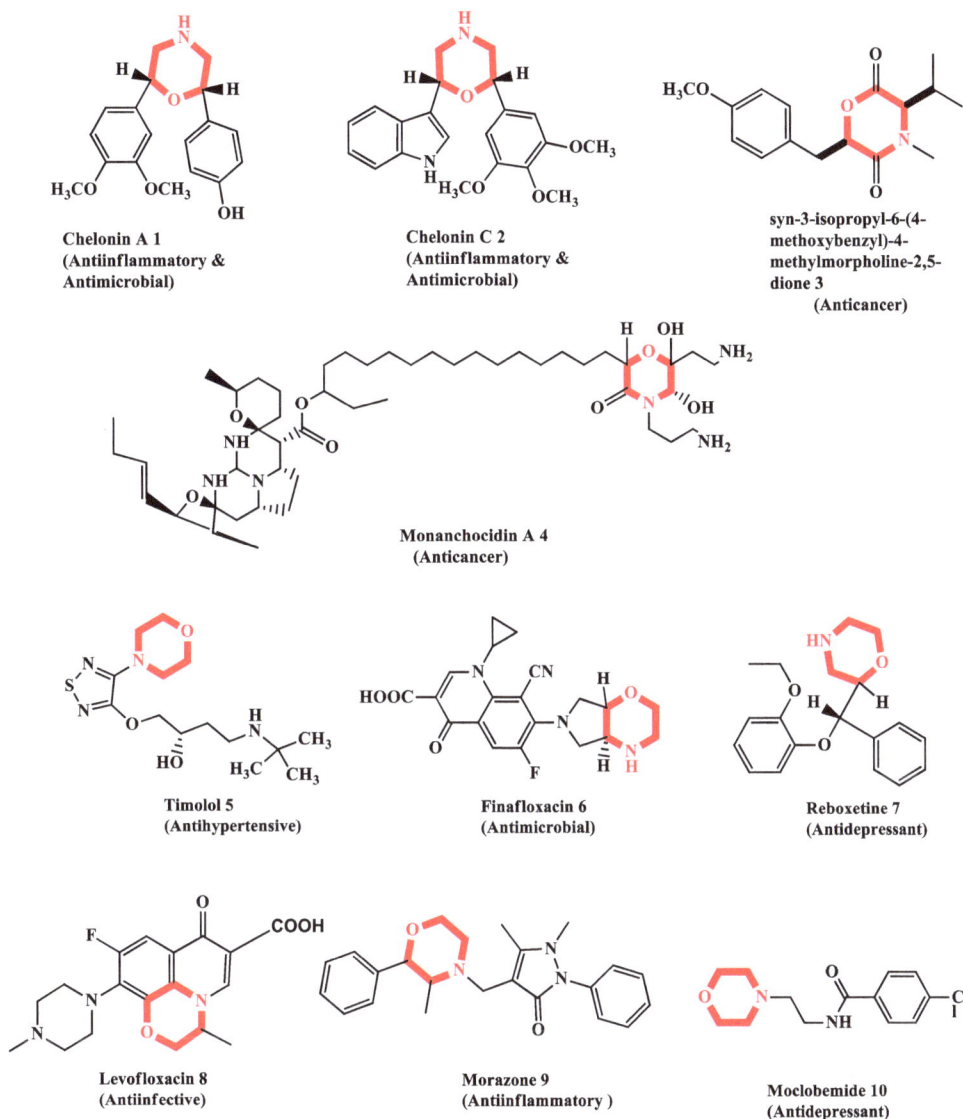

Fig. (1). Chemical structures of the natural compounds containing morpholine ring.

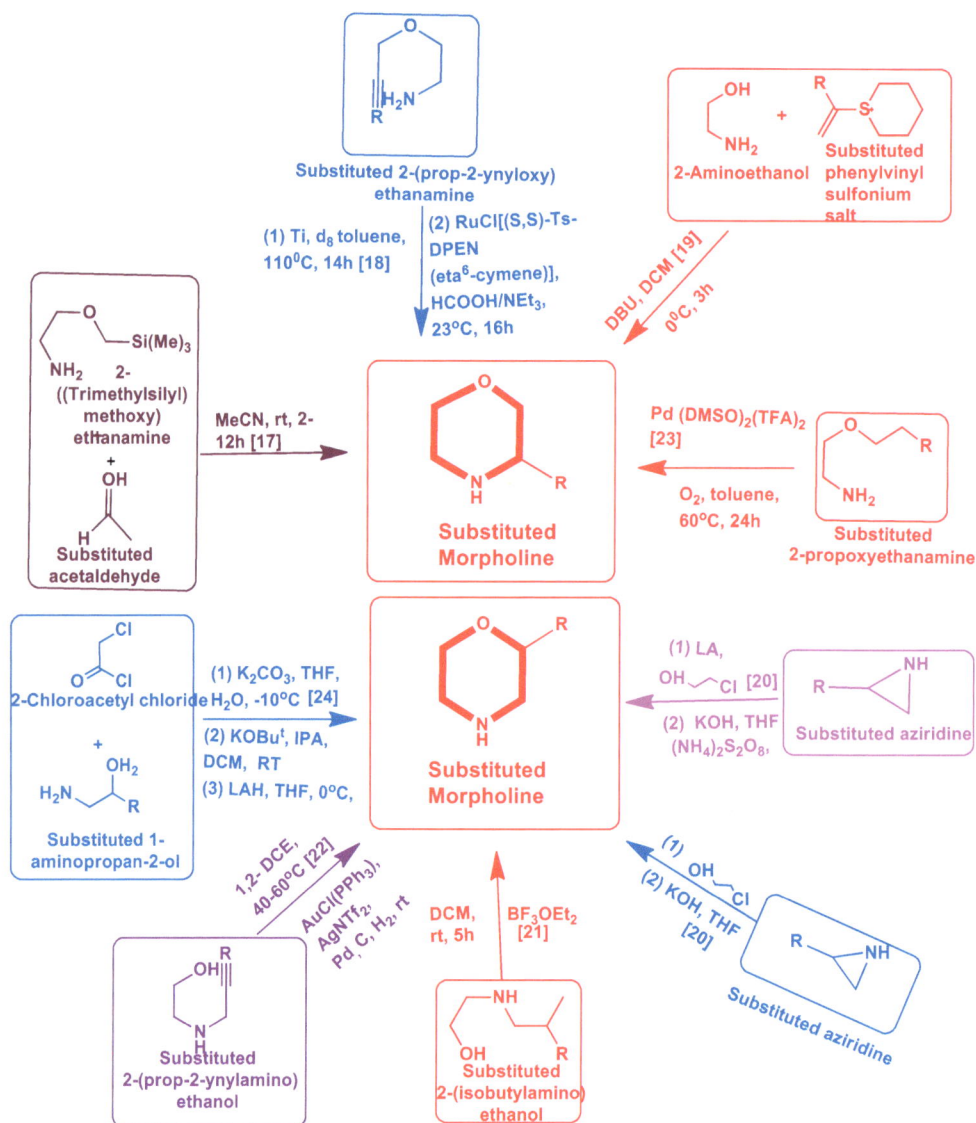

Scheme 2. Recent development of synthesized substituted morpholine rings.

ROLE OF MORPHOLINE RING IN MODULATING PHARMACOKINETIC PARAMETERS

In the drug discovery process, the early strategic optimization of physicochemical and pharmacokinetic parameters for promising pathways translates into the successful development of promising clinical candidates. From the pharmacokinetic point of view, morpholine can be seen as a more preferred molecule for various drugs. Due to the rapid oxidative metabolism of morpholine, there is the rapid removal of the drug from the body. Various metabolites of clinical drugs due to morpholine ring are presented in Fig. (**2**).

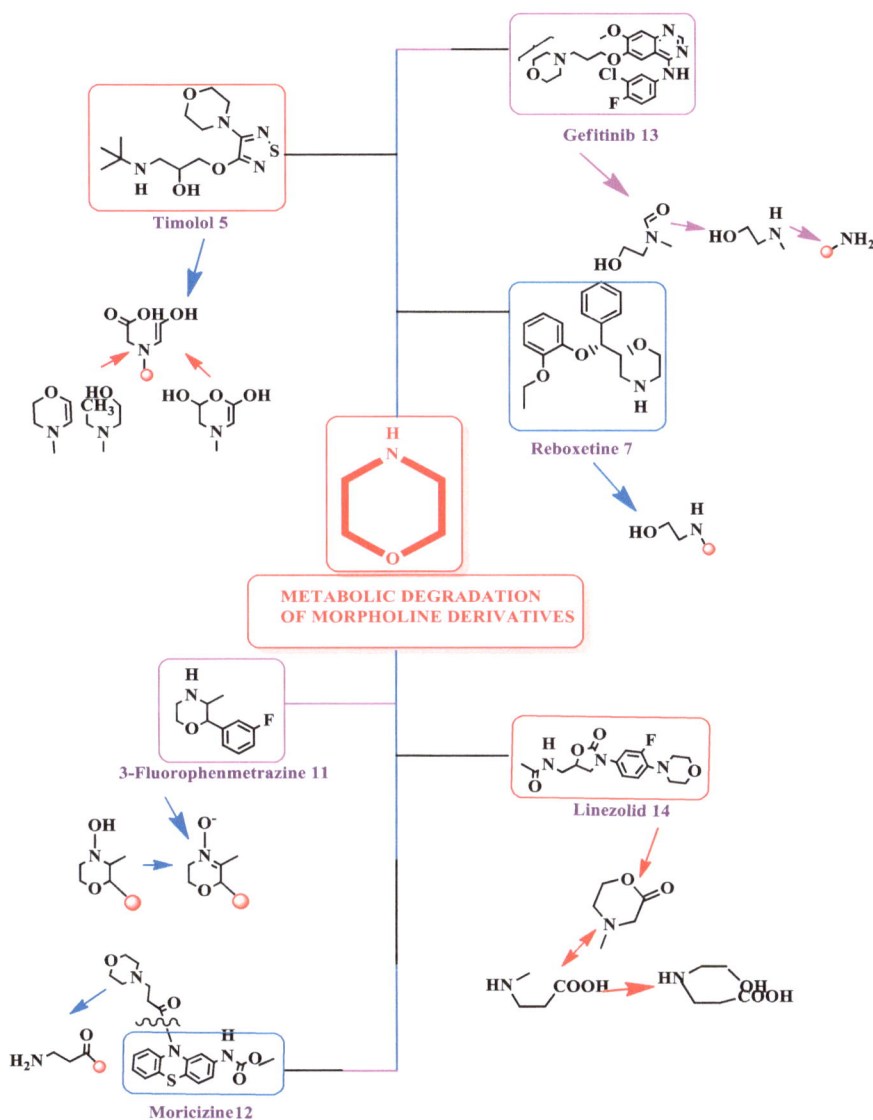

Fig. (2). Chemical structures of various morpholine metabolites **11-14.**

In case of Timolol 5, morpholine ring is metabolized by cytochrome P2C19 in the liver producing various metabolites, *i.e.* double bond formation, dihydroxylation and opening of morpholine ring [37]. 3-Fluorophenmetrazine 11 metabolism involves a series of *N*-oxidation, aryl hydroxylation and subsequent glucuronidation or sulfation pathway [38]. Hepatic cytochrome P-450 eliminates the 3-morpholin-4-yl propanoyl group and the morpholine ring in the metabolism of moricizine 12 [39]. Gefitinib 13 metabolism involves opening the morpholine ring and step-wise removing the propoxy side chain in the liver [40]. Reboxetine 7 is metabolism also includes the opening of morpholine ring involving [41]-oxidation of the morpholine cycle plays a role in the metabolism of linezolid 14, which forms an open metabolite of carboxylic acid (aminoethoxyacetic acid) and a hydroxyethyl metabolite of glycine [42].

IMPROVEMENT OF PHARMACOKINETIC PROPERTIES OF THE MORPHOLINE RING

Various researches reported the more conformationally preferred morpholine ring analogues having improved pharmacokinetic properties [43, 44]. Wuitschik and coworkers developed a more stable and less lipophilic oxetane ring. Hence, Spirocyclic oxetanes 15-26 shown in Fig. (**3**) may be taken as structural analogues of the morpholine ring for better results *i.e.*, increase in aqueous solubilty. Moreover, metabolic stability of the compounds was improved. In spirocycles 16–21, the oxetan unit and nitrogen atom are in close proximity to each other. This conformation makes the molecule more lipophilic and prone to the attack of CYP450 enzymes. Ultimately the rate of drug clearance increases from the body. Spirocyclic analogues, 17, are promising for other applications due to their reduced lipophilic properties, increased solubility, and reduced sensitivity to oxidative metabolic degradation [45]. Encouraged by the study, Andriy *et al.*, synthesized trifluoromethyl substituted amines 23 and 24 of the morpholine ring showing a further increase in the lipophilicity of the ring by efficiently reducing the basicity of the nitrogen atom [46]. Various spirocyclic amino acids were also synthesized by Kirichok *et al.*, and checked for the toxicity after incorporating into the drug Bupivacain. Spirocyclic compound 25 showed better results with similar properties of ADME, biological activity and toxicity five times lower than the marketed Bupivacaine [47]. Degorce *et al.*, designed a new conformationally restricted bridged morpholine ring **26** with modulated physicochemical properties of morpholine. Increased basicity and higher solvent-exposed polar surface area lead to reduced lipophilicity with increased selectivity for hERG enzyme [48].

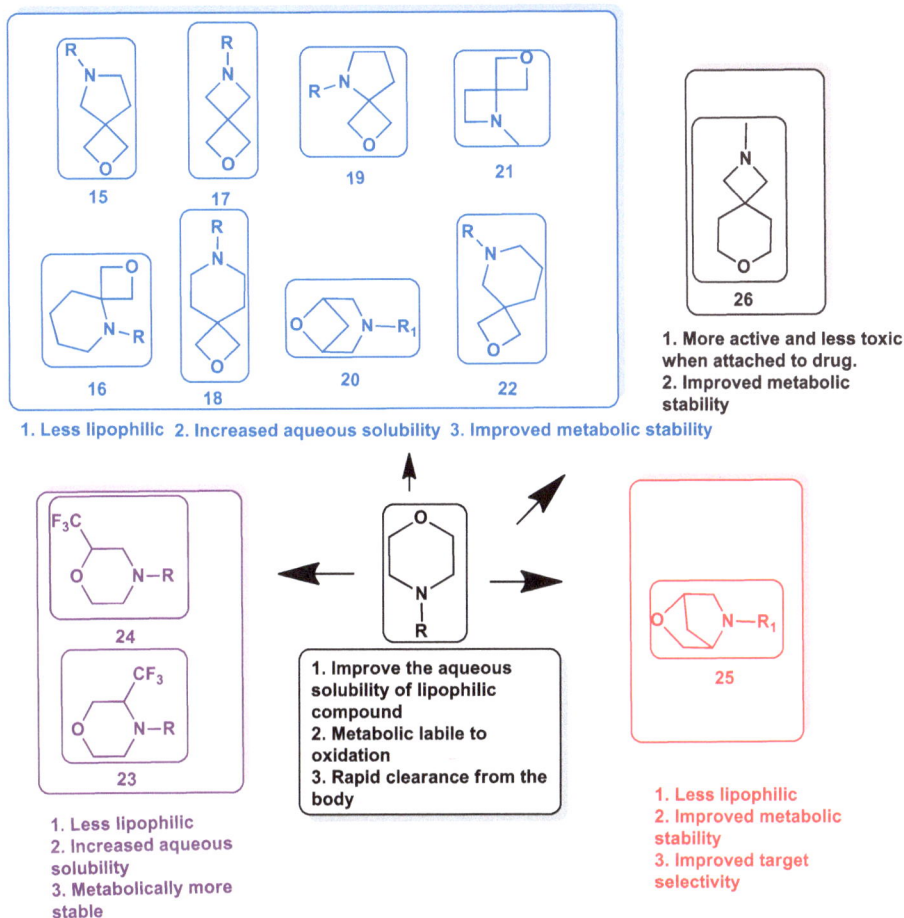

Fig. (3). Modified morphline rings 15-26 with improved pharmacokinetic properties.

ANTICANCER POTENTIAL OF MORPHOLINE DERIVATIVES

Cancer involves cellular invasions into various organs as a result of uncontrolled cell growth. Cell growth, cell proliferation and survival are affected by these mutations [49, 50]. In 2018, United States reported about 609,640 cancer deaths [51]. Hence, it is required to control cancerous conditions through different mechanisms. Varieties of anticancer drugs are reported by researchers having different mode of action [52, 53].

Inflammation process can be observed at the different levels of carcinogenesis as involving various proteins in mechanistic pathway *i.e.*, tumor-associated macrophages (TAM), reactive oxygen and nitrogen species (ROS and RNS respectively), tumor necrosis factor α (TNFα), interleukins (IL-1, IL-6, IL-8) *etc*.

[54]. Two processes Yin (apoptosis) and Yang (wound healing) are mainly involved in the maintenance of normal host immunity *i.e.*, inflammation associated chronic illness [55]. Reddy *et al.*, 2011, mentioned the inhibition of NO (nitric oxide) production due to morpholine derivatives [56].

The transmembrane receptor tyrosine kinase, controls growth, survival and differentiation of endothelial and tumor cells, present on the cell surface.

Gene expression controls the cellular function regulated by a signaling pathway activated on ligand binding. Abnormal cell growth, differentiation, metabolism and neoangiogenesis motility may be seen with over expression of RTKs. Aberrant RTKs signaling can be corrected by morpholine derivatives as reported in literature [57]. Previous studies have shown that the Akt/IKK/NF-κB chain regulates transcriptional activity through Akt [58].

Gefitinib **13,** a morpholine derivative, marketed by AstraZeneca and Teva as anticancer drug. It's mechanism of action involves the inhibition of Ras signaling pathway [59, 60]. Medicinal chemists and biologists are extensively studying morpholine derivatives as potential inhibitors of various important enzymes *i.e.*, PI3K and related enzymes, mTOR, which is also known as the mechanistic target of Rapamycin as involved in protein synthesis, cell proliferation, cell growth *etc*. The mTOR inhibitors have proven to be the biological and pharmacological tool and could be a significant class of anticancer agents (Fig. **4**) [61].

Morpholine Derivatives as mTOR Inhibitors

mTOR is mammalian target of Rapamycin, also called as mechanistic target of rapamycin and FK506-binding protein 12-rapamycin-associated protein 1. mTOR is a member of PIKKs encoded by mTOR gene. It regulates cellular cell growth, protein synthesis, cell motility, cell proliferation, cell survival, autophagy and transcription [62]. The mTORC1 and mTORC2 protein complexes are the key components of mTOR, where cell growth and metabolism are controlled by mTORC1 mainly and cell proliferation and survival are regulated by mTORC2. Active mTORC1 activates downstream targets, 4E-BP1 and p70 S6 kinase, Atg13 and ULK1, ribosome biogenesis, leads to the activation of transcription. Whereas, various targets such as, mTOR, Rictor, GβL, Sin1, PRR5/Protor-1 and DEPTOR induced by mTORC2. It promotes cell survival through the activation of Akt. mTOR gene mutations induces activation of mTOR signaling pathway and portray several types of cancer. Many heterocyclic derivatives are available as mTOR inhibitors to successfully treat human cancer and still few are under clinical trials [63, 64].

Arie Zask 2009 *et al.*, conducted molecular modeling on morpholine derivatives and concluded that morpholine derivatives significantly increases the selectivity of mammalian target of Rapamycin (mTOR) inhibitors [65]. Hence, to get better results, it is necessary to design novel morpholine derivatives as anticancer agents.

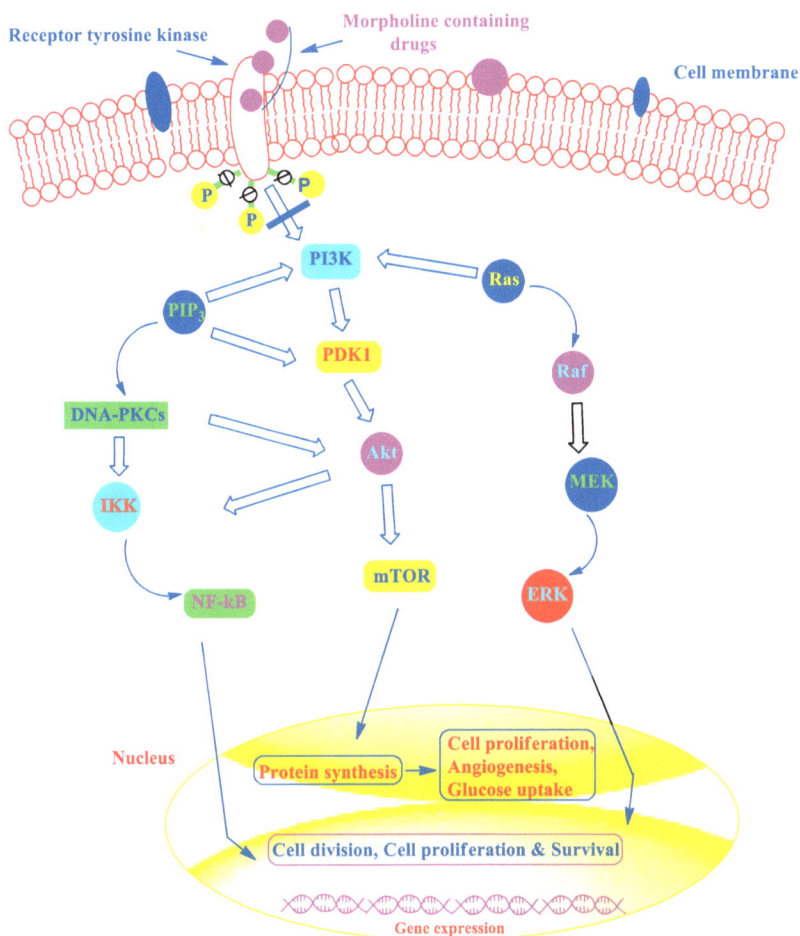

Fig. (4). Effect of morpholine derivatives on various signaling routes represented by mechanistic pathway. On ligand binding, PI3K is enabled by the generation of PIP3 in the membrane, which induces the proliferation of Akt to mTOR in a sequence. The signaling of the sequence of PI3K/Akt/mTOR leads to cell growth, proliferation and metabolism. mTOR, belongs to serine-threonine kinase family and is produced by soil bacteria. It induces the downstream regulation resulting in cancer-related consequences, *i.e.* protein translation, cellular differentiation, and cellular growth. A sérine/thréonine kinase activates Akt and also potentiates the chain. Many genes control cell signaling, stress responses, Ras-RAF-MEK-ERK (ERK) pathways. During cancer's pathogenesis, Ras oncogenes get commonly mutated or over expressed. Morpholine inhibiting this overall process of cell division, proliferation and survival by binding to the catalytic site of PI3K.

In 2017, synthesis and evaluation studies of imidazole-pyridine substituted morpholine derivatives against MCF-7 and A2780 cancer cell lines were conducted by Zang and colleagues. According to the SAR studies, 3rd position for alkyl substitution on morpholine ring is necessary for the anticancer activity. For good binding affinity with mTOR substituted morpholine is required. Among all the synthesized compounds, 27 and 28 (Fig. **5**) showed maximum activity [66]. The synthesis and designing of 2-ureidophenyltriazines-bridged morpholines as potent mTOR inhibitors is also mentioned in the literature. Molecular modeling suggested that maximum binding affinity in the pocket of mTOR is shown by bridged morpholine moiety. Among all the compounds, potent activity was shown by compound 29 (Fig. **5**) ($IC_{50}= 1.0 \pm 0.1$ nM) containing 3, 5-ethylene bridged morpholine [67].

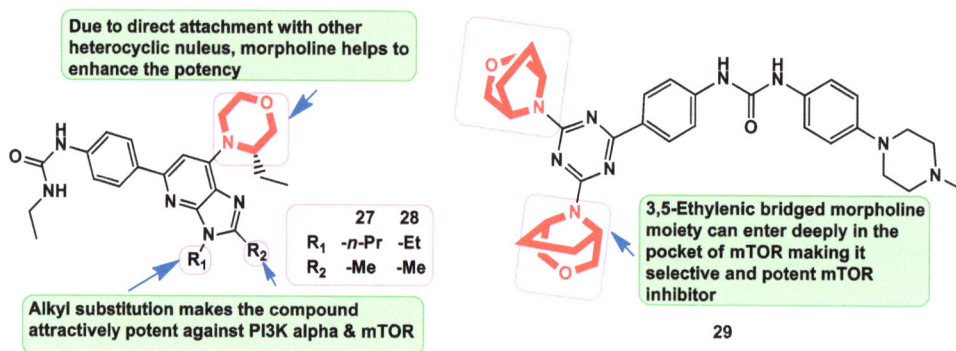

Fig. (**5**). Structure activity relationship (SAR) of morpholine derivatives **27-29** as mTOR inhibitors.

Morpholine Derivatives as Phosphoinositide 3-kinase (PI3K) Inhibitors

Human cancer is involved in performing various cellular functions such as cell proliferation, growth, differentiation, motility, and survival [68]. Phosphoinositide 3-kinases are a group of intracellular signal transducer enzymes. Abnormality in PI3K signaling leads to a variety of other disease conditions such as neurological disorders, immunological disorders, diabetes, and cardiovascular disease. PIP3 generation in membrane induces the activation of PI3K. It further activates proliferation by Akt to mTOR kinase sequence [69]. Cancer genomics reported that in human, tumors activating mutations in PI3K genes-PIK3CA gene encoding p110-α takes place [70]. The huge research on PI3K research by cancer biologists exposed various vital aspects of enzyme and its role in cellular functions and disease conditions (The PI3K pathway in human disease). Like mTOR inhibition, morpholine also showed a prominent role in PI3K enzyme inhibition. Due to morpholine moiety, bonding between the hinge regions in the ATP pocket of enzyme with the active valine site backbone occurs, leads to loss of its affinity

[71]. Occurrence of prostate cancer is also seen due serine/threonine kinase expression. Hence, it is also important to inhibit this kinase with novel anticancer drugs. In the literature, superior serine/threonine kinase inhibitory activity is shown by various morpholine derivatives [72, 73].

Rewcastle *et al.*, (2011) mentioned the study on various morpholine-benzimidazole derivatives and evaluation against PI3K inhibitors. *In vivo* studies were conducted on human glioblastoma cancer cell line-U87MG. Against PI3K isoforms, the most potent compounds were 30 (IC_{50}<0.9 nM) (Fig. **6**) and 31 (IC_{50}<1.4 µM) (Fig. **6**). According to the SAR studies, activity was due to the presence of 6-amino-4-methoxy group [74].

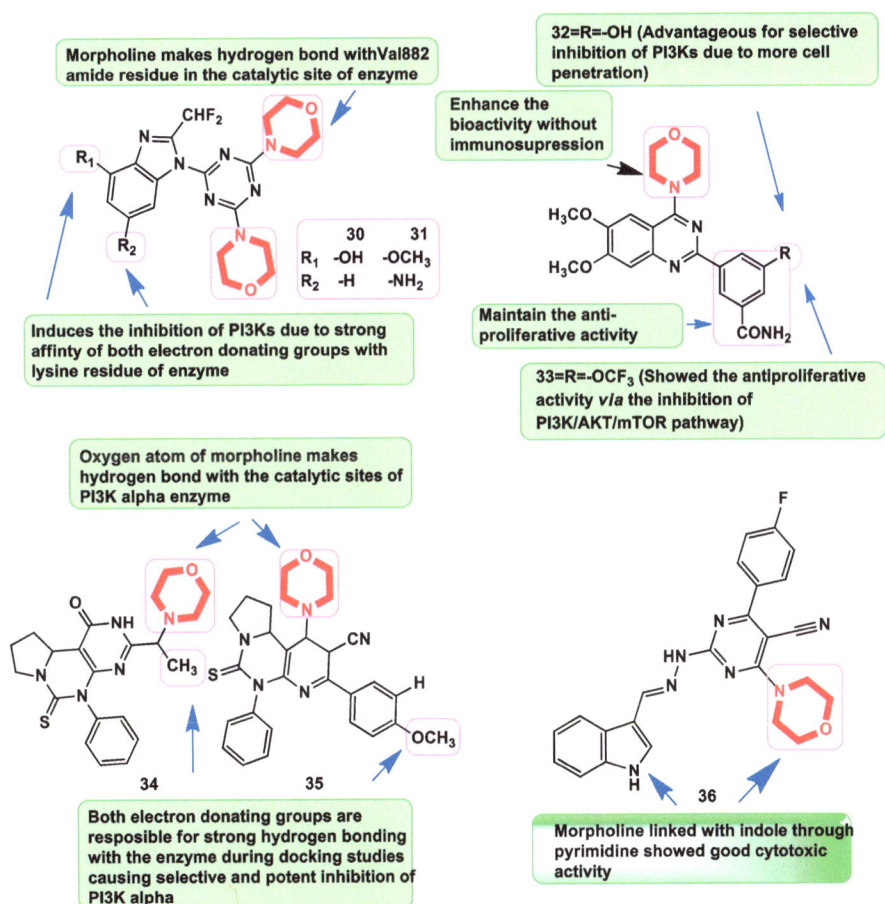

Fig. (6). Structure activity relationship (SAR) of morpholine derivatives **30-36** as phosphoinositide 3-kinase (PI3K) inhibitors.

The various heterocyclic combination as promising anticancer agents motivated researchers for designing hybrid compounds. Consequently, Wang and colleagues designed, synthesized and evaluated novel morpholine-benzamide derivatives as anticancer agents in 2015. Evaluation was conducted against human cancer cell lines *i.e.* MCF-7, HCT-116, A549 and U-87. Compound 32 (IC_{50}<17.18 ± 2.45 µM) (Fig. **6**), showed high activity whereas 33 (IC_{50}<1.68 ± 0.29 µM) (Fig. **6**) was active against the all the mentioned cell lines as compared with standard drug GDC0941, (IC_{50}<1.09 ± 0.15 µM). SAR studies revealed the importance of benzamide substitution for the activity.

Furthermore, an increase in potency can be seen with the attachment of trifluoromethoxy and hydroxyl substituted phenyl and methoxy at the 6th and 7th positions of quinazoline ring linked with morpholine ring. The oxygen atom of morpholine derivative showed prominent interaction with Val882, whereas aminopyridinyl group occupies Asp836 and Asp841 residues of the enzymes [75, 76].

Pyrrolo-pyrimidines suppress tumor angiogenesis through the inhibition of EGF and PDGF receptor. By considering this, potent anticancer derivatives, morpholine and pyrrolopyrimidine derivatives were synthesized by Ibrahim *et al.*, [77]. Compound, 34 (IC_{50}<1.34 µM) and 35 (IC_{50}<12.57 µM) (Fig. **6**) showed maximum potency as having maximum bonding at the active site of enzyme *i.e.*, morpholine showed hydrogen bonding with the Val851 residue and other substituent with Tyr836, Asp810, Lys802 residues of the p11α enzyme active site [78].

Helwa *et al.*, 2020 synthesized novel pyrimidine-5-carbonitriles substituted morpholine derivatives and evaluated against PI3K (α, β and δ) and a pool of cancer cell lines. SAR studies highlighted the importance of indole moiety. Among all compounds, 36 (Fig. **6**) was perceived to be most potent against CNS cancer SF-295, melanoma MALME-3M, M14 and UACC-257 and renal cancer 786-0 and RXF 393 cells (GI_{50}= 0.21µM -19.5 µM) [79].

Morpholine Derivatives as Potent TNF-α/IL-2 Dual Inhibitor

TNF-α, encoded by TNF-α gene, showing dual affinity for receptors-TNFR1 and TNFR2. It is a pro-inflammatory cytokine produced by various cells such as monocytes, macrophages, endothelial cells, adipocytes *etc.* TNF-α induces ERK (extracellular signal 2 regulated protein kinase), caspase protease, and JNK proteins [80, 81]. Prolonged and impaired TNF-α expression leads to a number of disease conditions, mainly autoimmune diseases such as ulcerative colitis, Crohn's disease, psoriasis arthritis, rheumatoid arthritis, psoriasis *etc.* [82].

Interleukin-2 (IL-2), is a type of protein regulating the activities of white blood cell. Pathways- JAK-STAT, PI3K/Akt/mTOR and MAPK/ERK can transduce IL-2. All of these three major pathways induces the cell activation, differentiation, proliferation, survival, and cytokine production in the immune cells involving IL-2. IL-2 is responsible for the induction of TNF-α as it can be inhibited by blocking IL-2 [83]. IL-2/TNF-α dual inhibition will be boon for cancer treatment.

Urea affects the cell proliferation, differentiation and survival by inhibiting TNF-α and IL-2. Urea substitution with morpholine ring enhances the potency [84, 85]. In 2012, Wang and coworker worked on various urea-morpholine derivatives and evaluated against various cancer cell lines using MTT assays and *in vivo* against H22 hepatocellular carcinoma cells. Compound **37** (% tumour inhibition = 44.10%) Fig. **(7)** was found to a potent. SAR studies concluded that most effective derivatives with least toxicity are due to morpholine substitution [86].

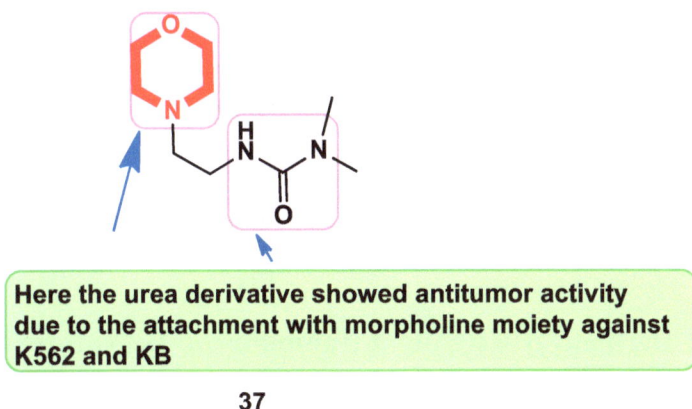

> **Here the urea derivative showed antitumor activity due to the attachment with morpholine moiety against K562 and KB**

37

Fig. (7). Structure activity relationship (SAR) of morpholine derivative **37** as potent TNF-α/IL-2 dual inhibitor.

Morpholine Derivatives as Dual PI3K and mTOR Inhibitors

PI3K and mTOR are central regulator in cell proliferation, angiogenesis and growth [83]. Additionally, mTOR is PI3K-related kinase having similar ATP site with PI3K. The mTOR could also be inhibited by numbers of PI3K inhibitors [87]. Hence, solving the problem of drug resistance of mTOR inhibitors. The inhibition of both enzymes can be a good strategy for cancer treatment. In literature, various morpholine derivatives are mentioned as powerful two-spot inhibitors. In fact, PI3K/mTOR dual mechanism is followed by most of the marketed and under clinical drug candidates.

Designing and synthesis of morpholine-thiopyrano pyrimidine derivatives are reported as potent mTOR inhibitors. SAR study highlighted that C-4 substituted phenyl and 4-OH substitutions are important for the activity in compound **38** (Fig. **8**) [88].

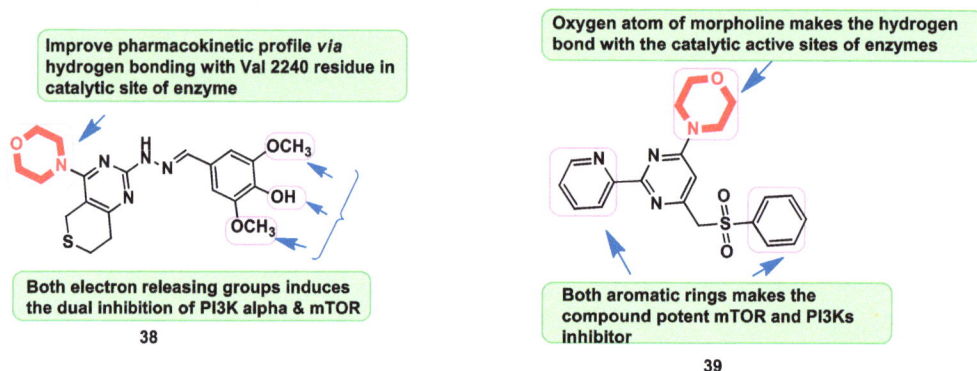

Fig. (8). Structure activity relationship (SAR) of morpholine derivatives **38-39** as dual PI3K and mTOR inhibitors.

In 2015, various chromone, quinoline and pyrazolopyrimidine substituted morpholine derivatives were reported by Andrs *et al.*, According to the SAR study, pyrazolopyrimidine substituent was found to be important. Compound **39** (IC_{50}=1.4 µM) (Fig. **8**) showed best activity [89].

Morpholine Derivatives as Potent Inhibitor of Dihydrofolate Reductase Enzyme

Dihydrofolate reductase, or DHFR, is an enzyme encoded by the DHFR gene expressed in all individuals. It converts the dihydrofolic acid to tetra hydrofolic acid in the presence of NADPH. Tetrahydrofolic acid is required for the synthesis of purines, thymidylic acid and certain amino acids [90]. Hence, the enzyme play key role in the production of nucleic acid involved in cell proliferation and growth. Low DHFR activity depletes THF pool inside the cell, causing stoppage of RNA and DNA synthesis and cell death. Hence, it's better to design antifolate drugs to treat human cancer. Various morpholine derivatives displayed anticancer effect through this mechanism. Antifolate drugs inhibit the DHFR action, hence, used to treat cancer and some inflammatory diseases [91].

In 2017, Muhammad and colleagues mentioned the synthesis and evaluation of thiouracil-morpholine derivatives and evaluation against A-549, HepG-2 cell lines. A docking study was also performed to estimate the binding affinity of derivatives with enzyme dihydrofolate reductase (DHFR). SAR studies confirmed that potency is due to morpholinylchalcones substitution as morpholine showed good binding affinity in the active site of the enzyme. Compound **40** was found to be most potent against HepG-2 cell line (IC_{50} = 3.54±1.11 µg/mL) and also moderate against A-549 (IC_{50}< 5.7±0.91 µg/mL) as compared with the standard drug cisplatin (IC_{50}<1.4±1.1 µg/ml) (Fig. **9**) [92].

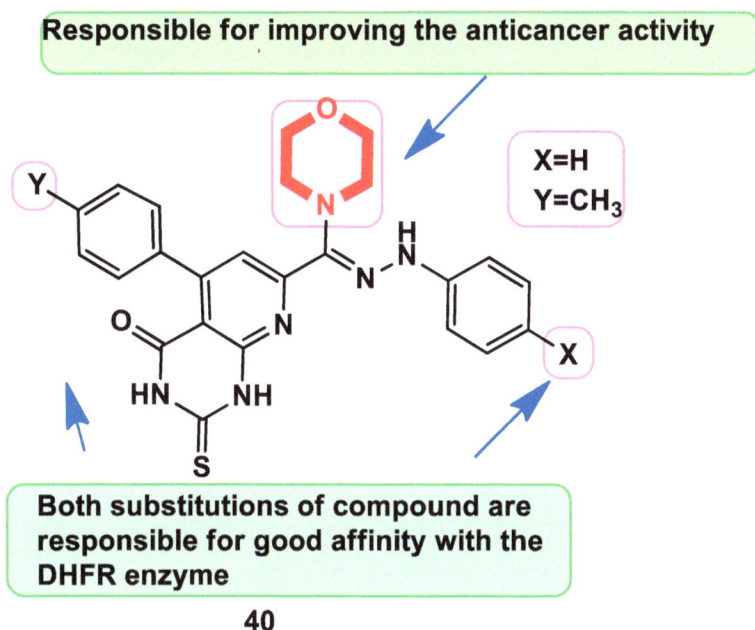

Fig. (9). Structure activity relationship (SAR) of morpholine derivative **40** as potent inhibitor of dihydrofolate reductase enzyme.

Morpholine Derivatives as Caspases Enzyme Inhibitors

Caspases (cysteine-aspartic acid protease) are a family of protease enzymes causing programmed cell death. Caspase 3 is a member of caspase family, encoded by *CASP3* gene. It is activated by FADD, caspase 8, BAX/BAK-dependent cytochrome c, and caspase 9 and plays an important role in cell apoptosis [93]. Caspase 3 belongs to caspase family with two types: initiator caspases and executioner caspases. Both intrinsic (death ligand) and extrinsic (mitochondrial) apoptotic pathways induces the activation of caspase 3 in apoptotic cell [94]. Caspase 3 inhibition by many morpholine derivatives is reported [95]. SAR studies confirm the importance of 4-methyl and 4-phenyl substituent and compound **41** (IC_{50}= 23±2 nM) (Fig. **10**) was found as most potent [96].

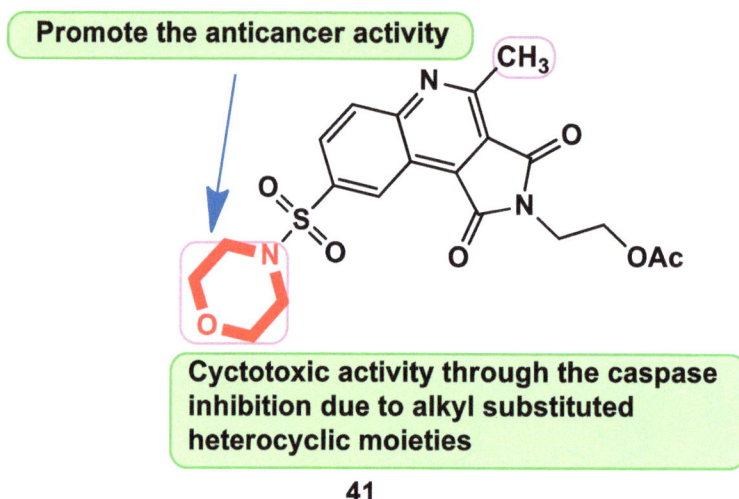

41

Fig. (10). Structure activity relationship (SAR) of morpholine derivative **41** as caspases enzyme inhibitor.

Miscellaneous Drugs

Aktar with colleagues designed, synthesized and evaluated chalcone-morpholine derivatives in 2018. Compound 42 (IC_{50}=7.36 µM and 68.27 µM for C6 and HeLa cell lines respectively) (Fig. **11**) showed activity almost equivalent to standard drug 5-fluoro uracil (IC_{50}= 5.80 µM and of 16.32 µM for C6 and HeLa cell lines respectively) [97].

In 2017, Kumar and coworkers designed, synthesized and evaluated pyrazoline-morpholine derivatives using cancer cell lines-HepG2, HeLa and MCSF-7. Compound 43 (Fig. **11**) showed average to good potency but most effective among all synthesized derivatives against cancer cell lines *i.e.*, HepG2 (GI_{50} = 12.2 µM), MCSF-7 (GI_{50} = 46.1 µm) and HeLa (GI_{50} = 51 µm) as compared with standard drug doxorubicin (GI_{50}< 0.05 µm). SAR studies confirmed that activity against HepG2 cell line is due to the morpholine with aromatic ring substituted halogen group [98]. In 2016, Doan *et al.*, reported a study on various *N*-substituted indolines and morpholine derivatives. The cytotoxic effect of indoline derivatives was more than compared to morpholine derivatives. The most potent derivative was compound, 44 (Fig. **11**) [99]. Benzamide nucleus was found to have important role in stopping cell cycle and apoptosis [100]. A benzisothiazole-morpholine derivatives series was also studied against the Jurkat T cell lines. From the SAR study point of view, 4-phenyl morpholine was favorable for the activity. Maximum potency showed by compound 45 (IC_{50} = 1.15 nM) (Fig. **11**) [101].

Rincy *et al.*, 2019, designed various novel morpholine analogues and conducted *in silico* studies against lung cancer, metastasis melanoma, and Non-Hodking's lymphoma. Biological activities were predicted by online software PASS (Prediction of Activity Spectra for Substances). Results concluded that synthesis and evaluation of morpholine derivatives as anticancer agents could be beneficial in the near future [102].

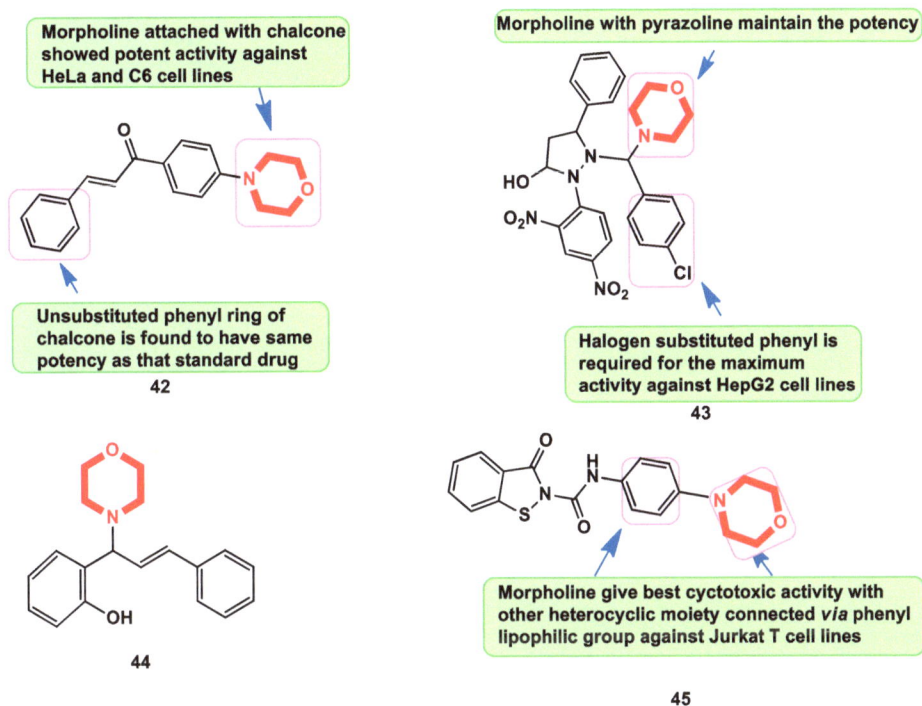

Fig. (11). Chemical structures and structure activity relationship (SAR) of morpholine derivatives **42-45**.

DRUGS UNDER CLINICAL TRIAL

A variety of drugs bearing the morpholine ring with advanced structural modification are under clinical trial with the hope of preventing complex disease conditions effectively in the future. The promising leads having morpholine ring under clinical trial are mentioned in Figs. (**12-14**) showing the mechanism of action, role and pharmacokinetic and pharmacodynamic properties of the compounds.

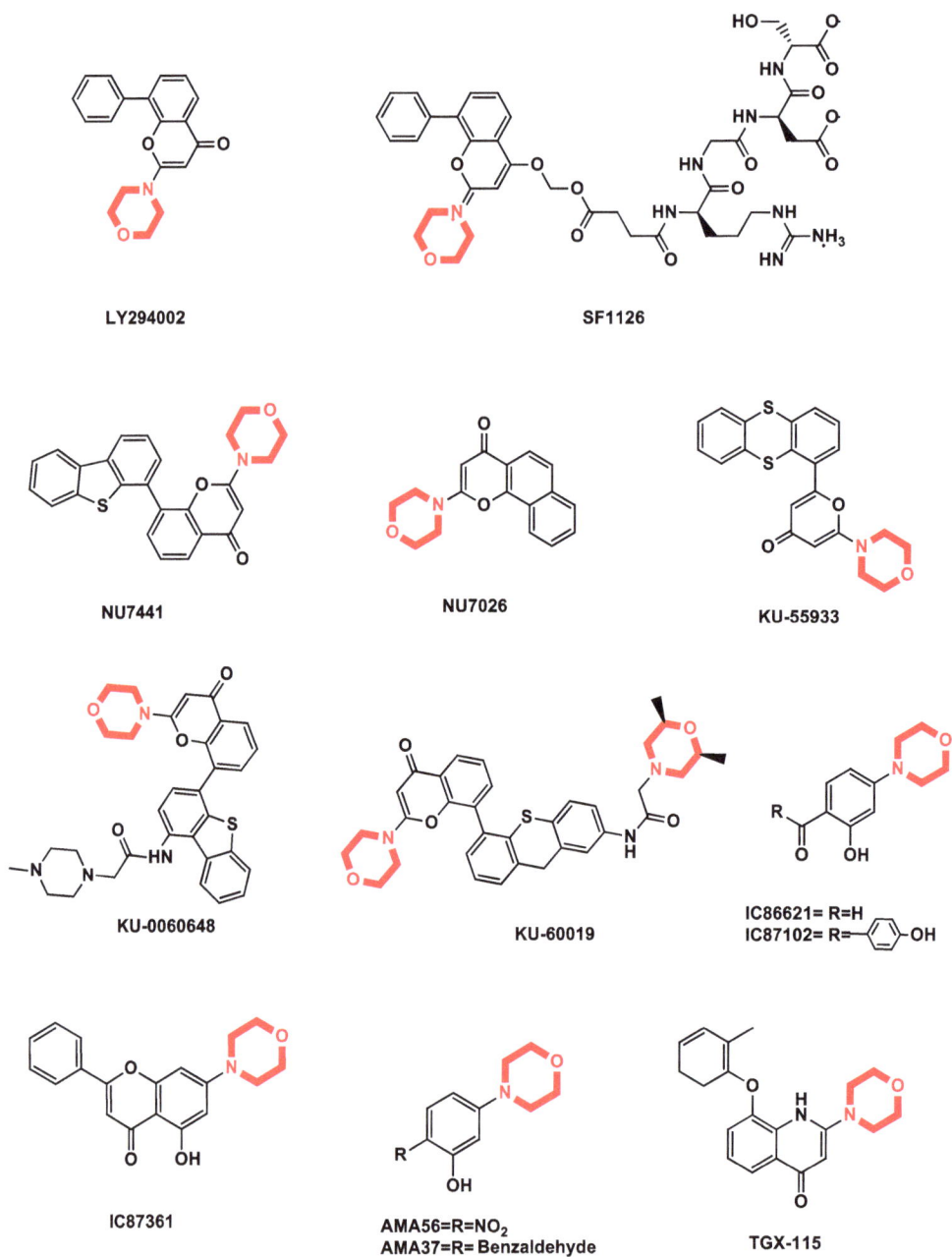

Fig. (12). Chemical structure of morpholine ring containing leads which are in advanced stages of development.

LY294002 active against ovarian cancer developed by (Lilly) in preclinical stage is a nonselective inhibitor of PI3K, DNA-PK, CK2, GSK3, therapeutically.

Morpholine showed good binding affinity with backbone amide of Val882 due to the presence of oxygen atom. However, replacement of oxygen with sulfur, nitrogen, hydroxymethyl or methylene causes decrease in activity. Further biological evaluation was not conducted due to poor solubility, bioavailability and rapid clearance [103].

To tackle the unfavourable pharmacokinetic properties of **LY294002**, prodrug, **SF1126** was developed by Semaphore which is in phase 1 clinical trial. **SF1126** has favourable antitumor, antiangiogenic efficacy and is involved in the treatment of chronic lymphocytic leukaemia [104].

The KuDOS developed **NU7441** [105] and **NU7026** [106] in treating liver cancer through similar mechanism and have good pharmacokinetic profile.

Another drug under the preclinical stage developed by KuDOS is **KU-55933** [107], which acts through potent and selective inhibition of ATM kinase, suppressing cell proliferation and apoptosis induction in cancer cells due to the binding affinity of morpholine for kinase's active site. Morpholine oxygen is required for ATM activity [107]. KuDOS also developed **KU-0060648** [108] to treat human breast and colon cancer by inhibiting DNA-PK and PI3K. At the molecular level, morpholine showed hydrogen bonding with Val-882 residue [108]. **KU-60019** [109] is another potent drug which acts through inhibiting a signaling pathway involving cell migration, invasion *via* Akt and MEK/ ERK through the inhibition of ATM kinase [109].

Eli Lilly company developed similar derivatives, **IC87102** [110], **IC87361** [111] as potent inhibitors of DNA-PK in which arylmorpholine is the main pharmacophore. The **IC87102, IC87361** are more potent than **IC86621** [112].

The University of California also developed potent inhibitors of DNA-PK arylmorpholine derivatives **AMA56** and **AMA37** [113] having arylmorpholine as a main pharmacophore which acts through the inhibition of DNA-PK. According to the SAR studies, hydrogen bond acceptor at the 1-position and hydrogen bond donor at the 2-position were vital for the activity. University of California also developed **TGX-115** [113], **TGX221** [114] and **MCA55** [115] as potent and selective inhibitor of PI3K-p110. The **TGX-115** and **TGX221** were used to treat prostate cancer, but **TGX221** was more potent than **TGX-115**.

Astra Zeneca developed **AZD6482** analogues of **TGX221** having anti-thrombotic activity which currently in phase I. It acts through the mechanism of ATP competitive inhibition of PI3K. Its lower plasma half-life and distribution suggested high metabolism clearance. The morpholine showed interaction with V882 residue of PI3Kγ [116].

GSK2636771 developed by GlaxoSmith Kline in Phase I/Ia is selective inhibitor of p110β and treats solid tumors. Good pharmacokinetic profile and bioavailability of drug is due to two point attachment of morpholine with receptor [117].

Sanofi produced **SAR260301** in Phase I/Ib. It is a potent compound having antineoplastic activity as it causes selective inhibition of PI3K-p110β. Binding of morpholine with the hinge Valine 848 region at catalytic site make it better pharmacokinetically *i.e.* having 70% oral bioavailability [118].

Piramed developed **PI-103** to treat human tumor xenografts by the inhibition of DNA-PK, PI3K, mTOR. Morpholine and phenol moieties show interaction with same residue valine 882. The metabolic process involves glucuronidation of the phenolic group and oxidation of the morpholine ring leads to rapid clearance [119].

GDC-0941 by Genetech in Phase I/II to treat breast cancer with the inhibition of PI3K. It displays improved solubility, oral bioavailability, nanomolar potency and metabolic stability [120]. Genetech gives similar derivatives **GNE-477** [121], **GDC-0980** those showed dual inhibition of PI3K and mTOR with improved pharmacokinetic properties and treated oncogenic malignancies [122].

The Spanish Experimental Therapeutic Program developed **ETP-46321** [123] and **ETP-46992** [124] in preclinical exhibited favourable pharmacokinetics. **ETP-46321** treats lung tumor with the inhibition of p110α and p110δ, whereas, **ETP-46992** treats skin cancer through the inhibition of PI3K and mTOR. **PKI-402** has good binding affinity with PI3K/mTOR. *i.e,* both nitrogens and carbonyl oxygen of urea moiety was responsible for hydrogen bonding with Asp810 and Lys802, respectively [125].

ZSTK474 by Zeynaku Kogyo in Phase I/II to treats inflammation through the inhibition of PI3K. Good binding affinity can be seen as showing two points of attachment *i.e.* hydrogen bonding of oxygen of one morpholine ring and nitrogen of benzimidazole moiety with Val828 and Lys779 respectively. Whereas, second morpholine oxygen enter the ATP-binding pocket of enzyme [126].

Shanghi Institute of Materia Medica developed **WDJ008** acts involving dual inhibition of PI3K/mTOR. Good bioavailability and pharmacokinetic profile can be seen in C-4 substituted morpholine [127].

NVP-BKM120 by Novartis in Phase II/III treats lung and gastric cancer through the inhibition of PI3K, treating lung and gastric cancer. Improved structural and pharmacokinetic properties of the compound is due to the presence of second morpholine group and presence of trifluoromethyl group on aminopyridine [128].

Wyeth provides structurally similar **PKI-587** (Phase II) [129] and **PKI-179** [130] (Phase I). Triazine nucleus is selected as having good pharmacokinetic properties due to hydrogen bonding of morpholine moiety with the backbone of Val851. In a viewpoint of metabolic oxidation, a second morpholine ring was added. Better results can be seen after IV administration as compared to oral administration as showing poor permeability, high molecular weight, low logP.

PKI-179 causes inhibition of both PI3K and mTOR to treat breast cancer. It is prepared by modifying **PKI-587**, *i.e.*, replacing benzamide moiety with a smaller heterocycle and one of the morpholine rings with bridged-morpholine analogue. It is more orally effective than **PKI-587**.

Chugai Pharmaceutical Co. developed **CH5132799** which is in Phase I. It treats prostate and breast cancer with the inhibition of PI3K showing excellent bioavailability with good microsomal stability also [131]. **VS-5584**, structurally similar to **CH5132799** in Phase I is developed by Verastem to treats breast cancer with the dual inhibition of PI3K and mTOR. Potent activity is due to the binding of morpholine with mTOR. It also showed better pharmacokinetic profile and oral bioavailability [132].

AstraZeneca Co., with KuDOS provides **KU-63794** (preclinical) [133], **AZD-8055** (Phase I) [134], **AZD-2014** (Phase I/II) having similar mechanism of action [135]. **KU-63794** is a potent compound acting through mTOR inhibition, inhibiting the growth of lymphoma, advanced solid tumors and endometrial carcinoma. SAR studies concluded that additional modified morpholine ring and C-7 substituted pyridopyrimidine are required for the activity. Better pharmacokinetic profile is due to the presence of morpholine ring and benzyl alcohol.

AZD-8055 has the same mechanism as **KU-63994**. Higher aqueous solubility and selectivity is due to the presence of 3,5-dimethyl morpholine. Benzyl alcohol and morpholine ring are the key moieties for high metabolism and liver clearance.

AZD-2014 follows the same mechanism as **KU-63994**. It treats ovarian, endometrial and breast cancer through the inhibition of mTOR. According to the SAR studies, activity is due to *N*-methylbenzamide moiety.

Wyeth developed **WAY-001** [18], **WAY-600** [136] and **WYE-687** [137] drugs with similar chemical structure and MOA. **WAY-001** have more potency against PI3K as compared to mTOR. Presence of phenolic group causes rapid clearance. Structurally, **WAY-600**, contain 5-indolyl and 3-pyridylmethyl substituted piperidine nitrogen in place of phenolic group as in **WAY-001**. Dealkylation of the piperidine ring leads to poor metabolic stability. It involves in the inhibition of PI3K, Akt and mTOR treating hepatocellular carcinoma. Morpholine inhibits the phosphorylation of S6K and 473 residues of Akt enzyme. In WYE-687 higher microsomal stability, selectivity and *in vivo* antitumor efficacy is due to the substitution at 4th position of the phenyl ring with methylcarbamate. **WYE-354** developed by Wyeth, Pfizer has methylcarbamate substitution at the 4th position of phenyl ring and carboxymethyl on piperidine nitrogen. However, potency is less but microsomal stability, selectivity, *in vivo* antitumor efficacy is high [138].

Shanghai Institute of Materia Medica produced **X-387,** involved in mTOR inhibition having antiproliferative activity [139]. Pfizer developed **PF-05139962** having better potency of mTOR and PI3Kα. As steric bulkiness and restricting conformation provided by methyl morpholine group, better potency is reported. Also, it declares good activity of S-methyl analogue as compared to R-methyl group.

Cyclic sulfones with restricted conformation provides higher potency to mTOR and lower selectivity for PI3K [140].

GDC-0349 (Phase I) synthesized by Genetech is involved in inhibiting mTOR showing antitumor activity. Docking studies highlighted that good bonding of morpholine oxygen with enzyme provides high oral bioavailability and low clearance [141].

AstraZeneca introduced **AZ20** in preclinical stage, is acts through the mechanism of ATR inhibition. The 3(R)-methyl modifications, 5-indolyl scaffold and cyclopropyl group in sulfone side chain were responsible for higher potency [142].

M3814 provided by Merck & Co. in Phase 1, treats Chronic Lymphocytic Leukaemia by acting through the inhibition of DNA-PK [143]. **PQR620** treats cancer and neurological disorders through selective mTOR inhibition. Presence of bridged morpholine provides more affinity towards mTOR over PI3K [144].

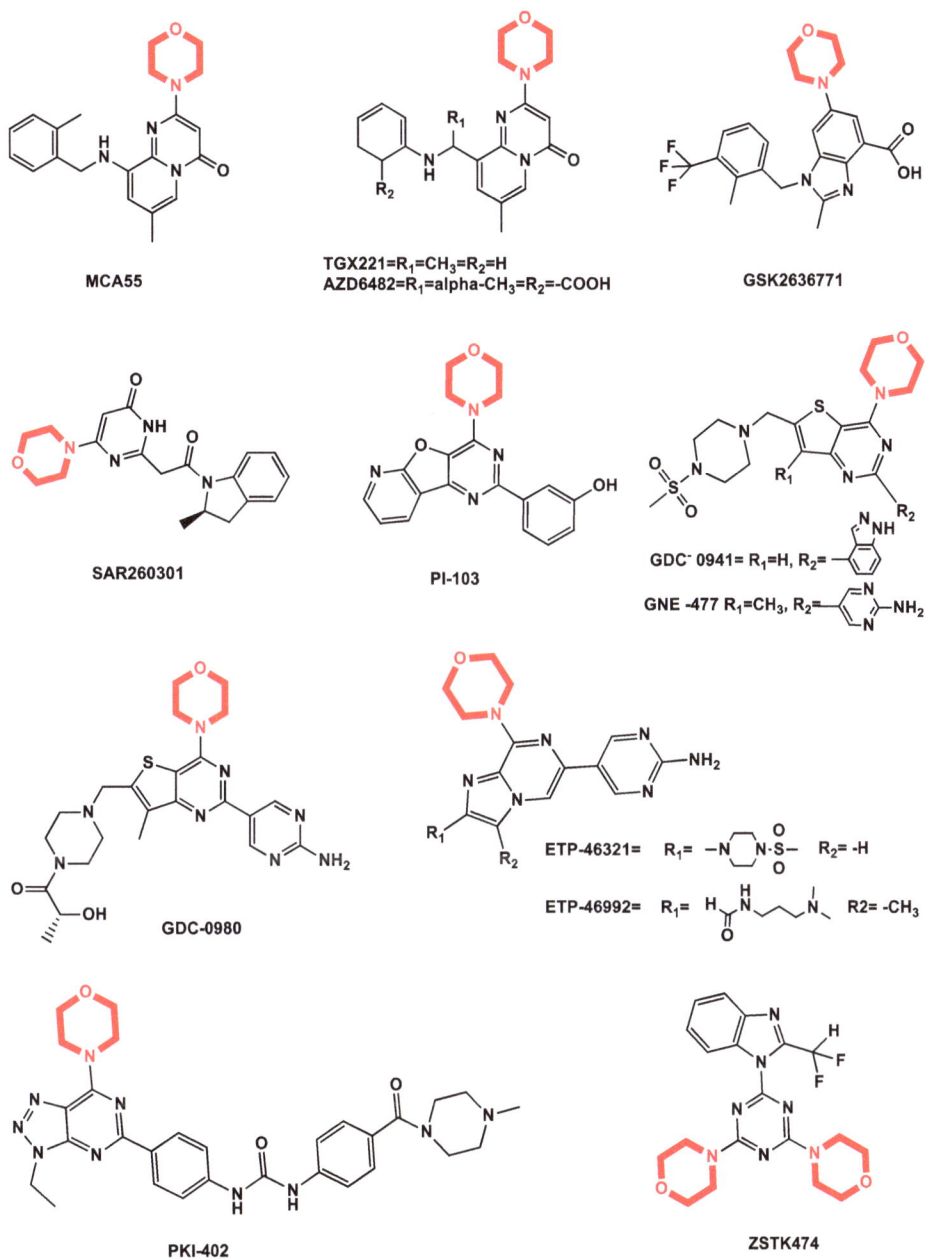

MCA55

TGX221=R$_1$=CH$_3$=R$_2$=H
AZD6482=R$_1$=alpha-CH$_3$=R$_2$=-COOH

GSK2636771

SAR260301

PI-103

GDC$^-$ 0941= R$_1$=H, R$_2$=

GNE -477 R$_1$=CH$_3$, R$_2$=

GDC-0980

ETP-46321=   R$_1$= ─N   N-S─   R$_2$= -H

ETP-46992=   R$_1$=   R2= -CH$_3$

PKI-402

ZSTK474

Fig. (13). Chemical structure of morpholine ring containing leads which are in advanced stages of development.

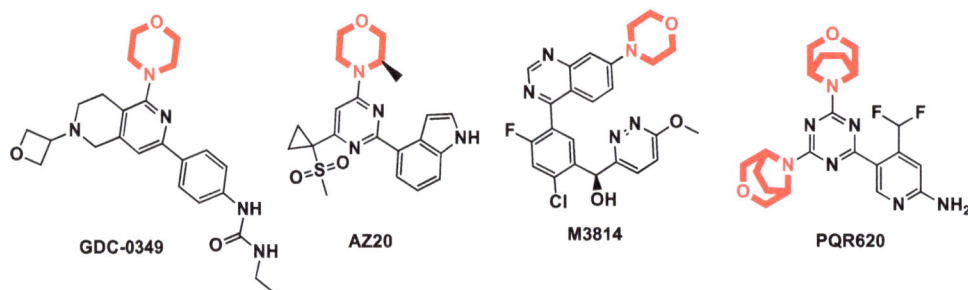

Fig. (14). Chemical structure of morpholine ring containing leads which are in advanced stages of development.

CONCLUSION AND FUTURE PERSPECTIVES

Heterocyclic compounds play the fantastic role from biological and industrial point of view. Among various heterocyclics, morpholine is considered to be the privileged moiety in drug discovery and development. It is marked out that FDA approved a large pool of morpholine ring containing drugs. Due to versatile nature of morpholine, it became the pivotal part of various drugs under clinical trial also. World Drug Index mentions more than 100 commercially available morpholine containing drugs. It is responsible for treating various disease conditions such as cancer, inflammation, viral and microbial infection, convulsion, tuberculosis, hyperlipidemia *etc.*, making it an attractive target for medicinal chemists and researchers. Natural and synthetic morpholine compounds make it an eye-catching moiety in the research area.

In the present chapter, SAR studies are included to understand the pharmacological effects and potency of drugs for cancer treatment. Apart from this, signaling pathway explained the mechanism of action at the molecular level. Changes in pharmacokinetic (metabolic liability) of some clinical drugs by morpholine ring have also been discussed. Different strategies to synthesize morpholine nucleus will be helpful for the researchers in drug discovery. Vast studies on the synthesis and pharmacological evaluation mentioned in the literature are still ongoing on this nucleus. Ultimately, this chapter will provide the maximum indispensable knowledge about morpholine derivatives as potential drug candidates for the cancer treatment.

CONSENT FOR PUBLICATION

Not applicable.

CONFLICT OF INTEREST

The author declares no conflict of interest, financial, or otherwise.

ACKNOWLEDGEMENTS

The author wishes to acknowledge the Management, Shivalik College of Pharmacy, Nangal and Management, Lovely Professional University, Phagwara for the constant encouragement and support.

REFERENCES

[1]   Gomtsyan, A. Heterocycles in drugs and drug discovery. *Chem. Heterocycl. Compd.,* **2012**, *48*(1), 7-10.
[http://dx.doi.org/10.1007/s10593-012-0960-z]

[2]   Martins, P; Jesus, J; Santos, S Heterocyclic anticancer compounds: Recent advances and the paradigm shift towards the use of nanomedicine's tool box. *Molecules,* **2015**, *20*(9), 16852-16891.
[http://dx.doi.org/10.3390/molecules200916852]

[3]   Sethi, N.S.; Prasad, D.N.; Singh, R.K. An insight into the synthesis and sar of 2,4-thiazolidinediones (2,4-TZD) as multifunctional scaffold: A review. *Mini Rev. Med. Chem.,* **2020**, *20*(4), 308-330.
[http://dx.doi.org/10.2174/1389557519666191029102838] [PMID: 31660809]

[4]   Kumari, A.; Singh, R.K. Medicinal chemistry of indole derivatives: Current to future therapeutic prospectives. *Bioorg. Chem.,* **2019**, *89*, 103021.
[http://dx.doi.org/10.1016/j.bioorg.2019.103021] [PMID: 31176854]

[5]   Kumari, A.; Singh, R.K. Morpholine as ubiquitous pharmacophore in medicinal chemistry: Deep insight into the structure-activity relationship (SAR). *Bioorg. Chem.,* **2020**, *96*, 103578.
[http://dx.doi.org/10.1016/j.bioorg.2020.103578] [PMID: 31978684]

[6]   Kumar, R.; Srinivasa, V.R.; Kapur, S. Emphasizing morpholine and its derivatives (MAID): Typical candidate of pharmaceutical importance. *Int. J. Chem. Sci.,* **2016**, *14*, 1777-1788.

[7]   Achari, B.; Sukhendu, B.M.; Dutta, P.; Chowdhury, C. Perspectives on 1, 4-benzo dioxions, 1, 4-benzoxazines and their 2, 3- dihydro derivatives. *Synlett,* **2014**, *14*, 2449-2467.

[8]   Gharpure, S.J.; Prasad, J.V.K. Stereoselective synthesis of C-substituted morpholine derivatives using reductive etherification reaction: Total synthesis of chelonin C. *J. Org. Chem.,* **2011**, *76*(24), 10325-10331.
[http://dx.doi.org/10.1021/jo201975b] [PMID: 22059866]

[9]   Dieckmann, H.; Stockmaier, M.; Kreuzig, R.; Bahadir, M. Simultaneous determination of fenpropimorph and the corresponding metabolite fenpropimorphic acid in soil. *Fresenius J. Anal. Chem.,* **1993**, *345*(12), 784-786.
[http://dx.doi.org/10.1007/BF00323011]

[10]   Burland, P.A.; Osborn, H.M.I.; Turkson, A. Synthesis and glycosidase inhibitory profiles of functionalised morpholines and oxazepanes. *Bioorg. Med. Chem.,* **2011**, *19*(18), 5679-5692.
[http://dx.doi.org/10.1016/j.bmc.2011.07.019] [PMID: 21862336]

[11]   Keldenich, J.; Michon, C.; Nowicki, A.; AgbossouNiedercorn, F. Synthesis of a chiral key intermediate of neurokinin antagonist SSR 240600 by asymmetric allylic alkylation. *Synlett,* **2011**, 2939-2942.

[12]   Amir, M.; Somakala, K.; Ali, S. p38 MAP kinase inhibitors as anti inflammatory agents. *Mini Rev. Med. Chem.,* **2013**, *13*(14), 2082-2096.
[http://dx.doi.org/10.2174/13895575113136660098] [PMID: 24107108]

[13]   Nepstad, I.; Hatfield, K.J.; Grønningsæter, I.S.; Reikvam, H. The PI3K-Akt-mTOR signaling pathway in human Acute Myeloid Leukemia (AML) cells. *Int. J. Mol. Sci.,* **2020**, *21*(8), 2907.
[http://dx.doi.org/10.3390/ijms21082907] [PMID: 32326335]

[14]   Brothers, S.P.; Wahlestedt, C. Therapeutic potential of neuropeptide Y (NPY) receptor ligands. *EMBO Mol. Med.,* **2010**, *2*(11), 429-439.
[http://dx.doi.org/10.1002/emmm.201000100] [PMID: 20972986]

[15]   Nishi, T.; Ishibashi, K.; Takemoto, T.; Nakajima, K.; Fukazawa, T.; Iio, Y.; Itoh, K.; Mukaiyama, O.; Yamaguchi, T. Combined tachykinin receptor antagonist: Synthesis and stereochemical structure–activity relationships of novel morpholine analogues. *Bioorg. Med. Chem. Lett.,* **2000**, *10*(15), 1665-1668.
[http://dx.doi.org/10.1016/S0960-894X(00)00324-3] [PMID: 10937720]

[16]   Pal'chikov, V.A. Morpholines. Synthesis and biological activity. *Russ. J. Org. Chem.,* **2013**, *49*(6), 787-814.
[http://dx.doi.org/10.1134/S1070428013060018]

[17]   Jackl, M.K.; Legnani, L.; Morandi, B.; Bode, J.W. Continuous flow synthesis of morpholines and oxazepanes with silicon amine protocol (slap) reagents and Lewis acid facilitated photoredox catalysis. *Org. Lett.,* **2017**, *19*(17), 4696-4699.
[http://dx.doi.org/10.1021/acs.orglett.7b02395] [PMID: 28813158]

[18]   Lau, Y.Y.; Zhai, H.; Schafer, L.L. Catalytic asymmetric synthesis of morpholines using mechanistic insights to realize the enantioselective synthesis of piperazines. *J. Org. Chem.,* **2016**, *81*(19), 8696-8709.
[http://dx.doi.org/10.1021/acs.joc.6b01884] [PMID: 27668321]

[19]   Matlock, J.V.; Svejstrup, T.D.; Songara, P.; Overington, S.; McGarrigle, E.M.; Aggarwal, V.K. Synthesis of 6- and 7-membered *N*-heterocycles using α-phenylvinylsulfonium salts. *Org. Lett.,* **2015**, *17*(20), 5044-5047.
[http://dx.doi.org/10.1021/acs.orglett.5b02516] [PMID: 26421884]

[20]   Sun, H.; Huang, B.; Lin, R.; Yang, C.; Xia, W. Metal-free one-pot synthesis of 2-substituted and 2,3-disubstituted morpholines from aziridines. *Beilstein J. Org. Chem.,* **2015**, *11*, 524-529.
[http://dx.doi.org/10.3762/bjoc.11.59] [PMID: 25977727]

[21]   Deka, M.J.; Indukuri, K.; Sultana, S.; Borah, M.; Saikia, A.K. Synthesis of five-, six-, and seven-membered 1,3-and 1,4-heterocyclic compounds *via* intramolecular hydrothioalkoxylation of alkenols/thioalkenols. *J. Org. Chem. Res.,* **2015**, *80*, 4349-4359.

[22]   Yao, L.F.; Wang, Y.; Huang, K.W. Synthesis of morpholine or piperazine derivatives through gold-catalyzed cyclization reactions of alkynylamines or alkynylalcohols. *Org. Chem. Front.,* **2015**, *2*(6), 721-725.
[http://dx.doi.org/10.1039/C5QO00060B]

[23]   Lu, Z.; Stahl, S.S. Intramolecular Pd(II)-catalyzed aerobic oxidative amination of alkenes: Synthesis of six-membered *N*-heterocycles. *Org. Lett.,* **2012**, *14*(5), 1234-1237.
[http://dx.doi.org/10.1021/ol300030w] [PMID: 22356620]

[24]   Choi, J.; Lee, J.O.; Kim, M.S.; Nam Shin, J.E.; Chun, K.H. Preparation of morpholine-2-one and 1,4-oxazepan-2-one derivatives by cyclization reaction between *N*-Bts amino alcohol and chloroacetyl chloride. *Bull. Korean Chem. Soc.,* **2008**, *29*(8), 1443-1444.
[http://dx.doi.org/10.5012/bkcs.2008.29.8.1443]

[25]   Handayani, D.; Artasasta, M.A.; Safirna, N.; Ayuni, D.F.; Tallei, T.E.; Hertiani, T. Fungal isolates from marine sponge Chelonaplysilla sp.: Diversity, antimicrobial and cytotoxic activities. *Biodiversitas (Surak.),* **2020**, *21*(5), 1954-1960.
[http://dx.doi.org/10.13057/biodiv/d210523]

[26]   Suntornchashwej, S.; Chaichit, N.; Isobe, M.; Suwanborirux, K. Hectochlorin and morpholine derivatives from the Thai sea hare, *Bursatella leachii. J. Nat. Prod.,* **2005**, *68*(6), 951-955.
[http://dx.doi.org/10.1021/np0500124] [PMID: 15974628]

[27]   Calcabrini, C.; Catanzaro, E.; Bishayee, A.; Turrini, E.; Fimognari, C. Marine sponge natural products

with anticancer potential: An updated review. *Mar. Drugs,* **2017**, *15*(10), 310.
[http://dx.doi.org/10.3390/md15100310] [PMID: 29027954]

[28]   Jakubowska, J.; Wasowska-Lukawska, M.; Czyz, M. STI571 and morpholine derivative of doxorubicin collaborate in inhibition of K562 cell proliferation by inducing differentiation and mitochondrial pathway of apoptosis. *Eur. J. Pharmacol.,* **2008**, *596*(1-3), 41-49.
[http://dx.doi.org/10.1016/j.ejphar.2008.08.021] [PMID: 18782571]

[29]   Nelson, W.L.; Fraunfelder, F.T.; Sills, J.M.; Arrowsmith, J.B.; Kuritsky, J.N. Adverse respiratory and cardiovascular events attributed to timolol ophthalmic solution, 1978-1985. *Am. J. Ophthalmol.,* **1986**, *102*(5), 606-611.
[http://dx.doi.org/10.1016/0002-9394(86)90532-5] [PMID: 3777080]

[30]   Food and Drug Administration. *FDA approves Xtoro to treat swimmer's ear.,* **2014**. https://www.biopharmadive.com/news/fda-approves-novartisalcons-xtoro-for-swimmers-ear/345399/

[31]   Eyding, D.; Lelgemann, M.; Grouven, U.; Härter, M.; Kromp, M.; Kaiser, T.; Kerekes, M.F.; Gerken, M.; Wieseler, B. Reboxetine for acute treatment of major depression: Systematic review and meta-analysis of published and unpublished placebo and selective serotonin reuptake inhibitor controlled trials. *BMJ,* **2010**, *341*(oct12 1), c4737.
[http://dx.doi.org/10.1136/bmj.c4737] [PMID: 20940209]

[32]   Ren, H.; Li, X.; Ni, Z.H.; Niu, J.Y.; Cao, B.; Xu, J.; Cheng, H.; Tu, X.W.; Ren, A.M.; Hu, Y.; Xing, C.Y.; Liu, Y.H.; Li, Y.F.; Cen, J.; Zhou, R.; Xu, X.D.; Qiu, X.H.; Chen, N. Treatment of complicated urinary tract infection and acute pyelonephritis by short-course intravenous levofloxacin (750 mg/day) or conventional intravenous/oral levofloxacin (500 mg/day): Prospective, open-label, randomized, controlled, multicenter, non-inferiority clinical trial. *Int. Urol. Nephrol.,* **2017**, *49*(3), 499-507.
[http://dx.doi.org/10.1007/s11255-017-1507-0] [PMID: 28108978]

[33]   Seyffart, G. *Drug Dosage in Renal Insufficiency*; Kluwer Academic Publishers: Boston, **1991**.
[http://dx.doi.org/10.1007/978-94-011-3804-8]

[34]   Siemer, H.; Doppstadt, A. Substituted 1-phenyl-2,3-dimethyl-4-morpholino methyl pyrazolone-(5) compounds and process of making same. US patent 2943022, 1960.

[35]   Entzeroth, M.; Ratty, A.K. Monoamine oxidase inhibitors—revisiting a therapeutic principle. *Open J. Depress.,* **2017**, *6*(2), 31-68.
[http://dx.doi.org/10.4236/ojd.2017.62004]

[36]   Al-Ghorbani, M.; Bushra, B.A.; Zabiulla, ; Mamatha, S.V.; Khanum, S.A. Piperazine and morpholine: Synthetic preview and pharmaceutical applications. *Res. J. Pharm. Technol,* **2015**, *8*(5), 611.
[http://dx.doi.org/10.5958/0974-360X.2015.00100.6]

[37]   Volotinen, M.; Turpeinen, M.; Tolonen, A.; Uusitalo, J.; Mäenpää, J.; Pelkonen, O. Timolol metabolism in human liver microsomes is mediated principally by CYP2D6. *Drug Metab. Dispos.,* **2007**, *35*(7), 1135-1141.
[http://dx.doi.org/10.1124/dmd.106.012906] [PMID: 17431033]

[38]   Mardal, M.; Miserez, B.; Bade, R.; Portolés, T.; Bischoff, M.; Hernández, F.; Meyer, M.R. 3-Fluorophenmetrazine, a fluorinated analogue of phenmetrazine: Studies on *in vivo* metabolism in rat and human, *in vitro* metabolism in human CYP isoenzymes and microbial biotransformation in Pseudomonas Putida and wastewater using GC and LC coupled to (HR)-MS techniques. *J. Pharm. Biomed. Anal.,* **2016**, *128*, 485-495.
[http://dx.doi.org/10.1016/j.jpba.2016.06.011] [PMID: 27372653]

[39]   Pieniaszek, H.J., Jr; Davidson, A.F.; Chaney, J.E.; Shum, L.; Robinson, C.A.; Mayersohn, M. Human moricizine metabolism. II. Quantification and pharmacokinetics of plasma and urinary metabolites. *Xenobiotica,* **1999**, *29*(9), 945-955.
[http://dx.doi.org/10.1080/004982599238182] [PMID: 10548454]

[40]   Mckillop, D.; Mccormick, A.D.; Miles, G.S.; Phillips, P.J.; Pickup, K.J.; Bushby, N.; Hutchison, M. *In vitro* metabolism of gefitinib in human liver microsomes. *Xenobiotica,* **2004**, *34*(11-12), 983-1000.

[http://dx.doi.org/10.1080/02772240400015222] [PMID: 15801543]

[41] Wienkers, L.C.; Allievi, C.; Hauer, M.J.; Wynalda, M.A. Cytochrome P-450-mediated metabolism of the individual enantiomers of the antidepressant agent reboxetine in human liver microsomes. *Drug Metab. Dispos.,* **1999**, *27*(11), 1334-1340.
[PMID: 10534319]

[42] Slatter, J.G.; Stalker, D.J.; Feenstra, K.L.; Welshman, I.R.; Bruss, J.B.; Sams, J.P.; Johnson, M.G.; Sanders, P.E.; Hauer, M.J.; Fagerness, P.E.; Stryd, R.P.; Peng, G.W.; Shobe, E.M. Pharmacokinetics, metabolism, and excretion of linezolid following an oral dose of [(14)C]linezolid to healthy human subjects. *Drug Metab. Dispos.,* **2001**, *29*(8), 1136-1145.
[PMID: 11454733]

[43] Wuitschik, G.; Rogers-Evans, M.; Müller, K.; Fischer, H.; Wagner, B.; Schuler, F.; Polonchuk, L.; Carreira, E.M. Oxetanes as promising modules in drug discovery. *Angew. Chem. Int. Ed.,* **2006**, *45*(46), 7736-7739.
[http://dx.doi.org/10.1002/anie.200602343] [PMID: 17013952]

[44] Wuitschik, G.; Carreira, E.M.; Wagner, B.; Fischer, H.; Parrilla, I.; Schuler, F.; Rogers-Evans, M.; Müller, K. Oxetanes in drug discovery: Structural and synthetic insights. *J. Med. Chem.,* **2010**, *53*(8), 3227-3246.
[http://dx.doi.org/10.1021/jm9018788] [PMID: 20349959]

[45] Wuitschik, G.; Rogers-Evans, M.; Buckl, A.; Bernasconi, M.; Märki, M.; Godel, T.; Fischer, H.; Wagner, B.; Parrilla, I.; Schuler, F.; Schneider, J.; Alker, A.; Schweizer, W.B.; Müller, K.; Carreira, E.M. Spirocyclic oxetanes: Synthesis and properties. *Angew. Chem. Int. Ed.,* **2008**, *47*(24), 4512-4515.
[http://dx.doi.org/10.1002/anie.200800450] [PMID: 18465828]

[46] Shcherbatiuk, A.V.; Shyshlyk, O.S.; Yarmoliuk, D.V.; Shishkin, O.V.; Shishkina, S.V.; Starova, V.S.; Zaporozhets, O.A.; Zozulya, S.; Moriev, R.; Kravchuk, O.; Manoilenko, O.; Tolmachev, A.A.; Mykhailiuk, P.K. Synthesis of 2- and 3-trifluoromethylmorpholines: Useful building blocks for drug discovery. *Tetrahedron,* **2013**, *69*(19), 3796-3804.
[http://dx.doi.org/10.1016/j.tet.2013.03.067]

[47] Kirichok, A.A.; Shton, I.O.; Pishel, I.M.; Zozulya, S.A.; Borysko, P.O.; Kubyshkin, V.; Zaporozhets, O.A.; Tolmachev, A.A.; Mykhailiuk, P.K. Synthesis of multifunctional spirocyclic azetidines and their application in drug discovery. *Chemistry,* **2018**, *24*(21), 5444-5449.
[http://dx.doi.org/10.1002/chem.201800193] [PMID: 29338097]

[48] Degorce, S.L.; Bodnarchuk, M.S.; Cumming, I.A.; Scott, J.S. Lowering lipophilicity by adding carbon: One-carbon bridges of morpholines and piperazines. *J. Med. Chem.,* **2018**, *61*(19), 8934-8943.
[http://dx.doi.org/10.1021/acs.jmedchem.8b01148] [PMID: 30189136]

[49] Tesfaye, T.; Ravichadran, Y.D. A review on anticancer activity of some plant-derived compounds and their mode of action. *Nat. Prod. Chem. Res.,* **2018**, *6*, 334.

[50] Singh, R.K.; Kumar, S.; Prasad, D.N.; Bhardwaj, T.R. Therapeutic journery of nitrogen mustard as alkylating anticancer agents: Historic to future perspectives. *Eur. J. Med. Chem.,* **2018**, *151*, 401-433.
[http://dx.doi.org/10.1016/j.ejmech.2018.04.001] [PMID: 29649739]

[51] Siegel, R.L.; Miller, K.D.; Jemal, A.; Jema, A. Cancer statistics, 2018. *CA Cancer J. Clin.,* **2018**, *68*(1), 7-30.
[http://dx.doi.org/10.3322/caac.21442] [PMID: 29313949]

[52] Arshad, F.; Khan, M.F.; Akhtar, W.; Alam, M.M.; Nainwal, L.M.; Kaushik, S.K.; Akhter, M.; Parvez, S.; Hasan, S.M.; Shaquiquzzaman, M. Revealing quinquennial anticancer journey of morpholine: A SAR based review. *Eur. J. Med. Chem.,* **2019**, *167*, 324-356.
[http://dx.doi.org/10.1016/j.ejmech.2019.02.015] [PMID: 30776694]

[53] Kourounakis, A.P.; Xanthopoulos, D.; Tzara, A. Morpholine as a privileged structure: A review on the medicinal chemistry and pharmacological activity of morpholine containing bioactive molecules. *Med. Res. Rev.,* **2019**.

[http://dx.doi.org/10.1002/med.21634] [PMID: 31512284]

[54]   Vendramini-Costa, D.B.; Carvalho, J.E. Molecular link mechanisms between inflammation and cancer. *Curr. Pharm. Des.,* **2012**, *18*(26), 3831-3852.
[http://dx.doi.org/10.2174/138161212802083707] [PMID: 22632748]

[55]   Khatami, M. 'Yin and Yang' in inflammation: Duality in innate immune cell function and tumorigenesis. *Expert Opin. Biol. Ther.,* **2008**, *8*(10), 1461-1472.
[http://dx.doi.org/10.1517/14712598.8.10.1461] [PMID: 18774915]

[56]   Reddy, M.V.B.; Hwang, T.L.; Leu, Y.L.; Chiou, W.F.; Wu, T.S. Inhibitory effects of Mannich bases of heterocyclic chalcones on NO production by activated RAW 264.7 macrophages and superoxide anion generation and elastase release by activated human neutrophils. *Bioorg. Med. Chem.,* **2011**, *19*(8), 2751-2756.
[http://dx.doi.org/10.1016/j.bmc.2011.02.038] [PMID: 21441032]

[57]   Patyna, S.; Laird, A.D.; Mendel, D.B.; O'Farrell, A.M.; Liang, C.; Guan, H.; Vojkovsky, T.; Vasile, S.; Wang, X.; Chen, J.; Grazzini, M.; Yang, C.Y.; Haznedar, J.Ö.; Sukbuntherng, J.; Zhong, W.Z.; Cherrington, J.M.; Hu-Lowe, D. SU14813: A novel multiple receptor tyrosine kinase inhibitor with potent antiangiogenic and antitumor activity. *Mol. Cancer Ther.,* **2006**, *5*(7), 1774-1782.
[http://dx.doi.org/10.1158/1535-7163.MCT-05-0333] [PMID: 16891463]

[58]   Yang, K.; Guo, Y.; Stacey, W.C.; Harwalkar, J.; Fretthold, J.; Hitomi, M.; Stacey, D.W. Glycogen synthase kinase 3 has a limited role in cell cycle regulation of cyclin D1 levels. *BMC Cell Biol.,* **2006**, *7*(1), 33.
[http://dx.doi.org/10.1186/1471-2121-7-33] [PMID: 16942622]

[59]   Scaltriti, M.; Baselga, J. The epidermal growth factor receptor pathway: A model for targeted therapy. *Clin. Cancer Res.,* **2006**, *12*(18), 5268-5272.
[http://dx.doi.org/10.1158/1078-0432.CCR-05-1554] [PMID: 17000658]

[60]   Takimoto, C.H.; Calvo, E. Principles of Oncologic Pharmacotherapy. In: *Cancer Management: A Multidisciplinary Approach,* 11th ed; Pazdur, R.; Wagman, L.D.; Camphausen, K.A.; Hoskins, W.J., Eds.; , **2008**.

[61]   Zheng, Y.; Jiang, Y. mTOR Inhibitors at a Glance. *Mol. Cell. Pharmacol.,* **2015**, *7*(2), 15-20.
[PMID: 27134695]

[62]   Kennedy, B.K.; Lamming, D.W. The mechanistic target of rapamycin: The grand conductor of metabolism and aging. *Cell Metab.,* **2016**, *23*(6), 990-1003.
[http://dx.doi.org/10.1016/j.cmet.2016.05.009] [PMID: 27304501]

[63]   Lipton, J.O.; Sahin, M. The Neurology of mTOR. *Neuron,* **2014**, *84*(2), 275-291.
[http://dx.doi.org/10.1016/j.neuron.2014.09.034] [PMID: 25374355]

[64]   Roohi, A.; Hojjat-Farsangi, M. Recent advances in targeting mTOR signaling pathway using small molecule inhibitors. *J. Drug Target.,* **2017**, *25*(3), 189-201.
[http://dx.doi.org/10.1080/1061186X.2016.1236112] [PMID: 27632356]

[65]   Zask, A.; Kaplan, J.; Verheijen, J.C.; Richard, D.J.; Curran, K.; Brooijmans, N.; Bennett, E.M.; Toral-Barza, L.; Hollander, I.; Ayral-Kaloustian, S.; Yu, K. Morpholine derivatives greatly enhance the selectivity of mammalian target of rapamycin (mTOR) inhibitors. *J. Med. Chem.,* **2009**, *52*(24), 7942-7945.
[http://dx.doi.org/10.1021/jm901415x] [PMID: 19916508]

[66]   Zhang, L.; Bu, T.; Bao, X.; Liang, T.; Ge, Y.; Xu, Y.; Zhu, Q. Design, synthesis and biological evaluation of novel 3 H -imidazole [4,5- b] pyridine derivatives as selective mTOR inhibitors. *Bioorg. Med. Chem. Lett.,* **2017**, *27*(15), 3395-3398.
[http://dx.doi.org/10.1016/j.bmcl.2017.06.010] [PMID: 28633896]

[67]   Zask, A.; Verheijen, J.C.; Richard, D.J.; Kaplan, J.; Curran, K.; Toral-Barza, L.; Lucas, J.; Hollander, I.; Yu, K. Discovery of 2-ureidophenyltriazines bearing bridged morpholines as potent and selective

ATP-competitive mTOR inhibitors. *Bioorg. Med. Chem. Lett.,* **2010**, *20*(8), 2644-2647.
[http://dx.doi.org/10.1016/j.bmcl.2010.02.045] [PMID: 20227881]

[68]   Janku, F.; Yap, T.A.; Meric-Bernstam, F. Targeting the PI3K pathway in cancer: Are we making
       headway? *Nat. Rev. Clin. Oncol.,* **2018**, *15*(5), 273-291.
       [http://dx.doi.org/10.1038/nrclinonc.2018.28] [PMID: 29508857]

[69]   Fruman, D.A.; Chiu, H.; Hopkins, B.D.; Bagrodia, S.; Cantley, L.C.; Abraham, R.T. The PI3K
       Pathway in Human Disease. *Cell,* **2017**, *170*(4), 605-635.
       [http://dx.doi.org/10.1016/j.cell.2017.07.029] [PMID: 28802037]

[70]   Samuels, Y.; Wang, Z.; Bardelli, A.; Silliman, N.; Ptak, J.; Szabo, S.; Yan, H.; Gazdar, A.; Powell,
       S.M.; Riggins, G.J.; Willson, J.K.V.; Markowitz, S.; Kinzler, K.W.; Vogelstein, B.; Velculescu, V.E.
       High frequency of mutations of the PIK3CA gene in human cancers. *Science,* **2004**, *304*(5670), 554.
       [http://dx.doi.org/10.1126/science.1096502] [PMID: 15016963]

[71]   Sele, A.M.; Rageot, D.; Beaufils, F.; Melone, A.; Bohnacker, T.; Jackson, E.; Langlois, J.B.; Hebeisen,
       P.; Fabbro, D.; Wymann, M.P. Abstract 153: Tricyclic fused pyrimidinopyrrolo-oxazines reveal
       conformational preferences of morpholine for PI3K hinge region binding. *Cancer Res.,* **2017**,
       77(13_Supplement), 153.
       [http://dx.doi.org/10.1158/1538-7445.AM2017-153]

[72]   Liu, P.; Cheng, H.; Roberts, T.M.; Zhao, J.J. Targeting the phosphoinositide 3-kinase pathway in
       cancer. *Nat. Rev. Drug Discov.,* **2009**, *8*(8), 627-644.
       [http://dx.doi.org/10.1038/nrd2926] [PMID: 19644473]

[73]   Cross, T.G.; Scheel-Toellner, D.; Henriquez, N.V.; Deacon, E.; Salmon, M.; Lord, J.M.
       Serine/threonine protein kinases and apoptosis. *Exp. Cell Res.,* **2000**, *256*(1), 34-41.
       [http://dx.doi.org/10.1006/excr.2000.4836] [PMID: 10739649]

[74]   Rewcastle, G.W.; Gamage, S.A.; Flanagan, J.U.; Frederick, R.; Denny, W.A.; Baguley, B.C.; Kestell,
       P.; Singh, R.; Kendall, J.D.; Marshall, E.S.; Lill, C.L.; Lee, W.J.; Kolekar, S.; Buchanan, C.M.;
       Jamieson, S.M.F.; Shepherd, P.R. Synthesis and biological evaluation of novel analogues of the pan
       class I phosphatidylinositol 3-kinase (PI3K) inhibitor 2-(difluoromethyl)-1-[4,6-di(4-morphol-
       nyl)-1,3,5-triazin-2-yl]-1*H*-benzimidazole (ZSTK474). *J. Med. Chem.,* **2011**, *54*(20), 7105-7126.
       [http://dx.doi.org/10.1021/jm200688y] [PMID: 21882832]

[75]   Wang, X.M.; Xin, M.H.; Xu, J.; Kang, B.R.; Li, Y.; Lu, S.M.; Zhang, S.Q. Synthesis and antitumor
       activities evaluation of *m-(*4-morpholinoquinazolin-2-yl)benzamides *in vitro* and *in vivo. Eur. J. Med.
       Chem.,* **2015**, *96*, 382-395.
       [http://dx.doi.org/10.1016/j.ejmech.2015.04.037] [PMID: 25911625]

[76]   Burger, M.T.; Pecchi, S.; Wagman, A.; Ni, Z.J.; Knapp, M.; Hendrickson, T.; Atallah, G.; Pfister, K.;
       Zhang, Y.; Bartulis, S.; Frazier, K.; Ng, S.; Smith, A.; Verhagen, J.; Haznedar, J.; Huh, K.; Iwanowicz,
       E.; Xin, X.; Menezes, D.; Merritt, H.; Lee, I.; Wiesmann, M.; Kaufman, S.; Crawford, K.; Chin, M.;
       Bussiere, D.; Shoemaker, K.; Zaror, I.; Maira, S.M.; Voliva, C.F. Identification of NVP-BKM120 as a
       potent, selective, orally bioavailable class I PI3 kinase inhibitor for treating cancer. *ACS Med. Chem.
       Lett.,* **2011**, *2*(10), 774-779.
       [http://dx.doi.org/10.1021/ml200156t] [PMID: 24900266]

[77]   Fekete, B.; Palkó, M.; Haukka, M.; Fülöp, F. Synthesis of pyrrolo[1,2-a]pyrimidine enantiomers *via*
       domino ring-closure followed by retrodiels-alder protocol. *Molecules,* **2017**, *22*(4), 613.
       [http://dx.doi.org/10.3390/molecules22040613] [PMID: 28406463]

[78]   Ibrahim, M.A.; Abou-Seri, S.M.; Hanna, M.M.; Abdalla, M.M.; El Sayed, N.A. Design, synthesis and
       biological evaluation of novel condensed pyrrolo[1,2-c]pyrimidines featuring morpholine moiety as
       PI3Kα inhibitors. *Eur. J. Med. Chem.,* **2015**, *99*, 1-13.
       [http://dx.doi.org/10.1016/j.ejmech.2015.05.036] [PMID: 26037808]

[79]   Helwa, A.A.; Gedawy, E.M.; Taher, A.T.; ED El-Ansary, A.K.; Abou-Seri, S.M. Synthesis and
       biological evaluation of novel pyrimidine-5-carbonitriles featuring morpholine moiety as antitumor

agents. *Future Med. Chem.,* **2020**, *12*(5), 403-421.
[http://dx.doi.org/10.4155/fmc-2019-0146] [PMID: 32027179]

[80] Lu, N.; Malemud, C.J. Extracellular Signal-Regulated Kinase: A Regulator of Cell Growth, Inflammation, Chondrocyte and Bone Cell Receptor-Mediated Gene Expression. *Int. J. Mol. Sci.,* **2019**, *20*(15), 3792.
[http://dx.doi.org/10.3390/ijms20153792] [PMID: 31382554]

[81] Kumari, A.; Prasad, D.N.; Kumar, S.; Singh, R.K. Clinical Benefits of Switching from Original Infliximab to its Biosimilar (CT-P13) as a Potential TNF-α Inhibitor. *Journal of Exploratory Research in Pharmacology,* **2020**, *000*(000), 1-9.
[http://dx.doi.org/10.14218/JERP.2020.00004]

[82] Berraondo, P.; Sanmamed, M.F.; Ochoa, M.C.; Etxeberria, I.; Aznar, M.A.; Pérez-Gracia, J.L.; Rodríguez-Ruiz, M.E.; Ponz-Sarvise, M.; Castañón, E.; Melero, I. Cytokines in clinical cancer immunotherapy. *Br. J. Cancer,* **2019**, *120*(1), 6-15.
[http://dx.doi.org/10.1038/s41416-018-0328-y] [PMID: 30413827]

[83] Bhatia, R.; Singh, R.K. Introductory Chapter: Protein Kinases as Promising Targets for Drug Design against Cancer. In: *Protein Kinases - Promising Targets for Anticancer Drug Research*; Singh, R.K., Ed.; IntechOpen: London, **2021**.
[http://dx.doi.org/10.5772/intechopen.100315]

[84] Zhu, W.; Sun, C.; Xu, S.; Wu, C.; Wu, J.; Xu, M.; Zhao, H.; Chen, L.; Zeng, W.; Zheng, P. Design, synthesis, anticancer activity and docking studies of novel 4-morpholino-7,8-dihydr--5H-thiopyrano[4,3-d]pyrimidine derivatives as mTOR inhibitors. *Bioorg. Med. Chem.,* **2014**, *22*(24), 6746-6754.
[http://dx.doi.org/10.1016/j.bmc.2014.11.003] [PMID: 25468038]

[85] Pratiksha, P.S.; Jagdish, K.; Sahu, J.K.; Mishra, A.K.; Hashim, S.R. Role of aryl urea containing compounds in medicinal chemistry. *Med. Chem.,* **2015**, *5*, 479-483.

[86] Wang, A.Y.; Lu, Y.; Zhu, H.L.; Jiao, Q.C. URD12: A urea derivative with marked antitumor activities. *Oncol. Lett.,* **2012**, *3*(2), 373-376.
[http://dx.doi.org/10.3892/ol.2011.474] [PMID: 22740914]

[87] Sabbah, D.A.; Brattain, M.G.; Zhong, H. Dual inhibitors of PI3K/mTOR or mTOR-selective inhibitors: Which way shall we go? *Curr. Med. Chem.,* **2011**, *18*(36), 5528-5544.
[http://dx.doi.org/10.2174/092986711798347298] [PMID: 22172063]

[88] Zhu, W.; Sun, C.; Xu, S.; Wu, C.; Wu, J.; Xu, M.; Zhao, H.; Chen, L.; Zeng, W.; Zheng, P. Design, synthesis, anticancer activity and docking studies of novel 4-morpholino-7,8-dihydro-5*H*-thiopyrano[4,3-d]pyrimidine derivatives as mTOR inhibitors. *Bioorg. Med. Chem.,* **2014**, *22*(24), 6746-6754.
[http://dx.doi.org/10.1016/j.bmc.2014.11.003] [PMID: 25468038]

[89] Andrs, M.; Korabecny, J.; Jun, D.; Hodny, Z.; Bartek, J.; Kuca, K. Phosphatidylinositol 3-Kinase (PI3K) and phosphatidylinositol 3-kinase-related kinase (PIKK) inhibitors: Importance of the morpholine ring. *J. Med. Chem.,* **2015**, *58*(1), 41-71.
[http://dx.doi.org/10.1021/jm501026z] [PMID: 25387153]

[90] Askari, B.S.; Krajinovic, M. Dihydrofolate reductase gene variations in susceptibility to disease and treatment outcomes. *Curr. Genomics,* **2010**, *11*(8), 578-583.
[http://dx.doi.org/10.2174/138920210793360925] [PMID: 21629435]

[91] Raimondi, M.; Randazzo, O.; La Franca, M.; Barone, G.; Vignoni, E.; Rossi, D.; Collina, S. DHFR Inhibitors: Reading the Past for Discovering Novel Anticancer Agents. *Molecules,* **2019**, *24*(6), 1140.
[http://dx.doi.org/10.3390/molecules24061140] [PMID: 30909399]

[92] Muhammad, Z.; Edrees, M.; Faty, R.; Gomha, S.; Alterary, S.; Mabkhot, Y. Synthesis, antitumor evaluation and molecular docking of new morpholine based heterocycles. *Molecules,* **2017**, *22*(7), 1211.

[http://dx.doi.org/10.3390/molecules22071211] [PMID: 28726760]

[93]   Cullen, S.P.; Martin, S.J. Caspase activation pathways: Some recent progress. *Cell Death Differ.*, **2009**, *16*(7), 935-938.
[http://dx.doi.org/10.1038/cdd.2009.59] [PMID: 19528949]

[94]   Belkacemi, L. Exploiting the Extrinsic and the Intrinsic Apoptotic Pathways for Cancer Therapeutics. *J. Cancer Cure*, **2018**, *1*(1), 1004.

[95]   Alnemri, E.S.; Livingston, D.J.; Nicholson, D.W.; Salvesen, G.; Thornberry, N.A.; Wong, W.W.; Yuan, J. Human ICE/CED-3 protease nomenclature. *Cell*, **1996**, *87*(2), 171.
[http://dx.doi.org/10.1016/S0092-8674(00)81334-3] [PMID: 8861900]

[96]   Kravchenko, D.V.; Kysil, V.M.; Tkachenko, S.E.; Maliarchouk, S.; Okun, I.M.; Ivachtchenko, A.V. Pyrrolo[3,4-c]quinoline-1,3-diones as potent caspase-3 inhibitors. Synthesis and SAR of 2-substituted 4-methyl-8-(morpholine-4-sulfonyl)-pyrrolo[3,4-c]quinoline-1,3-diones. *Eur. J. Med. Chem.*, **2005**, *40*(12), 1377-1383.
[http://dx.doi.org/10.1016/j.ejmech.2005.07.011] [PMID: 16169127]

[97]   Aktar, B.S.K.; Oruc-Emre, E.E.; Demirtas, I.; Yaglioglu, A.S.; Iyidogan, A.K.; Guler, C.; Adem, S. Synthesis and biological evaluation of novel chalcones bearing morpholine moiety as antiproliferative agents. *Turk. J. Chem.*, **2018**, *42*, 482-492.

[98]   Surendra Kumar, R.; Moydeen, M.; Al-Deyab, S.S.; Manilal, A.; Idhayadhulla, A. Synthesis of new morpholine - connected pyrazolidine derivatives and their antimicrobial, antioxidant, and cytotoxic activities. *Bioorg. Med. Chem. Lett.*, **2017**, *27*(1), 66-71.
[http://dx.doi.org/10.1016/j.bmcl.2016.11.032] [PMID: 27889456]

[99]   Doan, P.; Karjalainen, A.; Chandraseelan, J.G.; Sandberg, O.; Yli-Harja, O.; Rosholm, T.; Franzen, R.; Candeias, N.R.; Kandhavelu, M. Synthesis and biological screening for cytotoxic activity of *N*-substituted indolines and morpholines. *Eur. J. Med. Chem.*, **2016**, *120*, 296-303.
[http://dx.doi.org/10.1016/j.ejmech.2016.05.024] [PMID: 27214140]

[100] Abdelaziz, A.M.; Yu, M.; Li, P.; Zhong, L.; Singab, A.N.B.; Hanna, A.G.; Abouzid, K.A.; Maged, K.G.; Mekhael, M.K.G.; Wang, S. Synthesis and evaluation of 5-chloro-2-methoxy-*N*-(--sulphamoylphenyl)benzamide derivatives as anticancer agents. *Med. Chem.*, **2015**, *5*, 253-260.

[101] Wu, L.; Lu, M.; Yan, Z.; Tang, X.; Sun, B.; Liu, W.; Zhou, H.; Yang, C. 1,2-Benzisothiazol-3-one derivatives as a novel class of small-molecule caspase-3 inhibitors. *Bioorg. Med. Chem.*, **2014**, *22*(8), 2416-2426.
[http://dx.doi.org/10.1016/j.bmc.2014.03.002] [PMID: 24656804]

[102] Rincy, V.C.; Namitha, K.N.; Aswathy, J.; Binuja, S.S. An *in silico* study of novel morpholine derivatives for lung cancer, non-hodgkin's lymphoma and metastasis melanoma. *J. Pharm. Sci. & Res.*, **2019**, *11*(7), 2479-2484.

[103] Wang, Y.; Kuramitsu, Y.; Baron, B.; Kitagawa, T.; Tokuda, K.; Akada, J.; Maehara, S.I.; Maehara, Y.; Nakamura, K. PI3K inhibitor LY294002, as opposed to wortmannin, enhances AKT phosphorylation in gemcitabine-resistant pancreatic cancer cells. *Int. J. Oncol.*, **2017**, *50*(2), 606-612.
[http://dx.doi.org/10.3892/ijo.2016.3804] [PMID: 28000865]

[104] Wenqing, Q.; Amy, S.; Carla, M.; Laurence, S.C.; Joseph, R.G.; Donald, D.; Daruka, M. SF1126, a Pan-PI3K inhibitor has potent preclinical activity in aggressive B-cell non-Hodgkin lymphomas by inducing cell cycle arrest and apoptosis. *J. Cancer Sci. Ther.*, **2012**, *4*, 207-213.

[105] Zhao, Y.; Thomas, H.D.; Batey, M.A.; Cowell, I.G.; Richardson, C.J.; Griffin, R.J.; Calvert, A.H.; Newell, D.R.; Smith, G.C.M.; Curtin, N.J. Preclinical evaluation of a potent novel DNA-dependent protein kinase inhibitor NU7441. *Cancer Res.*, **2006**, *66*(10), 5354-5362.
[http://dx.doi.org/10.1158/0008-5472.CAN-05-4275] [PMID: 16707462]

[106] Nutley, B.P.; Smith, N.F.; Hayes, A.; Kelland, L.R.; Brunton, L.; Golding, B.T.; Smith, G.C.M.; Martin, N.M.B.; Workman, P.; Raynaud, F.I. Preclinical pharmacokinetics and metabolism of a novel

prototype DNA-PK inhibitor NU7026. *Br. J. Cancer,* **2005**, *93*(9), 1011-1018.
[http://dx.doi.org/10.1038/sj.bjc.6602823] [PMID: 16249792]

[107]   Chwastek, J.; Jantas, D.; Lasoń, W. The ATM kinase inhibitor KU-55933 provides neuroprotection against hydrogen peroxide-induced cell damage *via* a γH2AX/p-p53/caspase-3-independent mechanism: Inhibition of calpain and cathepsin D. *Int. J. Biochem. Cell Biol.,* **2017**, *87*, 38-53.
[http://dx.doi.org/10.1016/j.biocel.2017.03.015] [PMID: 28341201]

[108]   Munck, J.M.; Batey, M.A.; Zhao, Y.; Jenkins, H.; Richardson, C.J.; Cano, C.; Tavecchio, M.; Barbeau, J.; Bardos, J.; Cornell, L.; Griffin, R.J.; Menear, K.; Slade, A.; Thommes, P.; Martin, N.M.B.; Newell, D.R.; Smith, G.C.M.; Curtin, N.J. Chemosensitization of cancer cells by KU-0060648, a dual inhibitor of DNA-PK and PI-3K. *Mol. Cancer Ther.,* **2012**, *11*(8), 1789-1798.
[http://dx.doi.org/10.1158/1535-7163.MCT-11-0535] [PMID: 22576130]

[109]   Vecchio, D.; Daga, A.; Carra, E.; Marubbi, D.; Baio, G.; Neumaier, C.E.; Vagge, S.; Corvò, R.; Pia Brisigotti, M.; Louis Ravetti, J.; Zunino, A.; Poggi, A.; Mascelli, S.; Raso, A.; Frosina, G. Predictability, efficacy and safety of radiosensitization of glioblastoma-initiating cells by the ATM inhibitor KU-60019. *Int. J. Cancer,* **2014**, *135*(2), 479-491.
[http://dx.doi.org/10.1002/ijc.28680] [PMID: 24443327]

[110]   Shinohara, E.T.; Geng, L.; Tan, J.; Chen, H.; Shir, Y.; Edwards, E.; Halbrook, J.; Kesicki, E.A.; Kashishian, A.; Hallahan, D.E. DNA-dependent protein kinase is a molecular target for the development of noncytotoxic radiation-sensitizing drugs. *Cancer Res.,* **2005**, *65*(12), 4987-4992.
[http://dx.doi.org/10.1158/0008-5472.CAN-04-4250] [PMID: 15958537]

[111]   Salles, B.; Calsou, P.; Frit, P.; Muller, C. The DNA repair complex DNA-PK, a pharmacological target in cancer chemotherapy and radiotherapy. *Pathol. Biol. (Paris),* **2006**, *54*(4), 185-193.
[http://dx.doi.org/10.1016/j.patbio.2006.01.012] [PMID: 16563661]

[112]   Chandra, G.; Alexander, V.; Lee, H.W.; Jeong, L.S. Improved synthesis of a DNA-dependent protein kinase inhibitor IC86621. *Arch. Pharm. Res.,* **2012**, *35*(4), 639-645.
[http://dx.doi.org/10.1007/s12272-012-0407-1] [PMID: 22553056]

[113]   Knight, Z.A.; Chiang, G.G.; Alaimo, P.J.; Kenski, D.M.; Ho, C.B.; Coan, K.; Abraham, R.T.; Shokat, K.M. Isoform-specific phosphoinositide 3-kinase inhibitors from an arylmorpholine scaffold. *Bioorg. Med. Chem.,* **2004**, *12*(17), 4749-4759.
[http://dx.doi.org/10.1016/j.bmc.2004.06.022] [PMID: 15358300]

[114]   Yang, X.; Yang, J.A.; Liu, B.H.; Liao, J.M.; Yuan, F.E.; Tan, Y.Q.; Chen, Q.X. TGX-221 inhibits proliferation and induces apoptosis in human glioblastoma cells. *Oncol. Rep.,* **2017**, *38*(5), 2836-2842.
[http://dx.doi.org/10.3892/or.2017.5991] [PMID: 29048665]

[115]   Knight, Z.A.; Gonzalez, B.; Feldman, M.E.; Zunder, E.R.; Goldenberg, D.D.; Williams, O.; Loewith, R.; Stokoe, D.; Balla, A.; Toth, B.; Balla, T.; Weiss, W.A.; Williams, R.L.; Shokat, K.M. A pharmacological map of the PI3-K family defines a role for p110alpha in insulin signaling. *Cell,* **2006**, *125*(4), 733-747.
[http://dx.doi.org/10.1016/j.cell.2006.03.035] [PMID: 16647110]

[116]   Nylander, S.; Kull, B.; Björkman, J.A.; Ulvinge, J.C.; Oakes, N.; Emanuelsson, B.M.; Andersson, M.; Skärby, T.; Inghardt, T.; Fjellström, O.; Gustafsson, D. Human target validation of phosphoinositide 3-kinase (PI3K)β: Effects on platelets and insulin sensitivity, using AZD6482 a novel PI3Kβ inhibitor. *J. Thromb. Haemost.,* **2012**, *10*(10), 2127-2136.
[http://dx.doi.org/10.1111/j.1538-7836.2012.04898.x] [PMID: 22906130]

[117]   Mateo, J.; Ganji, G.; Lemech, C.; Burris, H.A.; Han, S.W.; Swales, K.; Decordova, S.; DeYoung, M.P.; Smith, D.A.; Kalyana-Sundaram, S.; Wu, J.; Motwani, M.; Kumar, R.; Tolson, J.M.; Rha, S.Y.; Chung, H.C.; Eder, J.P.; Sharma, S.; Bang, Y.J.; Infante, J.R.; Yan, L.; de Bono, J.S.; Arkenau, H.T. The first-time-in-humanstudy of gsk2636771, a phosphoinositide 3 kinase beta-selective inhibitor, in patients with advancedsolid tumours. *Clin. Cancer Res.,* **2017**, *23*(19), 5981-5992.
[http://dx.doi.org/10.1158/1078-0432.CCR-17-0725] [PMID: 28645941]

[118] Bédard, P.L.; Davies, M.A.; Kopetz, S.; Juric, D.; Shapiro, G.I.; Luke, J.J.; Spreafico, A.; Wu, B.; Castell, C.; Gomez, C.; Cartot-Cotton, S.; Mazuir, F.; Dubar, M.; Micallef, S.; Demers, B.; Flaherty, K.T. First-in-human trial of the PI3Kβ-selective inhibitor SAR260301 in patients with advanced solid tumors. *Cancer,* **2018,** *124*(2), 315-324.
[http://dx.doi.org/10.1002/cncr.31044] [PMID: 28976556]

[119] Djuzenova, C.S.; Fiedler, V.; Katzer, A.; Michel, K.; Deckert, S.; Zimmermann, H.; Sukhorukov, V.L.; Flentje, M. Dual PI3K- and mTOR-inhibitor PI-103 can either enhance or reduce the radiosensitizing effect of the Hsp90 inhibitor NVP-AUY922 in tumor cells: The role of drug-irradiation schedule. *Oncotarget,* **2016,** *7*(25), 38191-38209.
[http://dx.doi.org/10.18632/oncotarget.9501] [PMID: 27224913]

[120] Schöffski, P.; Cresta, S.; Mayer, I.A.; Wildiers, H.; Damian, S.; Gendreau, S.; Rooney, I.; Morrissey, K.M.; Spoerke, J.M.; Ng, V.W.; Singel, S.M.; Winer, E. A phase Ib study of pictilisib (GDC-0941) in combination with paclitaxel, with and without bevacizumab or trastuzumab, and with letrozole in advanced breast cancer. *Breast Cancer Res.,* **2018,** *20*(1), 109.
[http://dx.doi.org/10.1186/s13058-018-1015-x] [PMID: 30185228]

[121] Heffron, T.P.; Berry, M.; Castanedo, G.; Chang, C.; Chuckowree, I.; Dotson, J.; Folkes, A.; Gunzner, J.; Lesnick, J.D.; Lewis, C.; Mathieu, S.; Nonomiya, J.; Olivero, A.; Pang, J.; Peterson, D.; Salphati, L.; Sampath, D.; Sideris, S.; Sutherlin, D.P.; Tsui, V.; Wan, N.C.; Wang, S.; Wong, S.; Zhu, B. Identification of GNE-477, a potent and efficacious dual PI3K/mTOR inhibitor. *Bioorg. Med. Chem. Lett.,* **2010,** *20*(8), 2408-2411.
[http://dx.doi.org/10.1016/j.bmcl.2010.03.046] [PMID: 20346656]

[122] Powles, T.; Lackner, M.R.; Oudard, S.; Escudier, B.; Ralph, C.; Brown, J.E.; Hawkins, R.E.; Castellano, D.; Rini, B.I.; Staehler, M.D.; Ravaud, A.; Lin, W.; O'Keeffe, B.; Wang, Y.; Lu, S.; Spoerke, J.M.; Huw, L.Y.; Byrtek, M.; Zhu, R.; Ware, J.A.; Motzer, R.J. Randomized open-label phase II trial of Apitolisib (GDC-0980), a novel inhibitor of the PI3k/mammalian target of rapamycinpathway, *versus* everolimus in patients with metastatic renal cell carcinoma. *J. Clin. Oncol.,* **2016,** *34*(14), 1660-1668.
[http://dx.doi.org/10.1200/JCO.2015.64.8808] [PMID: 26951309]

[123] Granda, T.G.; Cebrián, D.; Martínez, S.; Anguita, P.V.; López, E.C.; Link, W.; Merino, T.; Pastor, J.; Serelde, B.G.; Peregrina, S.; Palacios, I.; Albarran, M.I.; Cebriá, A.; Lorenzo, M.; Alonso, P.; Fominaya, J.; López, A.R.; Bischoff, J.R. Biological characterization of ETP-46321 a selective and efficacious inhibitor of phosphoinositide-3-kinases. *Invest. New Drugs,* **2013,** *31*(1), 66-76.
[http://dx.doi.org/10.1007/s10637-012-9835-5] [PMID: 22623067]

[124] Martínez González, S.; Hernández, A.I.; Varela, C.; Lorenzo, M.; Ramos-Lima, F.; Cendón, E.; Cebrián, D.; Aguirre, E.; Gomez-Casero, E.; Albarrán, M.I.; Alfonso, P.; García-Serelde, B.; Mateos, G.; Oyarzabal, J.; Rabal, O.; Mulero, F.; Gonzalez-Granda, T.; Link, W.; Fominaya, J.; Barbacid, M.; Bischoff, J.R.; Pizcueta, P.; Blanco-Aparicio, C.; Pastor, J. Rapid identification of ETP-46992, orally bioavailable PI3K inhibitor, selective *versus* mTOR. *Bioorg. Med. Chem. Lett.,* **2012,** *22*(16), 5208-5214.
[http://dx.doi.org/10.1016/j.bmcl.2012.06.093] [PMID: 22819764]

[125] Mallon, R.; Hollander, I.; Feldberg, L.; Lucas, J.; Soloveva, V.; Venkatesan, A.; Dehnhardt, C.; Delos Santos, E.; Chen, Z.; dos Santos, O.; Ayral-Kaloustian, S.; Gibbons, J. Antitumor efficacy profile of PKI-402, a dual phosphatidylinositol 3-kinase/mammalian target of rapamycin inhibitor. *Mol. Cancer Ther.,* **2010,** *9*(4), 976-984.
[http://dx.doi.org/10.1158/1535-7163.MCT-09-0954] [PMID: 20371716]

[126] Singh, A.; Thatikonda, T.; Kumar, A.; Wazir, P.; v, V.; Nandi, U.; Singh, P.P.; Singh, S.; Gupta, A.P.; Tikoo, M.K.; Singh, G.; Vishwakarma, R. Determination of ZSTK474, a novel Pan PI3K inhibitor in mouse plasma by LC–MS/MS and its application to Pharmacokinetics. *J. Pharm. Biomed. Anal.,* **2018,** *149*, 387-393.
[http://dx.doi.org/10.1016/j.jpba.2017.11.031] [PMID: 29175554]

[127] Li, T.; Wang, J.; Wang, X.; Yang, N.; Chen, S.; Tong, L.; Yang, C.; Meng, L.; Ding, J. WJD008, a dual phosphatidylinositol 3-kinase (PI3K)/mammalian target of rapamycin inhibitor, prevents PI3K signaling and inhibits the proliferation of transformed cells with oncogenic PI3K mutant. *J. Pharmacol. Exp. Ther.,* **2010**, *334*(3), 830-838.
[http://dx.doi.org/10.1124/jpet.110.167940] [PMID: 20522531]

[128] Netland, I.A.; Førde, H.E.; Sleire, L.; Leiss, L.; Rahman, M.A.; Skeie, B.S.; Miletic, H.; Enger, P.Ø.; Goplen, D. Treatment with the PI3K inhibitor buparlisib (NVP-BKM120) suppresses the growth of established patient-derived GBM xenografts and prolongs survival in nude rats. *J. Neurooncol.,* **2016**, *129*(1), 57-66.
[http://dx.doi.org/10.1007/s11060-016-2158-1] [PMID: 27283525]

[129] Freitag, H.; Christen, F.; Lewens, F.; Grass, I.; Briest, F.; Iwaszkiewicz, S.; Siegmund, B.; Grabowski, P. Inhibition of mTOR's catalytic site by PKI-587 is a promising therapeutic option for gastro entero pancreatic neuroendocrine tumor disease. *Neuroendocrinology,* **2017**, *105*(1), 90-104.
[http://dx.doi.org/10.1159/000448843] [PMID: 27513674]

[130] Venkatesan, A.M.; Chen, Z.; Santos, O.D.; Dehnhardt, C.; Santos, E.D.; Ayral-Kaloustian, S.; Mallon, R.; Hollander, I.; Feldberg, L.; Lucas, J.; Yu, K.; Chaudhary, I.; Mansour, T.S. PKI-179: An orally efficacious dual phosphatidylinositol-3-kinase (PI3K)/mammalian target of rapamycin (mTOR) inhibitor. *Bioorg. Med. Chem. Lett.,* **2010**, *20*(19), 5869-5873.
[http://dx.doi.org/10.1016/j.bmcl.2010.07.104] [PMID: 20797855]

[131] Blagden, S.; Olmin, A.; Josephs, D.; Stavraka, C.; Zivi, A.; Pinato, D.J.; Anthoney, A.; Decordova, S.; Swales, K.; Riisnaes, R.; Pope, L.; Noguchi, K.; Shiokawa, R.; Inatani, M.; Prince, J.; Jones, K.; Twelves, C.; Spicer, J.; Banerji, U. First-in-human study of CH5132799, an oral class I PI3K inhibitor, studying toxicity, pharmacokinetics, and pharmacodynamics, in patients with metastatic cancer. *Clin. Cancer Res.,* **2014**, *20*(23), 5908-5917.
[http://dx.doi.org/10.1158/1078-0432.CCR-14-1315] [PMID: 25231405]

[132] Shao, Z.; Bao, Q.; Jiang, F.; Qian, H.; Fang, Q.; Hu, X. VS-5584, a Novel PI3K-mTOR Dual inhibitor, inhibits melanoma cell growth *in vitro* and *in vivo*. *PLoS One,* **2015**, *10*(7), e0132655.

[133] Shappley, R.K.H.; Spentzas, T. Differential role of rapamycin and torin/ku63794 in inflammatory response of 264.7 RAW macrophages stimulated by CA-MRSA. *Int. J. Inflamm.,* **2014**, *2014*, 1-9.
[http://dx.doi.org/10.1155/2014/560790] [PMID: 24800098]

[134] Willems, L.; Chapuis, N.; Puissant, A.; Maciel, T.T.; Green, A.S.; Jacque, N.; Vignon, C.; Park, S.; Guichard, S.; Herault, O.; Fricot, A.; Hermine, O.; Moura, I.C.; Auberger, P.; Ifrah, N.; Dreyfus, F.; Bonnet, D.; Lacombe, C.; Mayeux, P.; Bouscary, D.; Tamburini, J. The dual mTORC1 and mTORC2 inhibitor AZD8055 has anti-tumor activity in acute myeloid leukemia. *Leukemia,* **2012**, *26*(6), 1195-1202.
[http://dx.doi.org/10.1038/leu.2011.339] [PMID: 22143671]

[135] Guichard, S.M.; Curwen, J.; Bihani, T.; D'Cruz, C.M.; Yates, J.W.T.; Grondine, M.; Howard, Z.; Davies, B.R.; Bigley, G.; Klinowska, T.; Pike, K.G.; Pass, M.; Chresta, C.M.; Polanska, U.M.; McEwen, R.; Delpuech, O.; Green, S.; Cosulich, S.C. AZD2014, an inhibitor of mtorc1 and mTORC2, is highly effective in breast cancer when administered using intermittent or continuous schedules. *Mol. Cancer Ther.,* **2015**, *14*(11), 2508-2518.
[http://dx.doi.org/10.1158/1535-7163.MCT-15-0365] [PMID: 26358751]

[136] Yu, K.; Toral-Barza, L.; Shi, C.; Zhang, W.G.; Lucas, J.; Shor, B.; Kim, J.; Verheijen, J.; Curran, K.; Malwitz, D.J.; Cole, D.C.; Ellingboe, J.; Ayral-Kaloustian, S.; Mansour, T.S.; Gibbons, J.J.; Abraham, R.T.; Nowak, P.; Zask, A. Biochemical, cellular, and *in vivo* activity of novel ATP-competitive and selective inhibitors of the mammalian target of rapamycin. *Cancer Res.,* **2009**, *69*(15), 6232-6240.
[http://dx.doi.org/10.1158/0008-5472.CAN-09-0299] [PMID: 19584280]

[137] Pan, X.; Gu, D.; Mao, J.H.; Zhu, H.; Chen, X.; Zheng, B.; Shan, Y. Concurrent inhibition of mTORC1 and mTORC2 by WYE-687 inhibits renal cell carcinoma cell growth *in vitro* and *in vivo*. *PLoS One,* **2017**, *12*(3), e0172555.

[http://dx.doi.org/10.1371/journal.pone.0172555] [PMID: 28257457]

[138] Zask, A.; Verheijen, J.C.; Curran, K.; Kaplan, J.; Richard, D.J.; Nowak, P.; Malwitz, D.J.; Brooijmans, N.; Bard, J.; Svenson, K.; Lucas, J.; Toral-Barza, L.; Zhang, W.G.; Hollander, I.; Gibbons, J.J.; Abraham, R.T.; Ayral-Kaloustian, S.; Mansour, T.S.; Yu, K. ATP-competitive inhibitors of the mammalian target of rapamycin: Design and synthesis of highly potent and selective pyrazolopyrimidines. *J. Med. Chem.,* **2009**, *52*(16), 5013-5016.
[http://dx.doi.org/10.1021/jm900851f] [PMID: 19645448]

[139] Lisi, L.; Aceto, P.; Navarra, P.; Dello Russo, C. mTOR kinase: A possible pharmacological target in the management of chronic pain. *BioMed Res. Int.,* **2015**, *2015*, 1-13.
[http://dx.doi.org/10.1155/2015/394257] [PMID: 25685786]

[140] Liu, K.K.C.; Bailey, S.; Dinh, D.M.; Lam, H.; Li, C.; Wells, P.A.; Yin, M.J.; Zou, A. Conformationally-restricted cyclic sulfones as potent and selective mTOR kinase inhibitors. *Bioorg. Med. Chem. Lett.,* **2012**, *22*(15), 5114-5117.
[http://dx.doi.org/10.1016/j.bmcl.2012.05.104] [PMID: 22765900]

[141] Pei, Z.; Blackwood, E.; Liu, L.; Malek, S.; Belvin, M.; Koehler, M.F.T.; Ortwine, D.F.; Chen, H.; Cohen, F.; Kenny, J.R.; Bergeron, P.; Lau, K.; Ly, C.; Zhao, X.; Estrada, A.A.; Truong, T.; Epler, J.A.; Nonomiya, J.; Trinh, L.; Sideris, S.; Lesnick, J.; Bao, L.; Vijapurkar, U.; Mukadam, S.; Tay, S.; Deshmukh, G.; Chen, Y.H.; Ding, X.; Friedman, L.S.; Lyssikatos, J.P. Discovery and biological profiling of potent andselective mTOR inhibitor GDC-0349. *ACS Med. Chem. Lett.,* **2013**, *4*(1), 103-107.
[http://dx.doi.org/10.1021/ml3003132] [PMID: 24900569]

[142] Foote, K.M.; Blades, K.; Cronin, A.; Fillery, S.; Guichard, S.S.; Hassall, L.; Hickson, I.; Jacq, X.; Jewsbury, P.J.; McGuire, T.M.; Nissink, J.W.N.; Odedra, R.; Page, K.; Perkins, P.; Suleman, A.; Tam, K.; Thommes, P.; Broadhurst, R.; Wood, C. Discovery of 4-{4-[(3R)-3-methylmorpholin-4-l]-6-[1-(methylsulfonyl)cyclopropyl]pyrimidin-2-yl}-1h-indole (AZ20): A potent and selective inhibitor of ATR protein kinase with monotherapy *in vivo* antitumor activity. *J. Med. Chem.,* **2013**, *56*, 2125-2138.
[http://dx.doi.org/10.1021/jm301859s] [PMID: 23394205]

[143] Van Triest, B.; Damstrup, L.; Falkenius, J.; Budach, V.; Troost, E.; Samuels, M.; Debus, J.; Sørensen, M.M.; Berghoff, K.; Strotman, R.; van Bussel, M.; Goel, S.; Geertsen, P.F. A phase Ia/Ib trial of the DNA-PK inhibitor M3814 in combination with radiotherapy (RT) in patients (pts) with advanced solid tumors: Dose-escalation results. *J. Clin. Oncol.,* **2018**, *36*(15_suppl), 2518-2518.
[http://dx.doi.org/10.1200/JCO.2018.36.15_suppl.2518]

[144] Rageot, D.; Bohnacker, T.; Melone, A.; Langlois, J.B.; Borsari, C.; Hillmann, P.; Sele, A.M.; Beaufils, F.; Zvelebil, M.; Hebeisen, P.; Loscher, W.; Burke, J.; Fabbro, D.; Wymann, M.P. Discovery and Preclinical Characterization of 5-[4,6-Bis({3-oxa-8-azabicyclo[3.2.1]octan-8-yl})-1,3,5-tr-azin-2-yl]-4-(difluoromethyl)pyridin-2-amine (PQR620), a Highly Potent and Selective mTORC1/2 Inhibitor for Cancer and Neurological Disorders. *J. Med. Chem.,* **2018**, *61*, 10084-10105.
[http://dx.doi.org/10.1021/acs.jmedchem.8b01262] [PMID: 30359003]

CHAPTER 6

Natural Products as Anticancer Agents: Recent Advancement and Future Directions

Anurag Chaudhary[1], Kalpana Singh[2], Nishant Verma[3] and Alok Sharma[4,*]

[1] *Department of Pharmaceutical Technology, Meerut Institute of Engineering and Technology, NH-58, Baghpat Road Crossing, Bypass Road, Meerut-250005, India*

[2] *HIMT College of Pharmacy, 8, Institutional Area, Knowledge Park I, Greater Noida, Uttar Pradesh-201301, India*

[3] *Panchwati College of Pharmacy, Ghat Institutional Area, NH-58, Delhi-Haridwar Bypass Road, Meerut, Uttar Pradesh,- 250001, India*

[4] *Department of Pharmacognosy, ISF College of Pharmacy, Moga, G.T Road, Ghal Kalan, Moga, Punjab-142001, India*

Abstract: Cancer is one of the biggest health-care challenges to human race and requires an innovative treatment strategy for cure. Undesirable side effects and rapid development of resistance to the conventional therapy have made the scenario more alarming. The chemical diversity of the natural products is immense and therefore is an amazing reserve for the finding of novel anticancer agents. Further, natural products have played a significant role in providing the novel and effective treatment inputs in the field on anticancer research. The compounds obtained from these sources range from a simple peptide, Dolastatin 10, to a complex polyether, Halichonrin B. Natural products have been source of many anticancer agents that are being used in clinical or pre-clinical trials. Further, many compounds derived from natural products have shown potential to be future anticancer agents. Due to their actions on numerous targets natural products are considered ideal for anticancer drug development. Further, their selectivity towards cancer cells is more in comparison to conventional treatment, so their toxicity is lower. This chapter summarizes the progress and ongoing developments in natural products and their analogs as anticancer agents. The challenges and future prospects of natural products based anticancer agents are also discussed.

Keywords: Anticancer agents, Bioactive, Cancer, Natural products, Phytopharma-ceutical, Secondary metabolite.

---
* **Corresponding author Alok Sharma:** Department of Pharmacognosy, ISF College of Pharmacy, Moga, G.T Road, Ghal kalan,Moga, Punjab-142001, India ; Tel: +919718052888; E-mail: alokalok22@gmail.com

INTRODUCTION

Cancer remains the leading cause of death and a serious metabolic syndrome given its consequently advances in the methods of diagnosis, treatment, and prevention. It's the root cause of worldwide mortality and morbidity [1, 2]. The uncontrolled growth and proliferation of a normal cell that brings genetic instability, invades and makes tissues and cells around it metastasize. Such genetic instabilities include DNA mutations at various DNA repair genes (p21, p22, p27, p51, p53, and DNA toolbox), tumor suppressor genes (p53, NF1, NF2, RB, and biological breaks), oncogenes (BRCA1, BRCA2, BRAF, CDKN1B, MYC, Rad, Bcl-2, RAS) [3]. Due to no cure and regression of established cancer and new side effects are emerging after prolonged anticancer therapy, new anti-cancer therapy are severely needed to cure metastasis. There are various evidences seen from *in-vitro* and *in-vivo* preclinical studies that support the use of compounds derived from plant or chemically altered plant natural products [6]. Therefore, there is growing interest in anticancer agents which have low side effects and has targeted specific key signalling pathways that control the establishment and progression of the cancer [4, 5].

Nature has provided so many medicinal plants to help them achieve better health as a gift to humans. Since the ancient times, plants and their bioactive compounds have been used medically [6, 7]. Since ancient times the plants and their bioactive compounds have been in medical use. A wide variety of herbal phytochemicals compounds and their synthetic counterparts for cancer treatment have been discovered [8, 9]. The anticancer medicinal plants and their bioactive compounds use to inhibit the establishment and progression of the metastasis. Around 2.5 lakh plant species has been discovered yet and only 10% of plants have been examined for the treatment of various diseases world-wide. Phytochemicals and analogues derived from them are extracted from different parts of the plants like, flower, roots, fruits, sprouts, seeds, pericarp, stem, flower stigmas, leaf, embryo, bark, rhizomes. The bioactive from plant parts serves various pharmacological functions [1, 8, 9]. For centuries, many exemplary anticancer phytochemicals compounds and their derivatives having different biochemical mechanism.

The plant products like taxanes, terpenes, minerals, glycosides, vitamins, gums, oils, saponins, lignans, and other primary and secondary plant metabolites have shown major roles in activation of cancer cell activating genes, proteins, enzymes, signalling cascades which block initiation and progression of cancer [topoisomerase enzymes, cyclooxygenase-1 (COX-1) and cyclooxygenase-2 (COX-2), Bcl-2, cytokines, Cdc-2, CDK2 and CDK4 kinases, PI3K, Akt, TNK] as shown in Fig. (**1**), or by activating Bax proteins, DNA repair pathways (p53, p51, p27, p21 genes and their protein products) or invigorating the production of protective enzymes (Capase-3, 7, 8, 9, 10, 12) or induction of the antioxidant action (GSH, GST). Thus, the Fig. (**2**) shows mechanisms of different plant proteins in terms of either increasing the efficacy by inhibiting expression on the mentioned proteins, enzymes, genes or signalling cascades [10, 11].

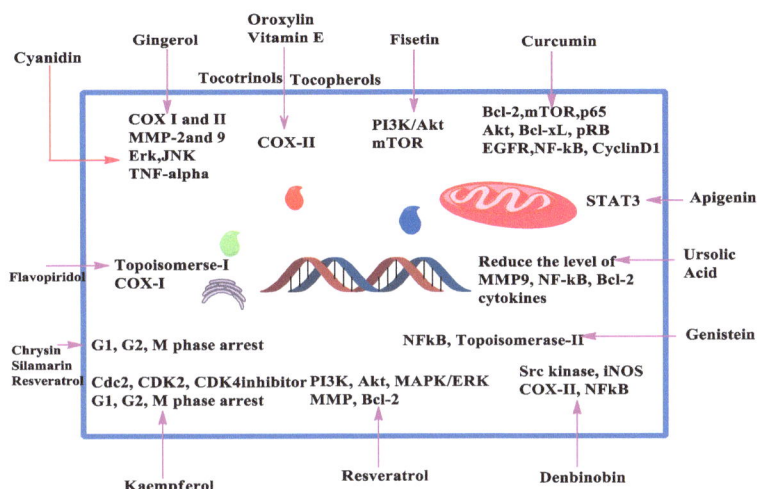

Fig. (1). Mechanism of anticancer action of various plant derived phytochemicals which act by activating expression of various enzymes, genes, proteins and different signalling cascades which result in inhibition of cancer initiation and progression.

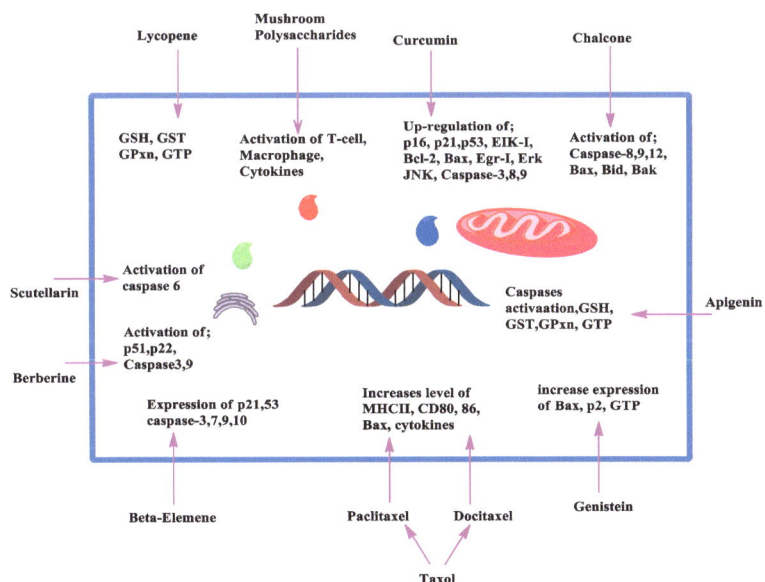

Fig. (2). Mechanism of anticancer action of various plant derived phytochemicals which act by inhibiting expression of various enzymes, genes, proteins and different signalling which result in inhibition of cancer initiation and progression.

The detailed information of anticancer medicinal plants, family, part used, phytochemicals, their mechanism of action against specific cancer cell lines and specific type of cancer suppressed by phytochemical is showed in Table **1**. The various literatures were reviewed on the effect of natural phytochemicals against cancer from 2010 to 2021.

Various plants and its parts used in suppressing cancer are shown in Table **1** below:

Table 1. Various plant and its parts used in supressing cancer.

Name of the Plant	Part Used	Phytochemical/s Responsible for the Activity	MOA of Phytochemical/s (Genes, Proteins and Signalling Cascade Activated to Block the Cancer Initiation and Progression)	Specific Cancer Suppressed	Refs.
Peganum harmala	Roots	Harmine	Bcl-2, cytokines, PI3K, Akt	Breast cancer (Both *in vitro* and *in vivo*)	[13]
Curcuma longa	Rhizomes	Curcumin, ascorbic acid	Bcl-2, EGFR, mTOR, p-65, NF-kB activated	Leukemia, glioblastoma and colon cancer (*In vitro*)	[13]
Allium wallichii	Whole plant	Steroids, terpenoids, flavonoids, reducing sugars and glycosides	Topoisomerase-1 and COX-1 activated	Prostate cancer, breast cancer, cervical cancer (*In vitro*)	[14]
Artemisia annua	Whole plant	Artemisinin	CDK-4, bcl-2	Liver, breast and pancreatic cancer (Both *in vitro* and *in vivo*)	[15]
Debregeasia saeneb	Stem	Tannins	EGFR, PI3K,AKt	Internal tumors (*In vitro*)	[16]
Camelia sinesis	Leaves	Epicatechingallate, picatechin, epigallocatechin	A431, 4TI cancer cell line	Lung, bladder, skin, prostate and breast cancer (Both *in vitro* and *in vivo*)	[16]

(Table 1) cont.....

Name of the Plant	Part Used	Phytochemical/s Responsible for the Activity	MOA of Phytochemical/s (Genes, Proteins and Signalling Cascade Activated to Block the Cancer Initiation and Progression)	Specific Cancer Suppressed	Refs.
Paeonia suffruticosa	Seed	Polysaccharides (HBSS, CHSS, DASS, and CASS)	MAPK family	Prostate, colon, human breast, and cervical cancer (*In vitro*)	[2]
Ocimum sanctum	Leaves	Eugenol, orientin, vicenin	P21, p53	Breast, liver and fibrosarcoma cancer (*In vitro*)	[17]
Ginkgo biloba	Leaves	Ginkgetin, ginkgolide A & B	EGb761, Topo II *gene*	Hepatocarcinoma, ovary, prostate, colon and liver cancer	[18]
Camellia sinensis	Leaves	Theabrownin		Lung cancer (*In vivo*)	[19]
Ziziphus mauritiana	Leaves, bark, fruit	a-linolenic acid, Methyl stearate	P21, P27 and P53 genes	Leukemia, human cervical and liver cancer (*In vitro*)	[20]
Solanum nigrum	Leaves	Solamargine, solasonine	NF-κB	Breast, liver, lung and skin cancer (*In vitro*)	[21]
Vigna unguiculata	Seeds Black-eyed-peas	trypsin/Chymotrypsin inhibitor	NF-kB	Human breast cancer (*In vitro*)	[22]
Ziziphus spina-christi	Flowers, leaves	Doxorubicin, spinanine-A, rutnine, quercetin	P21, P27 and P53 genes	Lung cancer and breast cancer (*In vivo*)	[23]
Glycyrrhiza glabra	Roots	Licochalcone-A, licoagrochalcone	HSP90 Gene, p27kip1 tumor suppressor gene	Prostate, brea st, lung, stomach and kidney cancer (*In vivo*)	[24]
Herba epimedii	Leaves	Icariin, icaritin, icariside II	Rac1	Prostate, lung, kidney and gastric cancer (Both *in vitro* and *in vivo*)	[25]

(Table 1) cont.....

Name of the Plant	Part Used	Phytochemical/s Responsible for the Activity	MOA of Phytochemical/s (Genes, Proteins and Signalling Cascade Activated to Block the Cancer Initiation and Progression)	Specific Cancer Suppressed	Refs.
Elusine coracana	Seeds	Ragi bifunctional inhibitor	K562 chronic myeloid gene	Myeloid leukemia cell and K562 cell line (Both *in vitro* and *in vivo*)	[26]
Psoralea corylifolia	Seeds	Psoralidin	cyclin D1 and CDK4	Stomach and prostate cancer	[27]
Peltophorum dubium	Seeds	Peltophorum dubium trypsin inhibitor	K562 chronic myeloid gene	Rat lymphoma cells, human leukemia cells	[28]
Vicia faba	Seeds	Field bean protease Inhibitors	IL-4	Skin cancer (Both *in vitro* and *in vivo*)	[28]
Xanthium strumarium	Fruit	Xanthatin	ATG4B	Lymphocytic leukemia and liver cancer (*In vitro*)	[29]
Nigella sativa	Seeds	Thymoquinone	STAT3-regulated gene	Colon, prostate, breast and pancreas cancer	[16]
Ocimum sanctum	Leaves	Eugenol, orientin, Vicenin	P21, p53	Breast, liver and fibrosarcoma	[31]
Moringa oleifera	Flowers, leaves	Hexadeconoic acid, Isopropyl isothiocyanate	BCL-2 and BCL-XL, AKt	Abdominal cancer (Both *in vitro* and *in vivo*)	[26]
Glycine max	Seeds	Proteins, flavonoids, phenolic compounds	PTK, topoisomerase II and matrix metalloprotein (MMP9)	Colorectal, prostate and colon cancer (Both *in vitro* and *in vivo*)	[26]
Bauhinia variegata	Flower	Kaempferol galactoside	-	Breast, lung and liver cancer (*In vivo*)	[30]
Withania somnifera	Roots	Withaferin A, D	-	Breast, cervix, prostate and colon cancer (*In vivo*)	[31]

(Table 1) cont.....

Name of the Plant	Part Used	Phytochemical/s Responsible for the Activity	MOA of Phytochemical/s (Genes, Proteins and Signalling Cascade Activated to Block the Cancer Initiation and Progression)	Specific Cancer Suppressed	Refs.
Aegle marmelos	Bark, root	Lupeol	-	Lymphoma, melanoma, leukemia and breast cancer (*In vitro*)	[32]
Zingiber officinale	Ginger	Gingerol	-	Ovary, cervix, colon, liver and urinary caner (*In vitro* and *in vivo*)	[33]
Sylibum marianum	Flower, leaves	Silibinin	CDK	Lung, liver, skin, colon and prostate cancer (Both *in vitro* and *in vivo*)	[34]
Capsicum annuum	Pepper	Luteolin	caspase-3, reactive oxygen species (ROS), Rac1, and HER-2	Colorectal cancer (Both *in vitro* and *in vivo*)	[35]
Colchicum autumnale	Leaves	Colchicine	-	Hodgkin's lymphoma, chronic granulocytic leukemia (Both *in vitro* and *in vivo*)	[36]
Aegle marmelos	Stem bark	Skimmianine	-	Liver cancer (Both *in vitro* and *in vivo*)	[37]
Boswellia serrata	Gum	Boswellic acid	Ki-67 and CD31	Prostate cancer (*In vitro*)	[38]
Sylibum marianum	Leaves, flowers	Silymarin	*blocking* NF-kappaB pathways	Colorectal cancer and colon cancer (Both *in vitro* and *in vivo*)	[39]
Curcuma longa	Dried rhizome	Curcumin	Bcl-2, EGFR, mTOR, p-65, NF-kB activated	Colon adenocarcinoma (*In vitro*)	[40]

Name of the Plant	Part Used	Phytochemical/s Responsible for the Activity	MOA of Phytochemical/s (Genes, Proteins and Signalling Cascade Activated to Block the Cancer Initiation and Progression)	Specific Cancer Suppressed	Refs.
Alstonia scholaris	Root, bark	O methylmacralstonine, talcarpine, villalstonine, pleiocarpamine, ursolic acid, betulinic acid, botulin	Stat3, FAK, MMPs inhibitor	Lung cancer (Both *in vitro* and *in vivo*)	[41]
Podophyllum peltatum	Leaves	Podophyllotoxin	-	Non-small cell lung carcinoma (Both *in vitro* and *in vivo*)	[42]
Andrographis paniculata	Whole plant	Andrographolide	-	Colon cancer (Both *in vitro* and *in vivo*)	[35]
Ziziphus jujuba	Fruits, seeds, leaves	Linoleic acids, triterpenoids	GCL	Breast cancer, human Jurkat leukemia T cells (Both *in vitro* and *in vivo*)	[43]
Podophyllum hexandrum	Leaves	Podophyllotoxin	GCL	Breast, ovary, lung, liver, bladder and testis cancer (*In vitro*)	[44]
Betula utilis	Bark	Betulinic acid	GCL	Melanomas (*In vitro*)	[45]
Panax ginseng	Roots	Panaxadiol	Phospho-EGF Receptor (Tyr1068), EGFR	Human colon cancer (Both *in vitro* and *in vivo*)	[46]
Panax pseudoginseng	Roots	Panaxadiol	EGFR	Human colon cancer (Both *in vitro* and *in vivo*)	[46]
Gossypium hirsutum	Cotton	Gossypol	-	Mice xenograft (HT-29) and colorectal cancer (Both *in vitro* and *in vivo*)	[47]
Passiflora caerulea	Flower	Chrysin	-	Colorectal cancer (*in vitro*)	[48]

(Table 1) cont.....

Name of the Plant	Part Used	Phytochemical/s Responsible for the Activity	MOA of Phytochemical/s (Genes, Proteins and Signalling Cascade Activated to Block the Cancer Initiation and Progression)	Specific Cancer Suppressed	Refs.
Plumbago zeylanica	Leaves	Plumbagin	BRCA1 gene	Liver, fibrosarcoma, leukemia and breast cancer (*In vitro*)	[49]
Capsicum annuum	Pepper	Luteolin	caspase-3, reactive oxygen species (ROS), Rac1, and HER-2	Colorectal cancer (Both *in vitro* and *in vivo*)	[35]
Zingiber officinale	Rhizomes	6-Shogaol		Ovary cancer (*In vitro*)	[50]
Curcuma longa	Root, rhizome	Curcumin	Bcl-2, EGFR, mTOR, p-65, NF-kB	Breast, lung, colon, prostate esophagus, liver and skin cancer (*In vitro*)	[51]
Oldenlandia diffusa	Stem bark, leaves, fruit peel	Ursolic acid	cyclin D1 and CDK4	Lungs, ovary, uterus, stomach, liver, colon, rectum and brain cancer (Both *in vitro* and *in vivo*)	[52]
Zingiber officinale	Ginger	6-Shogaol	-	Ovary cancer (*in vitro*)	[52]
Zingiber officinale	Root	Gingerol	-	Colon, breast and ovarian cancer (Both *in vitro* and *in vivo*)	[33]
Broussonetia papyrifera	Fruits, leaf, bark	2S-abyssinone, verubulin	AMPK inhibitor	Glioblastoma and brain cancer (*In vitro*)	[53]
Glycyrrhiza uralensis	Roots	Isoliquiritigenin	IL-7 gene	Human lung cancer (*In vitro*)	[54]
Boerrhavia diffusa	Roots	Punarnavine	IL-2 and IL-2R gene	Malignant melanoma cancer (*In vitro*)	[55]

(Table 1) cont.....

Name of the Plant	Part Used	Phytochemical/s Responsible for the Activity	MOA of Phytochemical/s (Genes, Proteins and Signalling Cascade Activated to Block the Cancer Initiation and Progression)	Specific Cancer Suppressed	Refs.
Vitis vinifera	Seeds extract	Procyanidins	COX gene	Human colon cancer (*In vitro*)	[56]
Polygonum cuspidatum	Whole plant	Resveratrol	-	Colorectal, skin and liver cancer (*In vitro*)	[57]
Morinda citrifolia	Roots	Damnacanthal	TNF-a and IL-6	Lung cancer, sarcomas (*In vitro*)	[58]
Biophytum sensitivum	Fruits and berries	Alcoholic extract	nm23, ERK-1, ERK-2, STAT-1	Dalton's lymphoma ascites, Ehrlich ascites carcinoma (*In vitro*)	[59]
Gossypium hirsutum	Whole plant	Gossypol	-	Breast, stomach, liver, prostate and bladder cancer (*In vitro*)	[60]
Aloe vera	Leaves	Alexin B, emodin	Bcl-2	Leukemia, stomach cancer (*In vivo*)	[61]
Vaccinium macrocarpon	Fruit	Hydroxycinnamoyl ursolic acid	-	Cervical, prostate cancer (*In vitro*)	[62]
Annona crassiflora	Leaves	Caffeic acid, sinapic acid, rutin	-	Glioma, renal, ovary cancer (*In vitro*)	[63]
Annona coriacea	Seeds	Ferulic and sinapic acid	-	Glioma, lymphoid melanoma, lung, renal and ovary cancer	[63]
Argemone gracilenta	Whole plant	Argemonine and berberine	-	B-cell lymphoma, leukemia (*In vitro*)	[64]

(Table 1) cont.....

Name of the Plant	Part Used	Phytochemical/s Responsible for the Activity	MOA of Phytochemical/s (Genes, Proteins and Signalling Cascade Activated to Block the Cancer Initiation and Progression)	Specific Cancer Suppressed	Refs.
Psoralea corylifolia	Seeds	Bavachanin, corylfolinin, psoralen	cyclin D1 and CDK4	Lung, osteosarcoma, fibrosarcoma and liver cancer (*In vitro*)	[65]
Moringa oliefera	Leaves	Niazinine A	cyclin D1 and CDK4	Blood cancer (*In vitro*)	[66]
Amoora rohituka	Stem bark	Amooranin	-	Lymphocytic leukemia (*In vitro*)	[67]
Conyza Canadensis	Roots	Conyzapyranone A and B	-	Epidermoid carcinoma (*In vitro*)	[68]
Ziziphus rugosa	Pericarp and seed	Betulinic acid	cyclin D1 and CDK4	Cytotoxicity against human melanoma cells (*In vivo*)	[69]
Panax ginseng	Leaves	Panaxadiol, panaxatriol	NK cell, VGEF	Breast, ovary, lung, prostate and colon cancer (*In vitro*)	[70]
C. roseus	Leaves	Vinblastine, Vincristine	transcription factor (TF) *genes*	Breast, ovary, cervix, lung, rectum and testis cancer (*In vitro*)	[71]
Centella asiatica	Leaves	Asiatic acid	human hepatoma HepG2 cells	Melanoma, glioblastoma, breast (*In vivo*)	[72]
Viscum album	Sprouts	Viscumin, digallic acid	SK-BR-3 cell line	Breast, cervix, ovary, stomach, colon, kidney, lung cancer (Both *in vitro* and *in vivo*)	[73]
Leea indica	Leaves	Gallic acid Ehrlich ascites	-	Carcinoma (*In vitro* and *in vivo*)	[74]

Name of the Plant	Part Used	Phytochemical/s Responsible for the Activity	MOA of Phytochemical/s (Genes, Proteins and Signalling Cascade Activated to Block the Cancer Initiation and Progression)	Specific Cancer Suppressed	Refs.
Liriodendron tulipifera	Stem	Costunolide, tulipinolide, liriodenine, germacranolide	NF-κB activation, Bcl-2 and COX-2 expression	KB (Oral cancer), HT29 cell line (Both *in vitro* and *in vivo*)	[75]
Viscum album	Fruits	Viscumin, digallic acid	Signalling casccade	Breast, ovary, lung, kidney, bladder and testis cancer (*In vitro*)	[73]
Cicer arietinum	Seeds	Lectin C-25	Bcl-2	Breast and prostate cancer (*In vitro*)	[76]
Crocus sativus	Dry stigmas	Crocetin	COX-2, Bcl-2	Hippocampal cell death and lung cancer (*In vivo*)	[77]
Centella asiatica	Leaves	Asiatic acid	Bcl-2	Melanoma, glioblastoma and breast cancer (*In vivo*)	[78]
Tylophora indica	Leaves	Tylophorine	-	Breast cancer (*In vivo*)	[79]
Dioscorea colletti	Rhizomes	Dioscin	Bcl-2	Liver and human gastric cancer (*In vitro*)	[80]
Croton macrobotrys	Leaves	Corydine, salutaridine	Bcl-2	Leukemia and lung cancer (*In vitro*)	[81]
Clausena lansium	Seeds	Clausenalansamid A and B	Bcl-2	Gastric, liver cancer (*In vitro*)	[82]
Bleekeria vitensis	Leaf	Elliptinium	Bcl-2	Myelogenous leukemia and breast cancer (*In vivo*)	[83]
Combretum caffrum	Bark, kernal and fruit	Combretastatins	Tubulin protein	Colon, and leukemia and lung cancer (*In vivo*)	[83]

(Table 1) cont.....

Name of the Plant	Part Used	Phytochemical/s Responsible for the Activity	MOA of Phytochemical/s (Genes, Proteins and Signalling Cascade Activated to Block the Cancer Initiation and Progression)	Specific Cancer Suppressed	Refs.
Solanum lycopersicum	Fruit	Lycopene	-	Prostate and colon cancer (*In vivo*)	[84]
Plumbago zeylanica	Roots	Plumbagin	-	Blood and skin cancer (*In vitro*)	[85]
Crocus sativus	Flower stigmas	Crocin, picrocrocin, crocetin, and safranal	-	Sarcoma and oral cancer (Both *in vitro* and *in vivo*)	[86]
Actaea racemosa	Rhizomes, roots	Actein	-	Liver and breast cancer (*In vivo*)	[87]
Peristrophe bicalyculata	Aerial parts	b-Caryophyllene, azingiberene	-	Breast cancer (*In vitro*)	[88]
Cannabis sativa	Leaf	Cannabinoid	-	Lung, pancreas, breast, prostate and colorectal cancer (Both *in vitro* and *in vivo*)	[89]
Sylibum marianum	Flower, leaves	Silymarin	-	Colorectal cancer (Both *in vitro* and *in vivo*)	[90]
Enterolobium contortisiliquum	Seeds	Trypsin inhibitor (EcTI)	-	Gastric and breast cancer (Both *in vitro* and *in vivo*)	[91]
Linum usitatissimum	Leaves, flowers	Cynogenetic glycosides	-	Breast cancer (*In vitro*)	[92]
Calvatia caelata	Fruiting bodies	Laccases (Enzymes)	-	Liver, breast cancer (*In vitro*)	[93]
Tylophora indica	Bark, Kernel fruit	Tylophorine	-	Breast cancer (*In vivo*)	[97]
Allium sativum	Buds, leaves	Allylmercaptocysteine, allicin	-	Lymphoma, cervix cancer (*In vivo*)	[94]
Hibiscus mutabilis	Pepper	Lectin	-	Liver, breast cancer (*In vitro*)	[95]

(Table 1) cont.....

Name of the Plant	Part Used	Phytochemical/s Responsible for the Activity	MOA of Phytochemical/s (Genes, Proteins and Signalling Cascade Activated to Block the Cancer Initiation and Progression)	Specific Cancer Suppressed	Refs.
Plumbago zeylanica	Roots	Plumbagin	Bcl-2	Blood cancer, skin cancers (*In vitro*)	[99]
Saffron crocus	Dry stigmas	Saffron	-	Liver, lung cancer and pancreatic cancer (*In vitro*)	[96]
Taxus brevifolia	Bark	nab-Paclitaxel	-	Ovarian and breast cancer (Both *in vitro* and *in vivo*)	[23]
Vitis vinifera	Fruit	Cyanidin	-	Colon cancer (*In vivo*)	[98]
Actaea racemosa	Rhizomes,roots	Actein	-	Liver and breast cancer (*In vivo*)	[101]
Pyrus malus	Bark, fruit	Quercetin, procyanidin	-	Colon cancer (Both *in vitro* and *in vivo*)	[99]
Betula Sp.	Leaves	Betulinic acid	Bcl-2, COX-2	Human melanoma xenografts and leukemia (*In vitro*)	[100]
Tabernaemontana divaricata	Leaves	Cononitarine B, Conophylline	-	Liver, lung, breast and colon cancer (*In vitro*)	[101]
Smilax chinensis	Rhizomes	Tannin, saponins and flavonoid	-	Sarcoma-180 and ascites sarcoma (Both *in vitro* and *in vivo*)	[99]
Allium sativum	Whole plant	Allin	-	Carcinoma of human (mammary) gland (Both *in vitro* and *in vivo*)	[102]

(Table 1) cont.....

Name of the Plant	Part Used	Phytochemical/s Responsible for the Activity	MOA of Phytochemical/s (Genes, Proteins and Signalling Cascade Activated to Block the Cancer Initiation and Progression)	Specific Cancer Suppressed	Refs.
Aloe vera	Whole plant	Aloesin, emodin	-	Anti-angiogenic activity (*In vitro*)	[103]
Curcuma longa	Roots	Curcumin	-	Stomach cancer (*In vitro*)	[104]
Emblica officinalis	Polyphenols	Tannins	-	Lymphoma and melanoma (*In vitro*)	[105]
Momordica charantia	Leaves, Roots	Charantin, cucurbitanetype triterpene	-	Colon cancer and breast cancer (*In vitro*)	[106]
Stevia rebaudiana	Leaves	Labdane sclareol properties	-	Anti-tumorous and cytotoxic (*In vitro*)	[107]
Camellia sinensis	Leaves	Epigallocatechin gallate	-	Brain, prostate, cervical and bladder cancer (*In vivo*)	[108]
Nelumbo nucifera	Embryo	Neferine	-	Liver cancer (*In vitro*)	[109]
Ocimum sanctum	Leaves	Caryophyllene, camphor	-	Sarcoma-180 solid tumor (*In vitro*)	[109]
Calvatia caelata	Fruiting bodies	Calcaelin	-	Breast and spleen cancer cells (*In vivo*)	[110]
Pleurotus sajor-caju	Fruiting bodies	Ribonucleases	-	Leukemia and liver cancer (*in vivo*)	[111]
Lentinus edodes	Fruiting bodies	Lentinan	-	Sarcoma-180 in mice (*In vivo*)	[111]
Schizophyllum commune	Fruiting bodies	Schizophyllan	-	Head and neck cancer (*In vivo*)	[112]
Matricaria chamomilla	Whole plant	Apigenin	-	Colorectal cancer (*in vivo*)	[113]

(Table 1) cont.....

Name of the Plant	Part Used	Phytochemical/s Responsible for the Activity	MOA of Phytochemical/s (Genes, Proteins and Signalling Cascade Activated to Block the Cancer Initiation and Progression)	Specific Cancer Suppressed	Refs.
Fagopyrum sculentum	Seeds	Buckwheat inhibitor-1 protein	*genes*, proteins, enzymes and signaling cascades	T-acute lymphoblastic leukemia (T-ALL) cells (*in vitro*)	[114]
Glycine max	Seeds	Soybean trypsin inhibitor	Inhibit ion channels and inhibit protein translation	Human ovarian cancer (*in vivo*)	[115]
Ipomoea batata	Roots	Trypsin inhibitor protein	Inhibit ion channels and inhibit protein translation	Promyelocytic leukemia cells (*In vitro* and *in vivo*)	[116]
Lavatera cashmeriana	Seeds	Lavatera cashmeriana protease inhibitors (LCpi I, II, III)	LCpi I, II, III)	Leukemia, lung, colon cancer (*In vitro*)	[117]
Lens culinaris	Seeds	Lentil (Lens culinaris trypsin inhibitor)	Inhibit ion channels and inhibit protein translation	Human colon cancer (Both *in vitro* and *in vivo*)	[118]
Medicago scutellata	Seeds	Medicago scutellata trypsin inhibitor		Human breast and cervical cancer (*In vitro*)	[119]
Phaseolus acutifolius	Seeds	Tepary bean protease inhibitor	MBL2, L1210	Leukemia L1210 and lymphoma MBL2 (*In vitro*)	[120]
Pisum sativum	Pea	Protease inhibitors, rTI1B, rTI2B	rTI1B	Human colorectal and colon cancer (*In vitro*)	[121]
Phaseolus vulgaris	Seeds	Tepary bean protease inhibitor	MBL2, L1210	Leukemia L1210 and lymphoma MBL2 (*In vitro*)	[122]
Coccinia grandis	Leaves		hTERT and c-Myc	(CG) protease inhibitors Colon cancer (*In vitro*)	[135]

(Table 1) cont.....

Name of the Plant	Part Used	Phytochemical/s Responsible for the Activity	MOA of Phytochemical/s (Genes, Proteins and Signalling Cascade Activated to Block the Cancer Initiation and Progression)	Specific Cancer Suppressed	Refs.
Ginkgo biloba	Leaves	EGb and bilobalide	Gas1 (growth arrest-specific 1)	Colon cancer (*In vivo*)	[123]
Curcuma zedoaria	Whole plant	Curcumin	B-16	Colorectal cancer and B-16 melanoma cells (*In vitro*)	[124]
Clematis manshrica	Flower, Leaves	1,4-benzoquinone,5-oethyl-embelin, 15- carbon isoprenoid	-	Liver cancer and blood cancer (*In vivo*)	[125]

A NOVEL APPROACH OF VARIOUS PHYTOCHEMICALS AGAINST CANCER

Nature has given humanity the gift of various medicinal plants. In ancient times, many plants and its bioactive compounds used to treat diseases. Among these occurred medicinal plants, several plants and its bioactive compounds used to inhibit initiation and progression of cancer. In past researches it has been occurred that there are about 250000 plant species out of which only 10% were studied against treatment of various diseases. The phytochemicals are extracted from various parts of plants like roots, stem, leaves, fruit, seeds, flowers, rhizomes, stigmas, pericarp, embryo, bark or whole plant which shows different pharmacological actions different diseases. The plant products like saponins, tannins, lignans, vitamins, minerals, terpenes, glycosides, taxanes, gums, or metabolites (primary and secondary) showed major effect in blocking cancer progression and development, genes, cell activating proteins, cell signalling cascade *etc.*. Various types of medicinal plants, their family, plant part used, phytochemical compounds and mechanism of action are discussed below (Fig. **3**):

Berberine

Berberine is isolated from the roots and rhizomes of *Tinospora cordifolia*, *Berberis vulgaris*, *Berberis aquifolium* and *Rhizoma coptidis*. It is a strong anticancer phytochemical compound. Various clinical trials were performed on berberine. It is used to treat various cancers like breast, prostrate, colorectal cancer. Its mechanism of action is to induce apoptosis and cell cycle arrest at G2/M phase in colorectal, liver and breast cancer. It also inhibits anti-apoptotic proteins bcl-2, and activates pro-apoptotic proteins (P21, p53, caspase-3 and caspase-9) [126, 127].

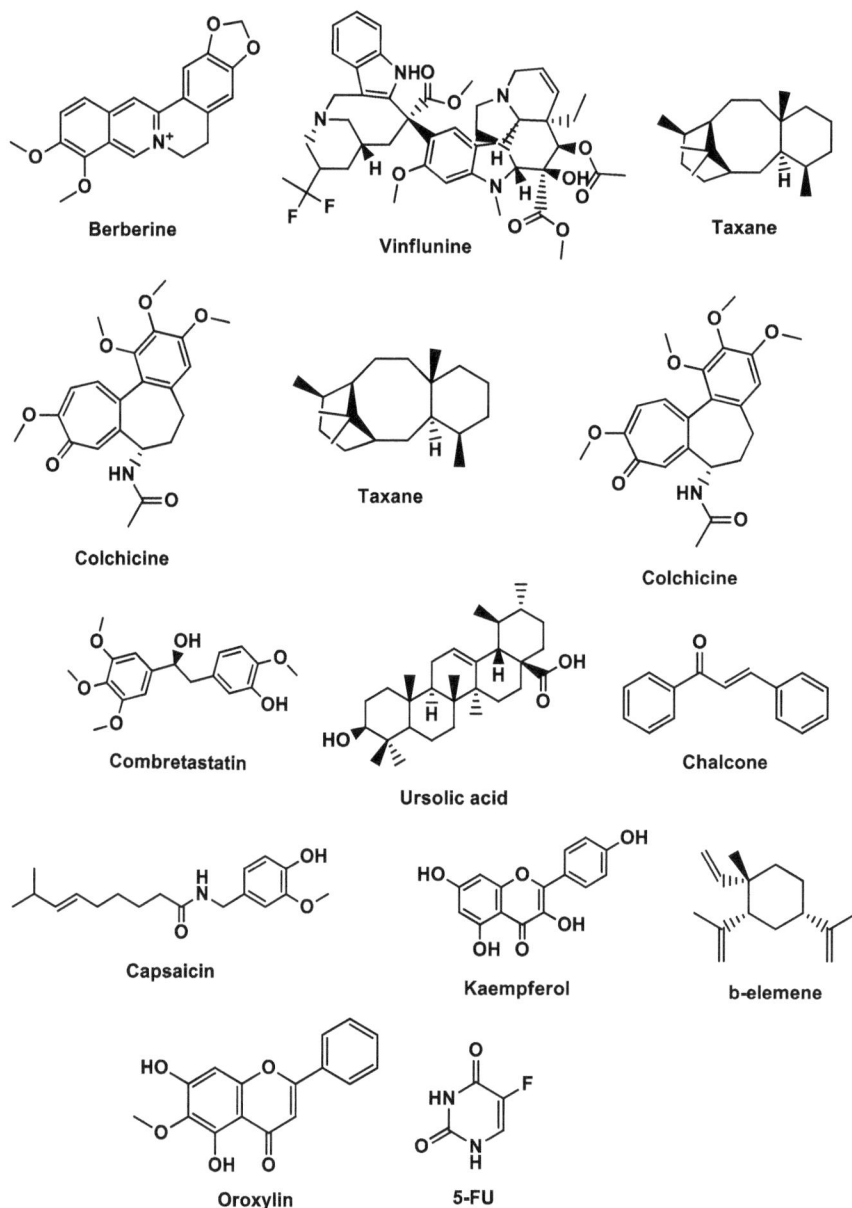

Fig. (3). Chemical structures of various phytochemicals having anticancer activity.

Vinca Alkaloids

It is an alkaloid obtained from *Catharanthus roseus* (*C. roseus*), family apocynaceae. It is used against various cancers like breast, liver, leukaemia, testes, and lung cancer. There are four main vinca alkaloids used extensively for cancer namely vinorelbine, vindesine, vincristine and vinblastine [128]. The vincristine and vinblastine showed anticancer activity by binding to tubulin heterodimers (vinca-binding site), thus disrupting the functions of microtubules or arrest cell cycle at metaphase [129]. The vinorelbine, vindesine are semisynthetic derivatives which arrest cell cycle at metaphase and inhibit the tubulin function. Vinflunine is synthesized from vinorelbine and it showed anticancer activity by binding to tubulin and microtubules, it disrupts newly formed blood vessels and decrease metastatic process. Clinically it is seen that it has potential role in treating mammary carcinoma and non-small cell lung cancer.

A monoterpene indole alkaloid namely catharoseumine isolated from whole plant of *C. roseus*, which showed moderate cytotoxic effect against HL-60 cell lines [130].

Taxanes

The national cancer institute discovered paclitaxel in 1960, it was isolated from barks of pacific yew tree named as *Taxus brevifolia Nutt*. It showed anticancer activity by bind to intermediate domain of β-tubulin within the interior lumen of microtubules, which decreases microtubule dynamics and results in cell arrest in mitosis. It used for the treatment of various cancer like lung, ovarian, breast cancer. Clinical trials of analogs of paclitaxel are undergoing which includes larotaxel, milataxel, ortataxel and tesetaxel. Among these analogs larotaxel is used to treat urethral cancer, pancreatic cancer, lung cancer, breast cancer [131].

Colchicine

Colchicine isolated from the bulbs and seeds of autumn crocus *Colchicum autumnale*. It is used as an immunosuppressant for the treatment of various diseases like gout, rheumatism, inflammation, Mediterranean fever, cancer [133]. It act as a microtubule destabilizing agent thus act by suppressing the formation of lateral connections between protofilaments. It binds interface between α and β-tubulins at a site different from the binding site of vinca alkaloids and taxanes [131, 132].

Combretastatin

Combretastatins were isolated from South African willow, *Combretum caffrum*. Combretastatin A-4 (CA-4) is water soluble analog and isolated from fruits, kernel and bark of Indian medicinal plant named *Terminalia bellerica* (Combretaceae). It has anticancer activity against leukaemia, lung cancer, colon cancer, thyroid cancer and anaplastic thyroid cancer [1]. It shows anticancer activity by selectively suppressing tumor angiogenesis and also suppresses cancer growth and metastasis [133].

Ursolic Acid

It is a triterpene obtained from herbal species like rosemary and basil plants. It showed anticancer activity by inducing pro-apoptotic effect on HCT116 cell lines and decrease the levels of pro-inflammatory NF-kB cytokine [134].

Chalcone

Chalcone is a natural flavonoid extracted from various edible fruits and vegetables. It has been used in cure of variety cancer like lung, breast, liver, colon, prostate cancer. It shows anticancer activity by activating caspases-8, 9, 12 enzyme, up-regulation of pro-apoptotic proteins (Bid, Bax, Bax proteins), anti-apoptotic Bcl-2 gene expression. It also showed apoptosis induction in MCF-7 cell. It also induced Ros generation and loss of mitochondrial membrane potential [135].

Taccalonanolide

In 1963, the taccalonanolide also known as taccalin extracted from the tubers of *Tacca leontopetaloides*. It has extremely bitter taste. Varieties of taccalonolides were obtained and taccolonolides A-M and W-Y isolated from *Tacca plantaginea*, and taccalonolides N and R V isolated from *Tacca paxiana*, and taccalonolides O-Q isolated from *Tacca subflabellata*. It has good anticancer activity with specific mechanism of action and acting as microtubule stabilizing agent [1].

Capsaicin

It is a natural occurring phytochemical isolated from red pepper. It is a good anticancer agent, anti-mutagenic, anti-metastatic, anti-angiogenic. It works against various cancer pancreatic, prostatic, liver, skin, leukaemia, lung, bladder, colon, and endothelial cells [136, 137]. It has been extensively studied against breast cancer and induced apoptosis at p53 gene, H-Ras, MCF10A and regulate various molecular targets caspase-3, reactive oxygen species (ROS), Rac1, and HER-2 *etc*., [138]. and induced signalling pathways in ROS and Rac-1 [139].

Kaempferol

Kaempferol is isolated from propolis, black tea, grapefruit, and broccoli. It shows significant anticancer activity against variety of cancer cells like colorectal cancer and HT-29 cancer cells. It target cancer cells by activating the expression of caspase-3 enzyme, p53 gene and arrest cell cycle at G1 and G2/M phase by inhibiting the activity of different enzymes (CDK2, Cdc2 and CDK4 [140 - 142].

Mushrooms Dietary Fibers

The mushrooms dietary fibers show anticancer activity. The cell wall of mushrooms contains high mol. wt. substances which cannot be absorbed by human intestine but it can absorb carcinogenic substances like free radicals, heavy metals. It targets molecular pathways in different cancers [143].

Mushroom Proteins

Mushroom proteins are isolated from different species of mushrooms like *Polyporus adusta and Ganoderma carpense, Pleurotus ostreatus, Pleurotus eryngii, Pleurotus nebrodensis, Amanita phalloides and Calvatia caelata.* The other bioactive compounds which extracted from above mentioned species are lectins, bolesatine, hemolysins, phallolysin, nebrodeolysin, laccases, calcaelin and ribonucleases and used against various cancer like lung cancer. The mushrooms proteins are most studied bioactive compound for protein engineering and pharmacological actions. Its mechanisms of action is increased the ratio of CD4+/CD8+/CD14+/CD16, T lymphocytes, increase the quantity and percentage of the B lymphocytes and CVP, induce apoptosis and cell cycle arrest [144 - 146].

β-elemene

β-elemene is obtained from Chinese plant *Curcuma wenyujin*. It is chemically a sesquiterpene which used against drug resistant tumors and treat different cancer like gastric, liver and induces apoptosis and cell death. Its mechanism of action is to inhibit the VEGF, down regulates Akt phosphorylation and CD34 expression, and suppressed PI3K/Akt/mTor/MAPK pathways. It attenuated angiogenesis and up regulated E3 ubiquitin ligases, cbl-b and c-cbl in human gastric cancer [147, 148].

Oroxylin Flavone

Oroxylin-A is a flavone isolated from the *Scutellariae radix*. The combination Oroxylin-A and 5-FU used to treat colorectal cancer by doubling action with COX-2 inhibition and increase ROS generation [156]. The mechanism of action of oroxylin- A is to down regulation of COX-2, and iNOS genes and block NF-kB, inhibit the activation of LPS-induced NF-kB by blocking IkB degradation [149, 150].

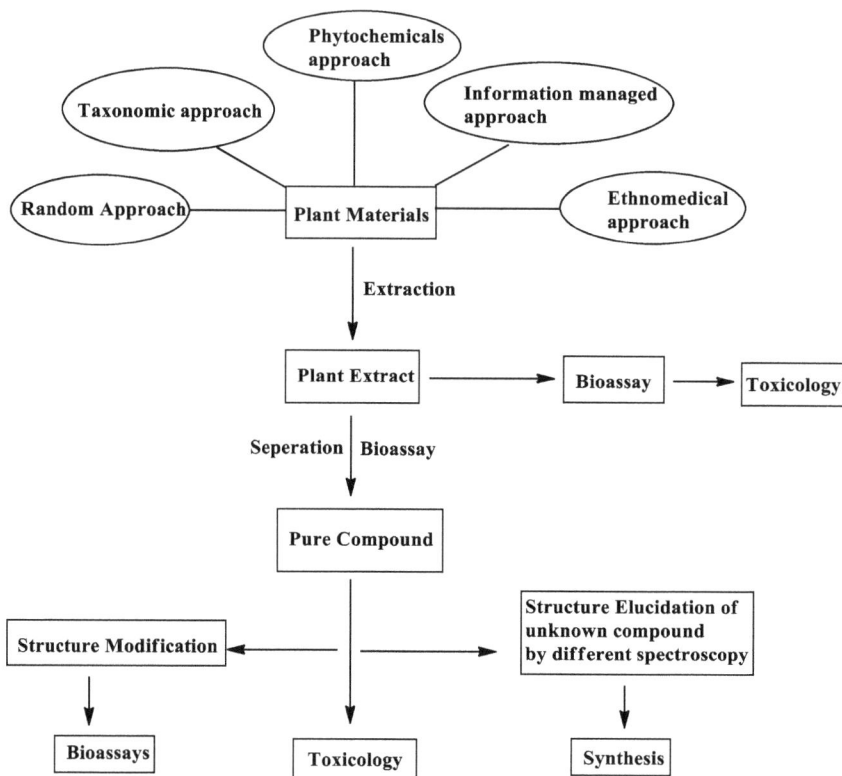

Fig. (4). Steps involve in phytochemicals screening of herbal drugs.

DIFFERENT STRATEGIES FOR THE DEVELOPMENT OF ANTICANCER PHYTOCHEMICALS

The potency of bioactive phytochemicals in the medicinal plants varies with latitude, longitude, age of plant, climate conditions from species to species [151]. Different plant part has different pharmacological activity. In current situation, the research for anticancer agent shift from synthetic agents to bioactive phytochemicals obtained from plants but this need extensive research in this area [152]. The various methods used for purification of bioactive phytochemicals like combinatorial chemistry, isolation assays, and bioassay-guided fractionation [153]. Different analytical techniques used to separate various bioactive compounds from the mixture of compounds [154]. The stepwise process involves from extracting of bioactive compound from plant to clinically approved pharmacological activity against various cancer is given above (Fig. 4).

FUTURE PROSPECTS

From the decades, bioactive phytochemicals has been used to cure the diseases. Various studies had been performed to evaluate the anticancer potential of the phytochemicals. Various plants bioactive compounds showed remarkable respond in curing the cancer [156]. Due to growing cost and high toxicity and increased incidences of cancer which challenged all the researchers to design and developed an alternative therapy which is cost effective, less toxic, targeted specific site. This review paper reflects light on the useful information about the medicinal plants and its bioactive phytochemicals used in targeting variety of cancers. On various bioactive compounds like curcumin, garcinol *etc.*, clinical trials are going on to evaluate its effectiveness and toxicity. Today's world demands extensive research work on different cancer either *in-vitro* or *in-vivo* using bioactive phytochemical compounds to evaluate pharmacological activity, toxicity and targeted specific sites.

CONSENT FOR PUBLICATION

Not applicable.

CONFLICT OF INTEREST

The author declares no conflict of interest, financial, or otherwise.

ACKNOWLEDGEMENTS

Declared none.

REFERENCES

[1]   Iqbal, J.; Abbasi, B.A.; Mahmood, T.; Kanwal, S.; Ali, B.; Shah, S.A.; Khalil, A.T. Plant-derived anticancer agents: A green anticancer approach. *Asian Pac. J. Trop. Biomed.,* **2017**, *7*(12), 1129-1150. [http://dx.doi.org/10.1016/j.apjtb.2017.10.016]

[2]   Zhang, L.Q.; Lv, R.W.; Qu, X.D.; Chen, X.J.; Lu, H.S.; Wang, Y. Aloesin suppresses cell growth and metastasis in ovarian cancer SKOV3 cells through the inhibition of the MAPK signalling pathway. *Anal. Cell. Pathol. (Amst.),* **2017**, *2017*, 1-6.

[3]   Krishnamurthi, K. 17-screening of natural products for anticancer and antidiabetic properties. *Cancer,* **2007**, *3*, 4.

[4]   Aung, T.; Qu, Z.; Kortschak, R.; Adelson, D. Understanding the effectiveness of natural compound mixtures in cancer through their molecular mode of action. *Int. J. Mol. Sci.,* **2017**, *18*(3), 656. [http://dx.doi.org/10.3390/ijms18030656] [PMID: 28304343]

[5]   Shaikh, R.; Pund, M.; Dawane, A.; Iliyas, S. Evaluation of anticancer, antioxidant, and possible anti-inflammatory properties of selected medicinal plants used in indian traditional medication. *J. Tradit. Complement. Med.,* **2014**, *4*(4), 253-257. [http://dx.doi.org/10.4103/2225-4110.128904] [PMID: 25379467]

[6]   Cragg, G.M.; Newman, D.J.; Yang, S.S. Natural product extracts of plant and marine origin having

antileukemia potential. The NCI experience. *J. Nat. Prod.,* **2006**, *69*(3), 488-498.
[http://dx.doi.org/10.1021/np0581216] [PMID: 16562862]

[7]   Khan, H. Medicinal plants in light of history: Recognized therapeutic modality. J Evid Based Complement. *J. Evid. Based Complementary Altern. Med.,* **2014**, *19*(3), 216-219.
[http://dx.doi.org/10.1177/2156587214533346] [PMID: 24789912]

[8]   Weaver, B.A. How Taxol/paclitaxel kills cancer cells. *Mol. Biol. Cell,* **2014**, *25*(18), 2677-2681.
[http://dx.doi.org/10.1091/mbc.e14-04-0916] [PMID: 25213191]

[9]   Singh, S.; Sharma, B.; Kanwar, S.S.; Kumar, A. Lead phytochemicals for anticancer drug development. *Front. Plant Sci.,* **2016**, *7*, 1667.
[http://dx.doi.org/10.3389/fpls.2016.01667] [PMID: 27877185]

[10]   Thakore, P.; Mani, R.K.; Kavitha, S.J. A brief review of plants having anti-cancer property. *Int J Pharm Res Dev,* **2012**, *3*, 129-136.

[11]   Tariq, A.; Sadia, S.; Pan, K.; Ullah, I.; Mussarat, S.; Sun, F.; Abiodun, O.O.; Batbaatar, A.; Li, Z.; Song, D.; Xiong, Q.; Ullah, R.; Khan, S.; Basnet, B.B.; Kumar, B.; Islam, R.; Adnan, M. A systematic review on ethnomedicines of anti-cancer plants. *Phytother. Res.,* **2017**, *31*(2), 202-264.
[http://dx.doi.org/10.1002/ptr.5751] [PMID: 28093828]

[12]   Ayoob, I.; Hazari, Y.M.; Lone, S.H.; Shakeel-u-Rehman, ; Khuroo, M.A.; Fazili, K.M.; Bhat, K.A. Phytochemical and cytotoxic evaluation of peganum harmala: Structure activity relationship studies of harmine. *ChemistrySelect,* **2017**, *2*(10), 2965-2968.
[http://dx.doi.org/10.1002/slct.201700232]

[13]   Ooko, E.; Kadioglu, O.; Greten, H.J.; Efferth, T. Pharmacogenomic characterization and isobologram analysis of the combination of ascorbic acid and curcumin-two main metabolites of Curcuma longa-in cancer cells. *Front. Pharmacol.,* **2017**, *8*, 38.
[http://dx.doi.org/10.3389/fphar.2017.00038] [PMID: 28210221]

[14]   Bhandari, J.; Muhammad, B.; Thapa, P.; Shrestha, B.G. Study of phytochemical, anti-microbial, anti-oxidant, and anti-cancer properties of Allium wallichii. *BMC Complement. Altern. Med.,* **2017**, *17*(1), 102.
[http://dx.doi.org/10.1186/s12906-017-1622-6] [PMID: 28178952]

[15]   Efferth, T. From ancient herb to versatile, modern drug: Artemisia annua and artemisinin for cancer therapy. *Semin Canc Biol,* **2017**.

[16]   Kumari, M.; Pattnaik, B.; Rajan, S.Y.; Shrikant, S.; Surendra, S.U. EGCG-A Promis anti-cancer. *Phytochemistry,* **2017**, *3*(2), 8-10.

[17]   Preethi, R.; Padma, P.R. Biosynthesis and bioactivity of silver nanobioconjugates from grape (vitis vinifera) seeds and its active component resveratrol. *Int. J. Pharm. Sci. Res.,* **2016**, *7*(10), 4253.

[18]   Xiong, M.; Wang, L.; Yu, H.L.; Han, H.; Mao, D.; Chen, J.; Zeng, Y.; He, N.; Liu, Z.G.; Wang, Z.Y.; Xu, S.J.; Guo, L.Y.; Wang, Y. Ginkgetin exerts growth inhibitory and apoptotic effects on osteosarcoma cells through inhibition of STAT3 and activation of caspase-3/9. *Oncol. Rep.,* **2016**, *35*(2), 1034-1040.
[http://dx.doi.org/10.3892/or.2015.4427] [PMID: 26573608]

[19]   Wu, F.; Zhou, L.; Jin, W.; Yang, W.; Wang, Y.; Yan, B.; Du, W.; Zhang, Q.; Zhang, L.; Guo, Y.; Zhang, J.; Shan, L.; Efferth, T. Antiproliferative and apoptosis-inducing effect of theabrownin against non-small cell lung adenocarcinoma A549 cells. *Front. Pharmacol.,* **2016**, *7*, 465.
[http://dx.doi.org/10.3389/fphar.2016.00465] [PMID: 27994550]

[20]   Beg, M.A.; Teotia, U.V.; Farooq, S. *In vitro* antibacterial and anticancer activity of Ziziphus. *Faslnamah-i Giyahan-i Daruyi,* **2016**, *4*(5), 230-233.

[21]   Al Sinani, S.S.; Eltayeb, E.A.; Coomber, B.L.; Adham, S.A. Solamargine triggers cellular necrosis selectively in different types of human melanoma cancer cells through extrinsic lysosomal mitochondrial death pathway. *Cancer Cell Int.,* **2016**, *16*(1), 11.

[http://dx.doi.org/10.1186/s12935-016-0287-4] [PMID: 26889092]

[22] Mehdad, A.; Brumana, G.; Souza, A.A.; Barbosa, J.A.R.G.; Ventura, M.M.; de Freitas, S.M. A Bowman–Birk inhibitor induces apoptosis in human breast adenocarcinoma through mitochondrial impairment and oxidative damage following proteasome 20S inhibition. *Cell Death Discov.,* **2016**, *2*(1), 15067.
[http://dx.doi.org/10.1038/cddiscovery.2015.67] [PMID: 27551492]

[23] Jaradat, N.A.; Al-Ramahi, R.; Zaid, A.N.; Ayesh, O.I.; Eid, A.M. Ethnopharmacological survey of herbal remedies used for treatment of various types of cancer and their methods of preparations in the West Bank-Palestine. *BMC Complement. Altern. Med.,* **2016**, *16*(1), 93.
[http://dx.doi.org/10.1186/s12906-016-1070-8] [PMID: 26955822]

[24] Zhang, Y.Y.; Huang, C.T.; Liu, S.M.; Wang, B.; Guo, J.; Bai, J.Q.; Fan, X-J.; Jia, Y-S. Licochalcone A exerts antitumor activity in bladder cancer cell lines and mice models. *Trop. J. Pharm. Res.,* **2016**, *15*(6), 1151-1157.
[http://dx.doi.org/10.4314/tjpr.v15i6.6]

[25] Yong, Y.L.; Tan, L.T.; Ming, L.C.; Chan, K.G.; Lee, L.H.; Goh, B.H. The effectiveness and safety of topical capsaicin in postherpetic neuralgia: A systematic review and meta-analysis. *Front Pharm,* **2017**.

[26] Srikanth, S.; Chen, Z. Plant protease inhibitors in therapeutics-focus on cancer therapy. *Front Pharma,* **2016**.
[http://dx.doi.org/10.3389/fphar.2016.00470]

[27] Pahari, P.; Saikia, U.P.; Das, T.P.; Damodaran, C.; Rohr, J. Synthesis of Psoralidin derivatives and their anticancer activity: First synthesis of Lespeflorin I[1]. *Tetrahedron,* **2016**, *72*(23), 3324-3334.
[http://dx.doi.org/10.1016/j.tet.2016.04.066] [PMID: 27698514]

[28] Amin, S.; Barkatullah, H.K.; Khan, H. Pharmacology of Xanthium species. A review. *J. Phytopharm,* **2016**, *5*(3), 126-127.
[http://dx.doi.org/10.31254/phyto.2016.5308]

[29] Thangapazham, R.L.; Sharad, S.; Maheshwari, R.K. Phytochemicals in wound healing. *Adv. Wound Care (New Rochelle),* **2016**, *5*(5), 230-241.
[http://dx.doi.org/10.1089/wound.2013.0505] [PMID: 27134766]

[30] Tu, L.Y.; Pi, J.; Jin, H.; Cai, J.Y.; Deng, S.P. Synthesis, characterization and anticancer activity of kaempferol-zinc(II) complex. *Bioorg. Med. Chem. Lett.,* **2016**, *26*(11), 2730-2734.
[http://dx.doi.org/10.1016/j.bmcl.2016.03.091] [PMID: 27080177]

[31] Lee, I.C.; Choi, B. WithaferinA-a natural anticancer agent with pleitropic mechanisms of action. *Int. J. Mol. Sci.,* **2016**, *17*(3), 290.
[http://dx.doi.org/10.3390/ijms17030290] [PMID: 26959007]

[32] Wal, A.; Srivastava, R.S.; Wal, P.; Rai, A.; Sharma, S. Lupeol as a magic drug. *Pharm Biol Eval,* **2015**, *2*, 142-151.

[33] Rastogi, N.; Duggal, S.; Singh, S.K.; Porwal, K.; Srivastava, V.K.; Maurya, R.; Bhatt, M.L.B.; Mishra, D.P. Proteasome inhibition mediates p53 reactivation and anti-cancer activity of 6-Gingerol in cervical cancer cells. *Oncotarget,* **2015**, *6*(41), 43310-43325.
[http://dx.doi.org/10.18632/oncotarget.6383] [PMID: 26621832]

[34] Tsai, C.C.; Chuang, T.W.; Chen, L.J.; Niu, H.S.; Chung, K.M.; Cheng, J.T.; Lin, K.C. Increase in apoptosis by combination of metformin with silibinin in human colorectal cancer cells. *World J. Gastroenterol.,* **2015**, *21*(14), 4169-4177.
[http://dx.doi.org/10.3748/wjg.v21.i14.4169] [PMID: 25892866]

[35] Osman, N.H.A.; Said, U.Z.; El-Waseef, A.M.; Ahmed, E.S.A. Luteolin supplementation adjacent to aspirin treatment reduced dimethylhydrazine-induced experimental colon carcinogenesis in rats. *Tumour Biol.,* **2015**, *36*(2), 1179-1190.

[http://dx.doi.org/10.1007/s13277-014-2678-2] [PMID: 25342594]

[36] Lin, X.; Peng, Z.; Su, C. Potential anti-cancer activities and mechanisms of costunolide and dehydrocostuslactone. *Int. J. Mol. Sci.,* **2015**, *16*(12), 10888-10906.
[http://dx.doi.org/10.3390/ijms160510888] [PMID: 25984608]

[37] Mukhija, M.; Singh, M.P.; Dhar, K.L.; Kalia, A.N. Cytotoxic and antioxidant activity of Zanthoxylum alatum stem bark and its flavonoid constituents. *J. Pharmacogn. Phytochem.,* **2015**, *4*, 86.

[38] Garg, P.; Deep, A. Anti-cancer potential of boswellic acid: A mini review. *Hygeia J D Med,* **2015**, *7*(2), 18-27.

[39] Ramasamy, K.; Agarwal, R. Multitargeted therapy of cancer by silymarin. *Cancer Lett.,* **2008**, *269*(2), 352-362.
[http://dx.doi.org/10.1016/j.canlet.2008.03.053] [PMID: 18472213]

[40] Vallianou, N.G.; Evangelopoulos, A.; Schizas, N.; Kazazis, C. Potential anticancer properties and mechanisms of action of curcumin. *Anticancer Res.,* **2015**, *35*(2), 645-651.
[PMID: 25667441]

[41] Monika Singh, J. Plants and phytochemicals as potential source of anticancer agents. *Int. J. Adv. Res. (Indore),* **2015**, *4*, 307-317.

[42] Choi, J.Y.; Hong, W.G.; Cho, J.H.; Kim, E.M.; Kim, J.; Jung, C.H.; Hwang, S.G.; Um, H.D.; Park, J.K. Podophyllotoxin acetate triggers anticancer effects against non-small cell lung cancer cells by promoting cell death *via* cell cycle arrest, ER stress and autophagy. *Int. J. Oncol.,* **2015**, *47*(4), 1257-1265.
[http://dx.doi.org/10.3892/ijo.2015.3123] [PMID: 26314270]

[43] Hoshyar, R.; Mollaei, H. A comprehensive review on anticancer mechanisms of the main carotenoid of saffron, crocin. *J. Pharm. Pharmacol.,* **2017**, *69*(11), 1419-1427.
[http://dx.doi.org/10.1111/jphp.12776] [PMID: 28675431]

[44] Liu, Y.Q.; Tian, J.; Qian, K.; Zhao, X.B.; Morris-Natschke, S.L.; Yang, L.; Nan, X.; Tian, X.; Lee, K.H. Recent progress on C-4-modified podophyllotoxin analogs as potent antitumor agents. *Med. Res. Rev.,* **2015**, *35*(1), 1-62.
[http://dx.doi.org/10.1002/med.21319] [PMID: 24827545]

[45] Król, S.K.; Kiełbus, M.; Rivero-Müller, A.; Stepulak, A. Comprehensive review on betulin as a potent anticancer agent. *BioMed Res. Int.,* **2015**, *2015*, 1-11.
[http://dx.doi.org/10.1155/2015/584189] [PMID: 25866796]

[46] Wang, C.Z.; Zhang, Z.; Wan, J.Y.; Zhang, C.F.; Anderson, S.; He, X.; Yu, C.; He, T.C.; Qi, L.W.; Yuan, C.S. Protopanaxadiol, an active ginseng metabolite, significantly enhances the effects of fluorouracil on colon cancer. *Nutrients,* **2015**, *7*(2), 799-814.
[http://dx.doi.org/10.3390/nu7020799] [PMID: 25625815]

[47] Lan, L.; Appelman, C.; Smith, A.R.; Yu, J.; Larsen, S.; Marquez, R.T.; Liu, H.; Wu, X.; Gao, P.; Roy, A.; Anbanandam, A.; Gowthaman, R.; Karanicolas, J.; De Guzman, R.N.; Rogers, S.; Aubé, J.; Ji, M.; Cohen, R.S.; Neufeld, K.L.; Xu, L. Natural product (−)-gossypol inhibits colon cancer cell growth by targeting RNA-binding protein Musashi-1. *Mol. Oncol.,* **2015**, *9*(7), 1406-1420.
[http://dx.doi.org/10.1016/j.molonc.2015.03.014] [PMID: 25933687]

[48] León, I.E.; Cadavid-Vargas, J.F.; Tiscornia, I.; Porro, V.; Castelli, S.; Katkar, P.; Desideri, A.; Bollati-Fogolin, M.; Etcheverry, S.B. Oxidovanadium(IV) complexes with chrysin and silibinin: Anticancer activity and mechanisms of action in a human colon adenocarcinoma model. *J. Biol. Inorg. Chem.,* **2015**, *20*(7), 1175-1191.
[http://dx.doi.org/10.1007/s00775-015-1298-7] [PMID: 26404080]

[49] Yan, C.H.; Li, F.; Ma, Y.C. Plumbagin shows anticancer activity in human osteosarcoma (MG-63) cells *via* the inhibition of S-Phase checkpoints and down-regulation of c-myc. *Int. J. Clin. Exp. Med.,* **2015**, *8*(8), 14432-14439.

[PMID: 26550431]

[50]   Ghasemzadeh, A.; Jaafar, H.Z.E.; Rahmat, A. Optimization protocol for the extraction of 6-gingerol and 6-shogaol from Zingiber officinale var. rubrum Theilade and improving antioxidant and anticancer activity using response surface methodology. *BMC Complement. Altern. Med.,* **2015**, *15*(1), 258.
[http://dx.doi.org/10.1186/s12906-015-0718-0] [PMID: 26223685]

[51]   Perrone, D.; Ardito, F.; Giannatempo, G.; Dioguardi, M.; Troiano, G.; Lo Russo, L.; De Lillo, A.; Laino, L.; Lo Muzio, L. Biological and therapeutic activities, and anticancer properties of curcumin. *Exp. Ther. Med.,* **2015**, *10*(5), 1615-1623.
[http://dx.doi.org/10.3892/etm.2015.2749] [PMID: 26640527]

[52]   Woźniak, Ł.; Skąpska, S.; Marszałek, K. Ursolic acid-a pentacyclic triterpenoid with a wide spectrum of pharmacological activities. *Molecules,* **2015**, *20*(11), 20614-20641.
[http://dx.doi.org/10.3390/molecules201119721] [PMID: 26610440]

[53]   Pang, S.Q.; Wang, G.Q.; Lin, J.; Diao, Y.; Xu, R. Cytotoxic activity of the alkaloids from *Broussonetia papyrifera* fruits. *Pharm. Biol.,* **2014**, *52*(10), 1315-1319.
[http://dx.doi.org/10.3109/13880209.2014.891139] [PMID: 24992202]

[54]   Jung, S.K.; Lee, M.H.; Lim, D.Y.; Kim, J.E.; Singh, P.; Lee, S.Y.; Jeong, C.H.; Lim, T.G.; Chen, H.; Chi, Y.I.; Kundu, J.K.; Lee, N.H.; Lee, C.C.; Cho, Y.Y.; Bode, A.M.; Lee, K.W.; Dong, Z. Isoliquiritigenin induces apoptosis and inhibits xenograft tumor growth of human lung cancer cells by targeting both wild type and L858R/T790M mutant EGFR. *J. Biol. Chem.,* **2014**, *289*(52), 35839-35848.
[http://dx.doi.org/10.1074/jbc.M114.585513] [PMID: 25368326]

[55]   Mishra, S.; Aeri, V.; Gaur, P.K.; Jachak, S.M. Phytochemical, therapeutic, and ethnopharmacological overview for a traditionally important herb: Boerhavia diffusa Linn. *BioMed Res. Int.,* **2014**, *2014*, 1-19.
[http://dx.doi.org/10.1155/2014/808302] [PMID: 24949473]

[56]   Cheah, K.Y.; Howarth, G.S.; Bindon, K.A.; Kennedy, J.A.; Bastian, S.E.P. Low molecular weight procyanidins from grape seeds enhance the impact of 5-Fluorouracil chemotherapy on Caco-2 human colon cancer cells. *PLoS One,* **2014**, *9*(6), e98921.
[http://dx.doi.org/10.1371/journal.pone.0098921] [PMID: 24905821]

[57]   Ali, I.; Braun, D.P. Resveratrol enhances mitomycin C-mediated suppression of human colorectal cancer cell proliferation by up-regulation of p21WAF1/CIP1. *Anticancer Res.,* **2014**, *34*(10), 5439-5446.
[PMID: 25275039]

[58]   Aziz, M.Y.A.; Omar, A.R.; Subramani, T.; Yeap, S.K.; Ho, W.Y.; Ismail, N.H.; Ahmad, S.; Alitheen, N.B. Damnacanthal is a potent inducer of apoptosis with anticancer activity by stimulating p53 and p21 genes in MCF-7 breast cancer cells. *Oncol. Lett.,* **2014**, *7*(5), 1479-1484.
[http://dx.doi.org/10.3892/ol.2014.1898] [PMID: 24765160]

[59]   Guruvayoorappan, C.; Kuttan, G. Immunomodulatory and antitumor activity of Biophytum sensitivum extract. *Asian Pac. J. Cancer Prev.,* **2007**, *8*(1), 27-32.
[PMID: 17477767]

[60]   Zhan, Y.; Jia, G.; Wu, D.; Xu, Y.; Xu, L. Design and synthesis of a gossypol derivative with improved antitumor activities. *Arch. Pharm. (Weinheim),* **2009**, *342*(4), 223-229.
[http://dx.doi.org/10.1002/ardp.200800185] [PMID: 19340835]

[61]   Shalabi, M.; Khilo, K.; Zakaria, M.M.; Elsebaei, M.G.; Abdo, W.; Awadin, W. Anticancer activity of Aloe vera and Calligonum comosum extracts separetely on hepatocellular carcinoma cells. *Asian Pac. J. Trop. Biomed.,* **2015**, *5*(5), 375-381.
[http://dx.doi.org/10.1016/S2221-1691(15)30372-5]

[62]   El-Shemy, H.; Aboul-Soud, M.; Nassr-Allah, A.; Aboul-Enein, K.; Kabash, A.; Yagi, A. Antitumor properties and modulation of antioxidant enzymes' activity by Aloe vera leaf active principles isolated

via supercritical carbon dioxide extraction. *Curr. Med. Chem.,* **2010**, *17*(2), 129-138.
[http://dx.doi.org/10.2174/092986710790112620] [PMID: 19941474]

[63]   Formagio, A.S.N.; Vieira, M.C.; Volobuff, C.R.F.; Silva, M.S.; Matos, A.I.; Cardoso, C.A.L.; Foglio, M.A.; Carvalho, J.E. *In vitro* biological screening of the anticholinesterase and antiproliferative activities of medicinal plants belonging to Annonaceae. *Braz. J. Med. Biol. Res.,* **2015**, *48*(4), 308-315.
[http://dx.doi.org/10.1590/1414-431x20144127] [PMID: 25714885]

[64]   Leyva-Peralta, M.A.; Robles-Zepeda, R.E.; Garibay-Escobar, A.; Ruiz-Bustos, E.; Alvarez-Berber, L.P.; Gálvez-Ruiz, J.C. *In vitro* anti-proliferative activity of Argemone gracilenta and identification of some active components. *BMC Complement. Altern. Med.,* **2015**, *15*(1), 13.
[http://dx.doi.org/10.1186/s12906-015-0532-8] [PMID: 25652581]

[65]   Wang, Y.; Hong, C.; Zhou, C.; Xu, D.; Qu, H. Screening antitumor compounds psoralen and isopsoralen from Psoralea corylifolia L. seeds. *Evid. Based Complement. Alternat. Med.,* **2011**, *2011*, 1-7.
[http://dx.doi.org/10.1093/ecam/nen087] [PMID: 19131395]

[66]   Mutasim, M.K.; Hussein, M.D.A.N.; Khalid, M.A.E.; Hany, A.E.S.; Eltayb, A.; Abdellatef, E. Dedifferentiation of leaf explants and antileukemia activity of an ethanolic extract of cell cultures of Moringa oleifera. *Afr. J. Biotechnol.,* **2011**, *10*(14), 2746-2750.
[http://dx.doi.org/10.5897/AJB10.2099]

[67]   Chan, LL; George, S; Ahmad, I; Gosangari, SL; Abbasi, A; Cunningham, BT Cytotoxicity effects of Amoora rohituka and chittagonga on breast and pancreatic cancer cells. *Evid base Compl Altern Med,* **2011**, *2011*, 860605.

[68]   Csupor-Löffler, B.; Hajdú, Z.; Zupkó, I.; Molnár, J.; Forgo, P.; Vasas, A.; Kele, Z.; Hohmann, J. Antiproliferative constituents of the roots of Conyza canadensis. *Planta Med.,* **2011**, *77*(11), 1183-1188.
[http://dx.doi.org/10.1055/s-0030-1270714] [PMID: 21294076]

[69]   Unnati, S.; Ripal, S.; Sanjeev, A.; Niyat, A. Novel anticancer agents from plant sources. *Chin. J. Nat. Med.,* **2013**, *11*, 16-23.

[70]   Du, G.J.; Wang, C.Z.; Qi, L.W.; Zhang, Z.Y.; Calway, T.; He, T.C.; Du, W.; Yuan, C.S. The synergistic apoptotic interaction of panaxadiol and epigallocatechin gallate in human colorectal cancer cells. *Phytother. Res.,* **2013**, *27*(2), 272-277.
[http://dx.doi.org/10.1002/ptr.4707] [PMID: 22566066]

[71]   Keglevich, P.; Hazai, L.; Kalaus, G.; Szántay, C. Modifications on the basic skeletons of vinblastine and vincristine. *Molecules,* **2012**, *17*(5), 5893-5914.
[http://dx.doi.org/10.3390/molecules17055893] [PMID: 22609781]

[72]   Heidari, M.; Heidari-Vala, H.; Sadeghi, M.R.; Akhondi, M.M. The inductive effects of Centella asiatica on rat spermatogenic cell apoptosis *in vivo. J. Nat. Med.,* **2012**, *66*(2), 271-278.
[http://dx.doi.org/10.1007/s11418-011-0578-y] [PMID: 21870191]

[73]   Bhouri, W.; Boubaker, J.; Skandrani, I.; Ghedira, K.; Chekir Ghedira, L. Investigation of the apoptotic way induced by digallic acid in human lymphoblastoid TK6 cells. *Cancer Cell Int.,* **2012**, *12*(1), 26.
[http://dx.doi.org/10.1186/1475-2867-12-26] [PMID: 22686580]

[74]   Raihan, M.O.; Tareq, S.M.; Brishti, A.; Alam, M.K.; Haque, A.; Ali, M.S. Evaluation of antitumor activity of Leea indica (Burm.f.) merr extract against Ehrlich ascites carcinoma (EAC) bearing mice. *Am. J. Biomed. Sci.,* **2012**, *4*, 143-152.
[http://dx.doi.org/10.5099/aj120200143]

[75]   Lan Wang, ; Xu, G.F.; Liu, X.X.; Chang, A.X.; Xu, M.L.; Ghimeray, A.K. *In vitro* antioxidant properties and induced G2/M arrest in HT-29 cells of dichloromethane fraction from Liriodendron tulipifera. *J. Med. Plants Res.,* **2012**, *6*(3), 424-432.
[http://dx.doi.org/10.5897/JMPR11.1125]

[76]   Magee, P.J.; Owusu-Apenten, R.; McCann, M.J.; Gill, C.I.; Rowland, I.R. Chickpea (Cicer arietinum) and other plant-derived protease inhibitor concentrates inhibit breast and prostate cancer cell proliferation *in vitro. Nutr. Cancer,* **2012**, *64*(5), 741-748.
[http://dx.doi.org/10.1080/01635581.2012.688914] [PMID: 22662866]

[77]   Hoshyar, R.; Mollaei, H. A comprehensive review on anticancer mechanisms of the main carotenoid of saffron, crocin. *J. Pharm. Pharmacol.,* **2017**, *69*(11), 1419-1427.
[http://dx.doi.org/10.1111/jphp.12776] [PMID: 28675431]

[78]   Arpita, R.; Navneeta, B. Centella asiatica: A pharmaceutically important medicinal plant. *Curr. Trends Biomed. Eng. Biosci.,* **2017**, *5*(3), 555661.

[79]   Kaur, R.; Karan, K.; Kaur, K. Plants as a source of anticancer agents. *J Nat Prod Plant Resour,* **2011**, *1*, 119-112.

[80]   Hu, M.; Xu, L.; Yin, L.; Qi, Y.; Li, H.; Xu, Y.; Han, X.; Peng, J.; Wan, X. Cytotoxicity of dioscin in human gastric carcinoma cells through death receptor and mitochondrial pathways. *J. Appl. Toxicol.,* **2013**, *33*(8), 712-722.
[http://dx.doi.org/10.1002/jat.2715] [PMID: 22334414]

[81]   Motta, L.B.; Furlan, C.M.; Santos, D.Y.A.C.; Salatino, M.L.F.; Duarte-Almeida, J.M.; Negri, G.; Carvalho, J.E.; Ruiz, A.L.T.G.; Cordeiro, I.; Salatino, A. Constituents and antiproliferative activity of extracts from leaves of Croton macrobothrys. *Rev. Bras. Farmacogn.,* **2011**, *21*(6), 972-977.
[http://dx.doi.org/10.1590/S0102-695X2011005000174]

[82]   Maneerat, W.; Thain, S.; Cheenpracha, S.; Prawat, U.; Laphookhieo, S. New amides from the seeds of Clausana lansium. *J. Med. Plants Res.,* **2011**, *5*, 2812-2815.

[83]   Lauritano, C.; Andersen, J.H.; Hansen, E.; Albrigtsen, M.; Escalera, L.; Esposito, F.; Helland, K.; Hanssen, K.Ø.; Romano, G.; Ianora, A. Bioactivity screening of microalgae for antioxidant, anti-inflammatory, anticancer, anti-diabetes, and antibacterial activities. *Front. Mar. Sci.,* **2016**, *3*, 68.
[http://dx.doi.org/10.3389/fmars.2016.00068]

[84]   Hahm, E.R.; Moura, M.B.; Kelley, E.E.; Van Houten, B.; Shiva, S.; Singh, S.V. Withaferin A-induced apoptosis in human breast cancer cells is mediated by reactive oxygen species. *PLoS One,* **2011**, *6*(8), e23354.
[http://dx.doi.org/10.1371/journal.pone.0023354] [PMID: 21853114]

[85]   Checker, R.; Sharma, D.; Sandur, S.K.; Subrahmanyam, G.; Krishnan, S.; Poduval, T.B.; Sainis, K.B. Plumbagin inhibits proliferative and inflammatory responses of T cells independent of ROS generation but by modulating intracellular thiols. *J. Cell. Biochem.,* **2010**, *110*(5), 1082-1093.
[http://dx.doi.org/10.1002/jcb.22620] [PMID: 20564204]

[86]   Bakshi, H.A.; Sam, S.; Feroz, A.; Ravesh, Z.; Shah, G.A.; Sharma, M. Crocin from Kashmiri saffron (Crocus sativus) induces *in vitro* and *in vivo* xenograft growth inhibition of Dalton's lymphoma (DLA) in mice. *Asian Pac. J. Cancer Prev.,* **2009**, *10*(5), 887-890.
[PMID: 20104983]

[87]   Einbond, L.S.; Soffritti, M.; Esposti, D.D.; Park, T.; Cruz, E.; Su, T.; Wu, H.; Wang, X.; Zhang, Y.J.; Ham, J.; Goldberg, I.J.; Kronenberg, F.; Vladimirova, A. Actein activates stress- and statin-associated responses and is bioavailable in Sprague-Dawley rats. *Fundam. Clin. Pharmacol.,* **2009**, *23*(3), 311-321.
[http://dx.doi.org/10.1111/j.1472-8206.2009.00673.x] [PMID: 19527300]

[88]   Ogunwande, I.A.; Walker, T.M.; Bansal, A.; Setzer, W.N.; Essien, E.E. Essential oil constituents and biological activities of Peristrophe bicalyculata and Borreria verticillata. *Nat. Prod. Commun.,* **2010**, *5*(11), 1934578X1000501.
[http://dx.doi.org/10.1177/1934578X1000501125] [PMID: 21213989]

[89]   Appendino, G.; Chianese, G.; Taglialatela-Scafati, O. Cannabinoids: Occurrence and medicinal chemistry. *Curr. Med. Chem.,* **2011**, *18*(7), 1085-1099.

[http://dx.doi.org/10.2174/092986711794940888] [PMID: 21254969]

[90]   Colombo, V.; Lupi, M.; Falcetta, F.; Forestieri, D.; D'Incalci, M.; Ubezio, P. Chemotherapeutic activity of silymarin combined with doxorubicin or paclitaxel in sensitive and multidrug-resistant colon cancer cells. *Cancer Chemother. Pharmacol.,* **2011**, *67*(2), 369-379.
       [http://dx.doi.org/10.1007/s00280-010-1335-8] [PMID: 20431887]

[91]   Nakahata, A.M.; Mayer, B.; Ries, C.; de Paula, C.A.A.; Karow, M.; Neth, P.; Sampaio, M.U.; Jochum, M.; Oliva, M.L.V. The effects of a plant proteinase inhibitor from Enterolobium contortisiliquum on human tumor cell lines. *Biol. Chem.,* **2011**, *392*(4), 327-336.
       [http://dx.doi.org/10.1515/bc.2011.031] [PMID: 21781023]

[92]   Sakarkar, D.M.; Deshmukh, V.N. Ethnopharmacological review of traditional medicinal plants for anti-cancer activity. *Int. J. Pharm. Tech. Res.,* **2011**, *3*, 298-308.

[93]   Xu, L.N.; Lu, B.N.; Hu, M.M.; Xu, Y.W.; Han, X.; Qi, Y.; Peng, J.Y. Mechanisms involved in the cytotoxic effects of berberine on human colon cancer HCT-8 cells. *Biocell,* **2012**, *36*(3), 113-120.
       [PMID: 23682426]

[94]   Karmakar, S.; Choudhury, S.R.; Banik, N.L.; Ray, S.K. Molecular mechanisms of anti-cancer action of garlic compounds in neuroblastoma. *Anticancer. Agents Med. Chem.,* **2011**, *11*(4), 398-407.
       [http://dx.doi.org/10.2174/187152011795677553] [PMID: 21521157]

[95]   Lam, S.K.; Ng, T.B. Novel galactonic acid-binding hexameric lectin from Hibiscus mutabilis seeds with antiproliferative and potent HIV-1 reverse transcriptase inhibitory activities. *Acta Biochim. Pol.,* **2009**, *56*(4), 649-654.
       [http://dx.doi.org/10.18388/abp.2009_2498] [PMID: 19956805]

[96]   Ververidis, F.; Trantas, E.; Douglas, C.; Vollmer, G.; Kretzschmar, G.; Panopoulos, N. Biotechnology of flavonoids and other phenylpropanoid-derived natural products. Part I: Chemical diversity, impacts on plant biology and human health. *Biotechnol. J.,* **2007**, *2*(10), 1214-1234.
       [http://dx.doi.org/10.1002/biot.200700084] [PMID: 17935117]

[97]   Caruso, M.; Colombo, A.L.; Fedeli, L.; Pavesi, A.; Quaroni, S.; Saracchi, M. Isolation of endophytic fungi and actinomycetes taxane producers. *Ann. Microbiol.,* **2000**, *50*, 3-14.

[98]   Lim, D.Y.; Park, J.H.Y. Induction of p53 contributes to apoptosis of HCT-116 human colon cancer cells induced by the dietary compound fisetin. *Am. J. Physiol. Gastrointest. Liver Physiol.,* **2009**, *296*(5), G1060-G1068.
       [http://dx.doi.org/10.1152/ajpgi.90490.2008]

[99]   Madhuri, S.; Pandey, G. Some anticancer medicinal plants of foreign origin. *Curr. Sci.,* **2009**, *96*, 6-25.

[100] Cragg, G.M.; Newman, D.J. Plants as a source of anti-cancer agents. *J. Ethnopharmacol.,* **2005**, *100*(1-2), 72-79.
       [http://dx.doi.org/10.1016/j.jep.2005.05.011] [PMID: 16009521]

[101] Bao, M.F.; Yan, J.M.; Cheng, G.G.; Li, X.Y.; Liu, Y.P.; Li, Y.; Cai, X.H.; Luo, X.D. Cytotoxic indole alkaloids from Tabernaemontana divaricata. *J. Nat. Prod.,* **2013**, *76*(8), 1406-1412.
       [http://dx.doi.org/10.1021/np400130y] [PMID: 23944995]

[102] Sabnis, M. *Chemistry and Pharmacology of Ayurvedic Medicinal Plants*; Prakashan: Chaukhambha Amarabharati, **2006**.

[103] Rahman, S.; Carter, P.; Bhattarai, N. Aloe vera for tissue engineering applications. *J. Funct. Biomater.,* **2017**, *8*(1), 6.
       [http://dx.doi.org/10.3390/jfb8010006] [PMID: 28216559]

[104] Aggarwal, B.B.; Kumar, A.; Bharti, A.C. Anticancer potential of curcumin: Preclinical and clinical studies. *Anticancer Res.,* **2003**, *23*(1A), 363-398.
       [PMID: 12680238]

[105] Merina, N.; Chandra, K.J.; Jibon, K. Medicinal plants with potential anticancer activities: A review.

Int Res J Phar, **2012**, *3*, 26-30.

[106] Weng, J.R.; Bai, L.Y.; Chiu, C.F.; Hu, J.L.; Chiu, S.J.; Wu, C.Y. Cucurbitane triterpenoid from Momordica charantia induces apoptosis and autophagy in breast cancer cells, in part, through peroxisome proliferator-activated receptor c activation. *Evid. Based Complement. Alternat. Med.,* **2013**, *2013*, 1-12.
[http://dx.doi.org/10.1155/2013/935675] [PMID: 23843889]

[107] Kaushik, R.; Narayanan, P.; Vasudevan, V.; Muthukumaran, G.; Usha, A. Nutrient composition of cultivated stevia leaves and the influence of polyphenols and plant pigments on sensory and antioxidant properties of leaf extracts. *J. Food Sci. Technol.,* **2010**, *47*(1), 27-33.
[http://dx.doi.org/10.1007/s13197-010-0011-7] [PMID: 23572597]

[108] Das, I.; Das, S.; Saha, T. Saffron suppresses oxidative stress in DMBA-induced skin carcinoma: A histopathological study. *Acta Histochem.,* **2010**, *112*(4), 317-327.
[http://dx.doi.org/10.1016/j.acthis.2009.02.003] [PMID: 19328523]

[109] Yoon, J.S.; Kim, H.M.; Yadunandam, A.K.; Kim, N.H.; Jung, H.A.; Choi, J.S.; Kim, C.Y.; Kim, G.D. Neferine isolated from Nelumbo nucifera enhances anti-cancer activities in Hep3B cells: Molecular mechanisms of cell cycle arrest, ER stress induced apoptosis and anti-angiogenic response. *Phytomedicine,* **2013**, *20*(11), 1013-1022.
[http://dx.doi.org/10.1016/j.phymed.2013.03.024] [PMID: 23746959]

[110] Ng, T.B.; Lam, Y.W.; Wang, H. Calcaelin, a new protein with translation-inhibiting, antiproliferative and antimitogenic activities from the mosaic puffball mushroom Calvatia caelata. *Planta Med.,* **2003**, *69*(3), 212-217.
[http://dx.doi.org/10.1055/s-2003-38492] [PMID: 12677523]

[111] Ngai, P.H.K.; Ng, T.B. A ribonuclease with antimicrobial, antimitogenic and antiproliferative activities from the edible mushroom Pleurotus sajor-caju. *Peptides,* **2004**, *25*(1), 11-17.
[http://dx.doi.org/10.1016/j.peptides.2003.11.012] [PMID: 15003351]

[112] Smith, J.E.; Zong, A.; Rowan, N.J. Medicinal mushrooms: Their therapeutic properties and current medical usage with special emphasis on cancer treatments. *Canc Res,* **2002**.

[113] Srivastava, J.K.; Gupta, S. Antiproliferative and apoptotic effects of chamomile extract in various human cancer cells. *J. Agric. Food Chem.,* **2007**, *55*(23), 9470-9478.
[http://dx.doi.org/10.1021/jf071953k] [PMID: 17939735]

[114] ALim, T,K. Edible medicinal and non-medicinal plants In: *Fruits*; Springer: Netherlands, **2013**.

[115] Suzuki, K.; Yano, T.; Sadzuka, Y.; Sugiyama, T.; Seki, T.; Asano, R. Restoration of connexin 43 by Bowman-Birk protease inhibitor in M5076 bearing mice. *Oncol. Rep.,* **2005**, *13*(6), 1247-1250.
[http://dx.doi.org/10.3892/or.13.6.1247] [PMID: 15870950]

[116] Huang, G.J.; Sheu, M.J.; Chen, H.J.; Chang, Y.S.; Lin, Y.H. Growth inhibition and induction of apoptosis in NB4 promyelocytic leukemia cells by trypsin inhibitor from sweet potato storage roots. *J. Agric. Food Chem.,* **2007**, *55*(7), 2548-2553.
[http://dx.doi.org/10.1021/jf063008m] [PMID: 17328557]

[117] Rakashanda, S.; Mubashir, S.; Qureshi, Y.; Hamid, A.; Masood, A.; Amin, S. Trypsin inhibitors from Lavatera cashmeriana camb. seeds: Isolation, characterization and *in-vitro* cytoxic activity. *Int. J. Pharm. Sci. Invent.,* **2013**, *2*, 55-65.

[118] Caccialupi, P.; Ceci, L.R.; Siciliano, R.A.; Pignone, D.; Clemente, A.; Sonnante, G. Bowman-Birk inhibitors in lentil: Heterologous expression, functional characterisation and anti-proliferative properties in human colon cancer cells. *Food Chem.,* **2010**, *120*(4), 1058-1066.
[http://dx.doi.org/10.1016/j.foodchem.2009.11.051]

[119] Lanza, A.; Tava, A.; Catalano, M.; Ragona, L.; Singuaroli, I.; Robustelli della Cuna, F.S.; Robustelli della Cuna, G. Effects of the Medicago scutellata trypsin inhibitor (MsTI) on cisplatin-induced cytotoxicity in human breast and cervical cancer cells. *Anticancer Res.,* **2004**, *24*(1), 227-233.

[PMID: 15015601]

[120] Sun, J.; Wang, H.; Ng, T.B. Trypsin isoinhibitors with antiproliferative activity toward leukemia cells from Phaseolus vulgaris cv "White Cloud Bean". *J. Biomed. Biotechnol.,* **2010**, *2010*, 1-8.
[http://dx.doi.org/10.1155/2010/219793] [PMID: 20617140]

[121] Jiraungkoorskul, W.; Rungruangmaitree, R. Pea, Pisum sativum, and its anticancer activity. *Pharmacogn. Rev.,* **2017**, *11*(21), 39-42.
[http://dx.doi.org/10.4103/phrev.phrev_57_16] [PMID: 28503053]

[122] Satheesh, L.S.; Murugan, K. Antimicrobial activity of protease inhibitor from leaves of Coccinia grandis (L.) Voigt. *Indian J. Exp. Biol.,* **2011**, *49*(5), 366-374.
[PMID: 21615062]

[123] Suzuki, R.; Kohno, H.; Sugie, S.; Sasaki, K.; Yoshimura, T.; Wada, K.; Tanaka, T. Preventive effects of extract of leaves of ginkgo (Ginkgo biloba) and its component bilobalide on azoxymethane-induced colonic aberrant crypt foci in rats. *Cancer Lett.,* **2004**, *210*(2), 159-169.
[http://dx.doi.org/10.1016/j.canlet.2004.01.034] [PMID: 15183531]

[124] Seo, W.G.; Hwang, J.C.; Kang, S.K.; Jin, U.H.; Suh, S.J.; Moon, S.K.; Kim, C.H. Suppressive effect of Zedoariae rhizoma on pulmonary metastasis of B16 melanoma cells. *J. Ethnopharmacol.,* **2005**, *101*(1-3), 249-257.
[http://dx.doi.org/10.1016/j.jep.2005.04.037] [PMID: 16023317]

[125] Zhao, Y.; Wang, C.M.; Wang, B.G.; Zhang, C.X. [Study on the anticancer activities of the Clematis manshrica saponins *in vivo.*]. *Zhongguo Zhongyao Zazhi,* **2005**, *30*(18), 1452-1453.
[PMID: 16381470]

[126] Mantena, S.K.; Sharma, S.D.; Katiyar, S.K. Berberine, a natural product, induces G1-phase cell cycle arrest and caspase-3-dependent apoptosis in human prostate carcinoma cells. *Mol. Cancer Ther.,* **2006**, *5*(2), 296-308.
[http://dx.doi.org/10.1158/1535-7163.MCT-05-0448] [PMID: 16505103]

[127] Barzegar, E.; Fouladdel, S.; Movahhed, T.K.; Atashpour, S.; Ghahremani, M.H.; Ostad, S.N.; Azizi, E. Effects of berberine on proliferation, cell cycle distribution and apoptosis of human breast cancer T47D and MCF7 cell lines. *Iran. J. Basic Med. Sci.,* **2015**, *18*(4), 334-342.
[PMID: 26019795]

[128] Singh, S.; Jarial, R.; Kanwar, S.S. Therapeutic effect of herbal medicines on obesity: Herbal pancreatic lipase inhibitors. *Wudpecker J Med Plants,* **2013**, *2*, 53-65.

[129] Moudi, M.; Go, R.; Yien, C.Y.S.; Nazre, M. Vinca alkaloids. *Int. J. Prev. Med.,* **2013**, *4*(11), 1231-1235.
[PMID: 24404355]

[130] Almagro, L.; Fernández-Pérez, F.; Pedreño, M. Indole alkaloids from Catharanthus roseus: Bioproduction and their effect on human health. *Molecules,* **2015**, *20*(2), 2973-3000.
[http://dx.doi.org/10.3390/molecules20022973] [PMID: 25685907]

[131] Ojima, I.; Lichtenthal, B.; Lee, S.; Wang, C.; Wang, X. Taxane anticancer agents: A patent perspective. *Expert Opin. Ther. Pat.,* **2016**, *26*(1), 1-20.
[http://dx.doi.org/10.1517/13543776.2016.1111872] [PMID: 26651178]

[132] Xie, S.; Zhou, J. Harnessing plant biodiversity for the discovery of novel anticancer drugs targeting microtubules. *Front. Plant Sci.,* **2017**, *8*, 720.
[http://dx.doi.org/10.3389/fpls.2017.00720] [PMID: 28523014]

[133] Xie, S.; Zhou, J. Harnessing plant biodiversity for the discovery of novel anticancer drugs targeting microtubules. *Front. Plant Sci.,* **2017**, *8*, 720.
[http://dx.doi.org/10.3389/fpls.2017.00720] [PMID: 28523014]

[134] Garon, E.B.; Neidhart, J.D.; Gabrail, N.Y.; de Oliveira, M.R.; Balkissoon, J.; Kabbinavar, F. A randomized Phase II trial of the tumor vascular disrupting agent CA4P (fosbretabulin tromethamine)

with carboplatin, paclitaxel, and bevacizumab in advanced nonsquamous non-small-cell lung cancer. *OncoTargets Ther.,* **2016**, *9*, 7275-7283.
[http://dx.doi.org/10.2147/OTT.S109186] [PMID: 27942221]

[135] Kim, S.H.; Ryu, H.G.; Lee, J.; Shin, J.; Harikishore, A.; Jung, H.Y.; Kim, Y.S.; Lyu, H.N.; Oh, E.; Baek, N.I.; Choi, K.Y.; Yoon, H.S.; Kim, K.T. Ursolic acid exerts anti-cancer activity by suppressing vaccinia-related kinase 1-mediated damage repair in lung cancer cells. *Sci. Rep.,* **2015**, *5*(1), 14570.
[http://dx.doi.org/10.1038/srep14570] [PMID: 26412148]

[136] Almagro, L.; Fernández-Pérez, F.; Pedreño, M. Indole alkaloids from Catharanthus roseus: Bioproduction and their effect on human health. *Molecules,* **2015**, *20*(2), 2973-3000.
[http://dx.doi.org/10.3390/molecules20022973] [PMID: 25685907]

[137] Venier, N.A.; Yamamoto, T.; Sugar, L.M.; Adomat, H.; Fleshner, N.E.; Klotz, L.H.; Venkateswaran, V. Capsaicin reduces the metastatic burden in the transgenic adenocarcinoma of the mouse prostate model. *Prostate,* **2015**, *75*(12), 1300-1311.
[http://dx.doi.org/10.1002/pros.23013] [PMID: 26047020]

[138] Clark, R.; Lee, S.H. Anticancer properties of capsaicin against human cancer. *Anticancer Res.,* **2016**, *36*(3), 837-843.
[PMID: 26976969]

[139] Chang, H.C.; Chen, S.T.; Chien, S.Y.; Kuo, S.J.; Tsai, H.T.; Chen, D.R. Capsaicin may induce breast cancer cell death through apoptosis-inducing factor involving mitochondrial dysfunction. *Hum. Exp. Toxicol.,* **2011**, *30*(10), 1657-1665.
[http://dx.doi.org/10.1177/0960327110396530] [PMID: 21300690]

[140] Kim, S.; Moon, A. Capsaicin-Induced apoptosis of h-ras-transformed human breast epithelial cells is rac-dependentvia ros generation. *Arch. Pharm. Res.,* **2004**, *27*(8), 845-849.
[http://dx.doi.org/10.1007/BF02980177] [PMID: 15460446]

[141] Brâkenhielm, E.; Cao, R.; Cao, Y. Suppression of angiogenesis, tumor growth, and wound healing by resveratrol, a natural compound in red wine and grapes. *FASEB J.,* **2001**, *15*(10), 1798-1800.
[http://dx.doi.org/10.1096/fj.01-0028fje] [PMID: 11481234]

[142] Jaswanth, A.; Vasanthi, H.R.; Rajamanickam, G.V.; Saraswathy, A. Tumoricidal effect of the red algae Acanthophora spicifera on Ehrlich's ascites carcinoma cellsutilization. *Seaweed Res,* **2004**, *26*(1–2), 217-223.

[143] Yuan, Y.V.; Carrington, M.F.; Walsh, N.A. Extracts from dulse (Palmaria palmata) are effective antioxidants and inhibitors of cell proliferation *in vitro. Food Chem. Toxicol.,* **2005**, *43*(7), 1073-1081.
[http://dx.doi.org/10.1016/j.fct.2005.02.012] [PMID: 15833383]

[144] Ivanova, T.S.; Krupodorova, T.A.; Barshteyn, V.Y.; Artamonova, A.B.; Shlyakhovenko, V.A. Anticancer substances of mushroom origin. *Exp. Oncol.,* **2014**, *36*(2), 58-66.
[PMID: 24980757]

[145] Mikiashvili, N.; Elisashvili, V.; Worku, M.; Davitashvili, E.; Isikhuemhen, O.S. Purification and characterization of a lectin isolated from the submerged cultivated mycelium of grey polypore Cerrena unicolor (Bull.) Murrill (Aphyllophoromycetideae). *Int. J. Med. Mushrooms,* **2009**, *11*(1), 61-68.
[http://dx.doi.org/10.1615/IntJMedMushr.v11.i1.70]

[146] Xu, W.; Huang, J.J.; Cheung, P.C.K. Extract of Pleurotus pulmonarius suppresses liver cancer development and progression through inhibition of VEGF-induced PI3K/AKT signaling pathway. *PLoS One,* **2012**, *7*(3), e34406.
[http://dx.doi.org/10.1371/journal.pone.0034406] [PMID: 22470568]

[147] Awadasseid, A.; Hou, J.; Gamallat, Y.; Xueqi, S.; Eugene, K.D.; Musa Hago, A.; Bamba, D.; Meyiah, A.; Gift, C.; Xin, Y. Purification, characterization, and antitumor activity of a novel glucan from the fruiting bodies of Coriolus Versicolor. *PLoS One,* **2017**, *12*(2), e0171270.
[http://dx.doi.org/10.1371/journal.pone.0171270] [PMID: 28178285]

[148] Jiang, Z.; Jacob, J.A.; Loganathachetti, D.S.; Nainangu, P.; Chen, B. belemene: Mechanistic studies on cancer cell interaction and its chemosensitization effect. *Front. Pharmacol.,* **2017**, *8*, 105.
[http://dx.doi.org/10.3389/fphar.2017.00105] [PMID: 28337141]

[149] Jiang, S.; Ling, C.; Li, W.; Jiang, H.; Zhi, Q.; Jiang, M. Molecular mechanisms of anti-cancer activities of b-elemene: Targeting hallmarks of cancer. Anti-cancer agents in medicinal chemistry. *Form Curr Med Chem AntiCancer Agent,* **2016**, *16*, 1426-1434.
[http://dx.doi.org/10.2174/1871520616666160211123424] [PMID: 26863884]

[150] Chen, Y.C.; Yang, L.L.; Lee, T.J.F. Oroxylin A inhibition of lipopolysaccharide-induced iNOS and COX-2 gene expression *via* suppression of nuclear factor-κB activation. *Biochem. Pharmacol.,* **2000**, *59*(11), 1445-1457.
[http://dx.doi.org/10.1016/S0006-2952(00)00255-0] [PMID: 10751555]

[151] Ha, J.; Zhao, L.; Zhao, Q.; Yao, J.; Zhu, B.B.; Lu, N.; Ke, X.; Yang, H.Y.; Li, Z.; You, Q.D.; Guo, Q.L. Oroxylin A improves the sensitivity of HT-29 human colon cancer cells to 5-FU through modulation of the COX-2 signaling pathway. *Biochem. Cell Biol.,* **2012**, *90*(4), 521-531.
[http://dx.doi.org/10.1139/o2012-005] [PMID: 22607196]

[152] Dey, A.; Nandy, S.; Mukherjee, A.; Modak, B.K. Sustainable utilization of medicinal plants and conservation strategies practiced by the aboriginals of Purulia district, India: A case study on therapeutics used against some tropical otorhinolaryngologic and ophthalmic disorders. *Environ. Dev. Sustain.,* **2020**, 1-38.

[153] Garcia-Oliveira, P.; Otero, P.; Pereira, A.G.; Chamorro, F.; Carpena, M.; Echave, J.; Fraga-Corral, M.; Simal-Gandara, J.; Prieto, M.A. Status and challenges of plant-anticancer compounds in cancer treatment. *Pharmaceuticals (Basel),* **2021**, *14*(2), 157.
[http://dx.doi.org/10.3390/ph14020157] [PMID: 33673021]

[154] Rolta, R.; Kumar, V.; Sourirajan, A.; Upadhyay, N.K.; Dev, K. Bioassay guided fractionation of rhizome extract of Rheum emodi wall as bio-availability enhancer of antibiotics against bacterial and fungal pathogens. *J. Ethnopharmacol.,* **2020**, *257*, 112867.
[http://dx.doi.org/10.1016/j.jep.2020.112867] [PMID: 32302716]

[155] Ingle, K.P.; Deshmukh, A.G.; Padole, D.A.; Dudhare, M.S.; Moharil, M.P.; Khelurkar, V.C. Phytochemicals: Extraction methods, identification and detection of bioactive compounds from plant extracts. *J. Pharmacogn. Phytochem.,* **2017**, *6*(1), 32-36.

[156] Redondo-Blanco, S.; Fernández, J.; Gutiérrez-del-Río, I.; Villar, C.J.; Lombó, F. New insights toward colorectal cancer chemotherapy using natural bioactive compounds. *Front. Pharmacol.,* **2017**, *8*, 109.
[http://dx.doi.org/10.3389/fphar.2017.00109] [PMID: 28352231]

SUBJECT INDEX

www.ingramcontent.com/pod-product-compliance
Lightning Source LLC
Chambersburg PA
CBHW050837220326
41598CB00006B/385